Current Concepts in Bone Pathology

Guest Editor

JOHN D. REITH, MD

SURGICAL PATHOLOGY CLINICS

surgpath.theclinics.com

Consulting Editor
JOHN R. GOLDBLUM, MD

March 2012 • Volume 5 • Number 1

SAUNDERS an imprint of ELSEVIER, Inc.

W.B. SAUNDERS COMPANY
A Division of Elsevier Inc.

1600 John F. Kennedy Boulevard • Suite 1800 • Philadelphia, Pennsylvania 19103-2899

http://www.surgpath.theclinics.com

SURGICAL PATHOLOGY CLINICS Volume 5, Number 1
March 2012 ISSN 1875-9181, ISBN-13: 978-1-4557-1156-7

Editor: Joanne Husovski

Surgical Pathology Clinics (ISSN 1875-9181) is published quarterly by Elsevier Inc., 360 Park Avenue South, New York, NY 10010. Months of issue are March, June, September, and December. Business and Editorial Office: Elsevier Inc., 1600 John F. Kennedy Blvd., Ste. 1800, Philadelphia, PA 19103-2899. Accounting and Circulation Offices: Elsevier Inc., 3251 Riverport Lane, Maryland Heights, MO 63043. Periodicals postage paid at New York, NY and at additional mailing offices. Subscription prices are $184.00 per year (US individuals), $212.00 per year (US institutions), $91.00 per year (US students/residents), $230.00 per year (Canadian individuals), $240.00 per year (Canadian Institutions), $230.00 per year (foreign individuals), $240.00 per year (foreign institutions), and $112.00 per year (international & Canadian students/residents). Foreign air speed delivery is included in all *Clinics'* subscription prices. All prices are subject to change without notice. **POSTMASTER:** Send address changes to *Surgical Pathology Clinics*, Elsevier, 3251 Riverport Lane, Maryland Heights, MO 63043. Customer Service: 1-800-654-2452 (US). From outside the United States, call 1-314-447-8871. Fax: 1-314-447-8029. E-mail: JournalsCustomerServiceusa@elsevier.com (for print support) and JournalsOnlineSupport-usa@elsevier.com (for online support).

Reprints. For copies of 100 or more, of articles in this publication, please contact the Commercial Reprints Department, Elsevier Inc., 360 Park Avenue South, New York, NY 10010-1710. Tel. (212) 633-3812; Fax: (212) 462-1935; E-mail: reprints@elsevier.com.

Printed and bound by CPI Group (UK) Ltd, Croydon, CR0 4YY

Transferred to Digital Print 2012

Contributors

CONSULTING EDITOR

JOHN R. GOLDBLUM, MD
Chairman, Department of Anatomic Pathology;
Professor of Pathology, Cleveland Clinics,
Lerner College of Medicine, Cleveland Clinic,
Cleveland, Ohio

GUEST EDITOR

JOHN D. REITH, MD
Professor, Director of Anatomic Pathology
and Unit of Bone and Soft Tissue Pathology,
Departments of Pathology, Immunology,
and Laboratory Medicine and Orthopaedics
and Rehabilitation, University of Florida
College of Medicine, Gainesville, Florida

AUTHORS

THOMAS W. BAUER, MD, PhD
Departments of Pathology, Orthopedic
Surgery and the Spine Center, The Cleveland
Clinic, Cleveland, Ohio

SHEFALI BHUSNURMATH, MD
Department of Pathology, University of
Washington, Seattle, Washington

CHARLES H. BUSH, MD
Department of Radiology, University of Florida
College of Medicine, Gainesville, Florida

DIANA M. CARDONA, MD
Assistant Professor of Pathology, Department
of Pathology, Duke University Medical Center,
Durham, North Carolina

JUSTIN M.M. CATES, MD, PhD
Associate Professor of Pathology, Department
of Pathology, Microbiology and Immunology,
Vanderbilt University School of Medicine,
Nashville, Tennessee

ANDREA T. DEYRUP, MD, PhD
Associate Professor of Clinical Pathology,
Department of Orthopaedic Surgery,
University of South Carolina School of
Medicine - Greenville; Pathology Consultants
of Greenville, Greenville, South Carolina

EDWARD F. DICARLO, MD
Associate Pathologist and Chief Surgical
Pathologist, Department of Pathology and
Laboratory Medicine, Hospital for Special
Surgery; Associate Professor of Clinical
Pathology, Joan and Sanford Weill College
of Medicine of Cornell University, New York,
New York

LESLIE G. DODD, MD
Associate Professor of Pathology, Department
of Pathology, Duke University Medical Center,
Durham, North Carolina

LIZETTE VILA DUCKWORTH, MD
Department of Pathology, Immunology, and
Laboratory Medicine, University of Florida
College of Medicine, Gainesville, Florida

C. PARKER GIBBS, MD
Department of Orthopaedics and Rehabilitative
Medicine, Division of Oncology, University
of Florida, Gainesville, Florida

ADRIANA L. GONZALEZ, MD
Former Assistant Professor of Pathology,
Department of Pathology, Microbiology and
Immunology, Vanderbilt University School
of Medicine, Nashville, Tennessee

RIKU HAYASHI, MD, PhD
Department of Orthopaedic Surgery,
Yokohama City University School of Medicine,
Yokohama, Japan

BENJAMIN HOCH, MD
Department of Pathology, University of
Washington, Seattle, Washington

CARRIE Y. INWARDS, MD
Consultant, Division of Anatomic Pathology;
Associate Professor, Department of
Laboratory Medicine and Pathology,
Mayo Clinic, Rochester, Minnesota

SCOTT E. KILPATRICK, MD
President, Pathologists Diagnostic Services,
Forsyth Medical Center, Winston-Salem,
North Carolina

MICHAEL J. KLEIN, MD
Pathologist-in-Chief and Director, Department
of Pathology and Laboratory Medicine,
Hospital for Special Surgery; Professor of
Pathology and Laboratory Medicine, Joan
and Sanford Weill College of Medicine of
Cornell University; Consultant in Pathology,
Memorial Sloan-Kettering Cancer Center
and Memorial Hospital for Cancer and
Allied Diseases, New York, New York

JACQUELYN A. KNAPIK, MD
Clinical Assistant Professor, Department of
Pathology, University of Florida, Gainesville,
Florida

DAVID R. LUCAS, MD
Professor and Director of Surgical Pathology,
Department of Pathology, University
of Michigan, Ann Arbor, Michigan

EDWARD F. MCCARTHY, MD
Professor of Pathology and Orthopaedic
Surgery, Department of Pathology,
Johns Hopkins Hospital, Baltimore,
Maryland

RAJIV RAJANI, MD
Department of Orthopaedics and Rehabilitative
Medicine, Division of Oncology,
University of Florida, Gainesville,
Florida

JOHN D. REITH, MD
Professor, Director of Anatomic Pathology
and Unit of Bone and Soft Tissue Pathology,
Departments of Pathology, Immunology,
and Laboratory Medicine and Orthopaedics
and Rehabilitation, University of Florida
College of Medicine, Gainesville, Florida

JUSTIN L. SENINGEN, MD
Resident, Department of Laboratory Medicine
and Pathology, Mayo Clinic, Rochester,
Minnesota

Contents

This review discusses how certain imaging features of bone tumors can give valuable clues as to their histology. The author emphasizes the clinical presentation of the patient, and how close cooperation among the radiologist, pathologist, and orthopedic surgeon are paramount in achieving an accurate diagnosis of bone tumors as well as optimizing their management.

The pathologic examination of failed joints, whether natural or artificial, is an indispensable part of the understanding of arthritis, as it is the last, and still best opportunity to determine or verify the correct diagnosis. Accuracy in pathologic diagnosis, based on a firm understanding of the various disease processes, provides reliable data for use in clinical registries, provides an opportunity to explain the "unusual" clinical presentation, and ultimately gives the "best evidence" for basing further treatments and prognosis for the individual patient.

Most patients who undergo total joint arthroplasty experience dramatic relief of pain and improved ambulation for many years, but some eventually develop pain, often accompanied by radiographic evidence of bone resorption around their implants. The most frequent cause of device failure is osteolysis, but infection is another important cause of pain and arthroplasty failure. The distinction between infection and aseptic loosening is important because the 2 conditions are treated very differently. The purpose of this article is to summarize the role of the anatomic and clinical pathologist in helping distinguish aseptic loosening from infection.

This article presents the use of bone cytology for diagnosis of bone tumors. It discusses critical factors and considerations of fine-needle aspiration and bone cytology and presents diagnostic options and differential diagnosis for benign and malignant bone lesions. Osteomyelitis, chrondroblastoma, Langerhans cell histiocytosis, chondromyxoid fibromas, enchondromas, giant cell tumor of bone, osteosarcoma, chondrosarcoma and variants, Ewing sarcoma, chordoma, plasmacytoma, multiple myeloma, lymphoma, and metastatic bone disease are presented.

The diagnosis of benign bone-forming tumors continues to be based on the traditional approach to bone tumor diagnosis using knowledge of the spectrum of histopathologic features seen in these tumors in combination with clinical and radiological correlation. This review emphasizes the pathologic features and the clinical and radiological features that the surgical pathologist must have a working understanding of to make an accurate diagnosis and avoid confusion with other lesions, particularly osteosarcoma. New and persistent challenges facing the practicing pathologist and our current understanding of the cytogenetic and molecular abnormalities involved in the pathogenesis of these tumors are discussed.

Accurate diagnosis of bone-forming tumors, including correct subclassification of osteogenic sarcoma is critical for determination of appropriate clinical management and prediction of patient outcome. The morphologic spectrum of osteogenic sarcoma is extensive, however, and its histologic mimics are numerous. This review focuses on the major differential diagnoses of the specific subtypes of osteosarcoma, presents summaries of various diagnoses, and provides tips to overcoming pitfalls in diagnosis.

Well-differentiated hyaline cartilage tumors are among the most common tumors encountered in the skeleton; their radiographic and pathologic classification and clinical management can be challenging. Pathologists find cartilage tumors difficult because their precise classification is as dependent on the clinical and radiographic findings as the histologic features; the distinction between benign and malignant cartilage neoplasms demands good communication and teamwork between pathologists, orthopedic surgeons, and radiologists. This review focuses on the necessary clinical, radiographic, and pathologic features that allow distinction between enchondroma and low-grade central chondrosarcoma and interpretation of lesions encountered in the enchondromatosis syndromes.

This article presents a review of chondrosarcoma variants, with a focus on the extraordinarily rare variants of chondrosarcoma in which hyaline cartilage is not the dominant feature and, in fact, in most cases of myxoid chondrosarcoma (chordoid sarcoma), is absent. Discussed are the differential diagnoses for these neoplasms, radiologic studies, gross and microscopic features, and prognosis. Summaries are provided of the key features for the major variants.

This article provides an overview of giant cell tumor, including the typical clinical, radiographic, and pathologic findings, as well as some unusual features, such as multifocality and metastases. The article addresses recent advances in the molecular biology of giant cell tumor, particularly receptor activator of nuclear factor kappa B (RANK)-ligand signaling, in addition to novel anti–RANK-ligand therapy, the use of which seems promising for unresectable and metastatic tumors.

Surgical Pathology Clinics

THE CLINICS ARE NOW AVAILABLE ONLINE!

Access your subscription at:
www.theclinics.com

Bone Pathology: Pathology, Radiology, and Orthopedics

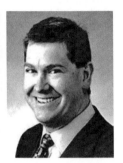

John D. Reith, MD
Guest Editor

Bone pathology, like most fields within surgical pathology, has evolved significantly in recent years. The field has benefited not only from advances in immunohistochemistry and molecular diagnostics, but from improvements in radiographic techniques, particularly the cross-sectional imaging modalities of CT and MRI scans. And yet the diagnoses of many of the cornerstones of bone pathology, including the cartilaginous, bone-forming, and giant cell-rich neoplasms, remain grounded in vigilant examination of hematoxylin and eosin-stained slides coupled with careful radiographic and clinical correlation. In fact, the interaction among pathologists, radiologists, and orthopedic surgeons is just one of several factors that makes the practice of orthopedic pathology so enjoyable as well as effective. Likewise, failure to utilize all information pertinent to a given case—particularly the radiographic findings—can make the practice of orthopedic pathology fraught with danger.

In selecting topics for this issue of *Surgical Pathology Clinics*, the goal was to include concepts relative to the everyday practice of bone pathology—such as arthritis, the evaluation of peri-prosthetic tissues for infection, and the practical workup of metastases in bone—in addition to the more esoteric subjects, namely, the evaluation of primary neoplastic processes. Toward the latter goal, topics such as giant cell-rich neoplasms, bone and cartilage matrix-producing neoplasms, small cell neoplasms, fibro-osseous lesions, and reactive bone lesions are covered in detail, including the necessary clinical and radiographic information necessary to formulate a thoughtful differential diagnosis. Where applicable, information on ancillary immunohistochemical and molecular diagnostic testing is also included. Additionally, articles introducing basic concepts of bone radiology and an update on the treatment of bone sarcomas have been included to reinforce the concept of the multidisciplinary team approach to the diagnosis of bone lesions and to assist the reader in understanding the most important points to include in a pathology report. Finally, because pathologists are increasingly being asked to provide more and more information with smaller and smaller tissue samples, an article on the application of cytology to the diagnosis of bone lesions has been included.

The completion of this edition of *Surgical Pathology Clinics* would not have been possible without the hard work of many individuals. I'd like to express heartfelt thanks to Joanne Husovski for both her continual support and her patience

Surgical Pathology 5 (2012) ix–x
doi:10.1016/j.path.2011.12.002

while this edition was being completed. Without her wisdom and guidance, this work would not have been possible. I'd also like to express my gratitude to all of the authors for lending their expertise to this journal. It was truly a pleasure to interact with such a talented group of experts in this field. Finally, I'd like to acknowledge my mentors from the world of mesenchymal pathology, Tom Bauer, John Goldblum, Sharon Weiss, and Howard Dorfman, whose guidance over the years has been absolutely invaluable to my career.

John D. Reith, MD
Unit of Bone and Soft Tissue Pathology
Department of Pathology, Immunology
and Laboratory Medicine
University of Florida College of Medicine
1600 SW Archer Road
PO Box 100275
Gainesville, FL 32610-0275, USA

E-mail address:
reith@pathology.ufl.edu

BONE TUMOR RADIOLOGY 101 FOR PATHOLOGISTS

Charles H. Bush, MD

KEYWORDS

• Bone tumor • Radiology • Pathologic-radiologic • Orthopedic • Diagnosis

ABSTRACT

This review discusses how certain imaging features of bone tumors can give valuable clues as to their histology. The author emphasizes the clinical presentation of the patient, and how close cooperation among the radiologist, pathologist, and orthopedic surgeon are paramount in achieving an accurate diagnosis of bone tumors as well as optimizing their management.

OVERVIEW: BONE IMAGING

The imaging of osseous neoplasia has undergone nothing short of a revolution since the 1970s. From a diagnostic armamentarium that previously consisted only of radiography, angiography, and nuclear medicine, today's radiologist now has computed tomography (CT), magnetic resonance imaging (MRI), and positron emission tomography (PET) to preoperatively stage, and sometimes non-invasively assess, the histology of bone tumors. With the increased sophistication of imaging, however, comes complexity: Which modality to use for a given tumor? This brief article summarizes the imaging of some of the more common bone tumors, emphasizing the paramount importance of close cooperation among the pathologist, radiologist, oncologist, and surgeon in the management of these lesions.

The role of imaging in the evaluation of bone tumors was summarized in memorable fashion in the age before cross-sectional imaging by Jaffe,[1] who likened the roentgenographic picture of a bone tumor to a blueprint of the gross pathology of the lesion. The analogy of the radiograph as a blueprint serves to identify the location of the lesion in relation to the host bone, reveals the effect of the lesion on its bone of origin, shows the response of that bone to the lesion, and often reveals a great deal of information of the character of the lesion itself. This approach is even more applicable to CT, MRI, and radionuclide imaging, with the first 2 modalities providing depiction of both bone and regional soft tissues, and the latter often providing a glimpse of the physiology of the lesion, as well as adjacent structures.

INITIAL ASSESSMENT

The workup of a patient with a bone tumor should start with a complete history and physical examination. Valuable information can be gleaned as

Key Points
BONE RADIOLOGY FOR PATHOLOGISTS

- Processes other than neoplasms can cause mass effect in the extremities: eg, osteomyelitis, hematoma, and some arthritides.

- The pathologist and radiologist should initially consider both tumor location and age of the patient in the formulation of a differential diagnosis of a bone tumor on radiography.

- Bone tumors, by virtue of their effect on the host bone, lend themselves naturally to conventional radiography: lesion size and margins, periosteal reaction, matrix mineralization, and the presence of a soft tissue component are often readily apparent.

Department of Radiology, University of Florida College of Medicine, 1600 SW Archer Road, PO Box 100374, Gainesville, FL 32610, USA

E-mail address: bushch@radiology.ufl.edu

Surgical Pathology 5 (2012) 1–13

doi:10.1016/j.path.2011.07.007

to the duration and growth rate of the lesion, as well as alerting the clinician to associated trauma, recent prior infection, or fever. It is important to keep in mind that processes other than neoplasms can cause mass effect in the extremities. Osteomyelitis can present as a bony mass. Traumatic masses, such as hematoma and myositis ossificans, can arise from a subperiosteal location, and large erosions in some arthritides can be confused with neoplasia in orthopedic practice.

One important distinguishing feature about many non-neoplastic bone lesions is their frequent polyostotic occurrence. Paget disease of bone, osteomyelitis, and some metabolic bone diseases that can present with bone destruction, such as the brown tumor of hyperparathyroidism, frequently present with more than one site of involvement (Fig. 1). In such cases, radionuclide bone scintigraphy can sometimes be a useful secondary imaging modality in detecting other osseous sites of involvement.

CONVENTIONAL RADIOGRAPHY OF BONE

Today, the venerable radiograph remains the initial imaging tool in the evaluation of a suspected osseous mass lesion in almost all cases. In this day of high technology, it is easy to dismiss the radiograph as an unnecessary relic of an older, simpler time, but this modality is still an indispensable tool in orthopedic oncology. Bone tumors, by virtue of their effect on the host bone, lend themselves naturally to conventional radiography. In the radiographic evaluation of bone tumors, the importance of lesion size, margins, periosteal reaction, matrix mineralization, and presence of a soft tissue component must be emphasized, and these factors are often readily apparent. An excellent review of the utility of conventional radiography in bone tumors has been written by Miller,[2] which draws on older, but no less readable sources.[3–5] Such tumor features as lesion margins, periosteal reaction, matrix mineralization, and often soft tissue extension can be seen radiographically. At a minimum, the radiograph can guide the selection of appropriate additional imaging. Conversely, sometimes using a cross-sectional imaging modality for the initial evaluation of some bone tumors can be misleading, particularly in the case of MRI (Fig. 2).

The information that the pathologist and radiologist should initially use in the formulation of a differential diagnosis of a bone tumor on radiography is identical, and comes neither from specimens nor imaging, but from patient demographics. The 2 most important facts about a bone tumor are its location and the age of the patient. A central,

lucent, intramedullary lesion of the intertrochanteric region of the proximal femur has far more ominous connotation in a 67-year-old smoker than in a 12-year-old, healthy adolescent. Such factors as patient age, past medical history, gender, and symptoms at presentation should always be kept in mind as initial radiographs of osseous mass lesions are examined.

In radiologic pathologic correlation, attention should be focused on those imaging features that correlate with a particular type of tissue. Optimally, radiography is capable of distinguishing 5 basic tissue densities:

1. Gas
2. Fat
3. Soft tissue
4. Bone (mineralization)
5. Metal.

Radiography has always had inherently poor contrast resolution, being unable to distinguish fluid from solid tissue. Low-kilovoltage radiography (<50 kVp) can improve the detection of subtle radiographic density differences between soft tissues, but this is not usually used in routine practice. Where radiography has excelled, even in the days of analog film screen radiographs, is spatial resolution, giving the radiologist the ability to detect signs of the biologic activity of bone tumors, such as lesion margins, character of matrix mineralization, and soft tissue extension.

It is in the area of characterizing mineralization that radiography excels (Fig. 3). All too often, mineralization on radiographs is described as "calcification," without the radiologist giving attention to the character of the mineralization, which can give valuable clues to its identity. Radiography is capable of distinguishing multiple types of mineralization. Ossification is distinguished by cortication, as well as frequently visible trabeculation. The most common causes of ossification are heterotopic bone, and the related entity of myositis ossificans. The pedicle of an osteochondroma is ossified. Some parosteal osteosarcomas can produce tumor bone indistinguishable radiographically from mature ossification. Amorphous calcification occurs in several instances. The ossification seen in conventional osteosarcoma can appear amorphous on radiography. Calcium hydroxyapatite deposition, which occasionally can mimic a juxtacortical mass, is typically amorphous on radiography. The bizarre trabecular bone seen in many lesions of fibrous dysplasia can be so small as to be below the resolution of conventional radiography, appearing as a vague, opalescent increase in density of the matrix of the lesion, often likened to ground glass. Last, the

Fig. 1. (*A*) This 47-year-old man presented with a pathologic fracture through a minimally expansile, lucent lesion of the left proximal humerus. T1-weighted (*B*) and T2-weighted (*C*) coronal MRI images through the left shoulder revealed additional small lesions in the glenoid. A radiograph of the hands (not shown) revealed prominent subperiosteal bone resorption from hyperparathyroidism, identifying the shoulder lesions as brown tumors. Further workup revealed a parathyroid adenoma.

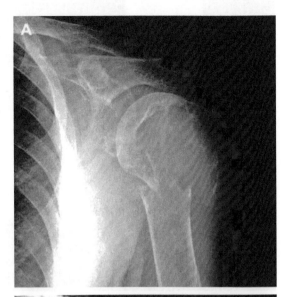

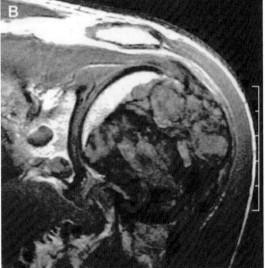

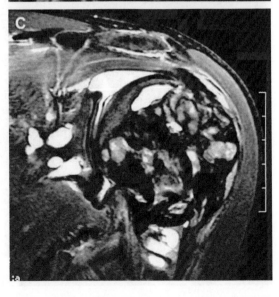

4

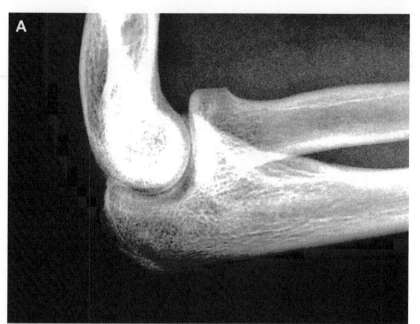

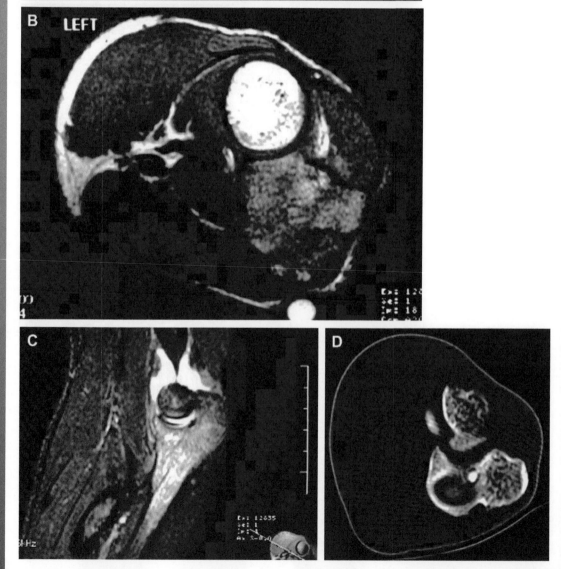

Fig. 2. A 20-year-old man with 8 months of left elbow pain. Radiography of the left elbow (*A*) is remarkable only for a small joint effusion. T1-weighted image (*B*) and STIR (*C*) revealed diffusely altered marrow signal in the proximal ulna. A CT image (*D*) revealed a tiny intracortical nidus of an osteoid osteoma.

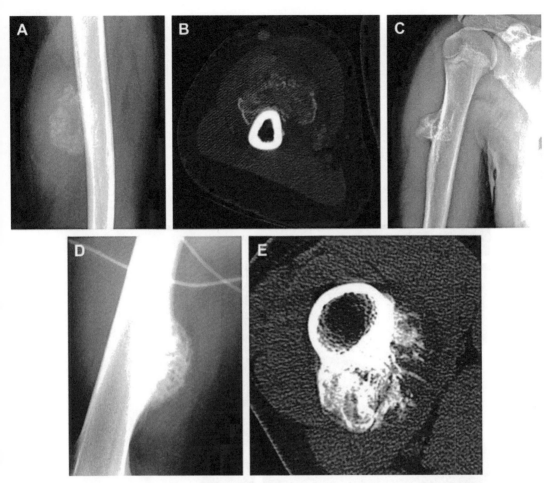

Fig. 3. Various types of mineralization encountered on imaging: ossification on myositis ossificans on radiography (*A*) and CT (*B*), ossification in the stalk of an osteochondroma on radiography (*C*), and ossification in a parosteal osteosarcoma on radiography (*D*) and CT (*E*).

mineralization in a chondroid matrix neoplasm is often quite characteristic on radiography, with mineralization at the periphery of cartilage lobules giving a "rings and arcs" appearance.

Radiography often furnishes valuable clues to the biologic activity of bone tumors. One of the simplest features that can predict the behavior of a bone tumor is its size. Large lesions are much more likely to prove malignant than small ones. Lesion margins are another indicator of behavior. The concepts devised by Lodwick and coworkers,[6–8] which predated the advent of cross-sectional imaging, are still relevant today. The Lodwick method logically evaluates both the pattern of bone destruction by the lesion, as well as the reaction of the host bone to the lesion. When considered together, the

biologic activity of the lesion can be estimated by imaging.

Bone destruction can be classified as geographic, moth eaten, or permeative, with the latter 2 categories often being difficult to distinguish. Geographic margins of a lucent lesion of bone can be further subclassified by the presence or absence of a thin rim of reactive bone, as well as cortical remodeling. A very thin margin of reactive bone, typified by a fibrous cortical defect (**Fig. 4**) is a good sign of a lesion of low biologic activity, in that the host bone has ample time to "wall off" the lesion from the adjacent normal cancellous trabeculae by producing a thin rim of cortical bone. In contrast, giant cell tumor of epiphysis, an often locally aggressive lesion, has margins

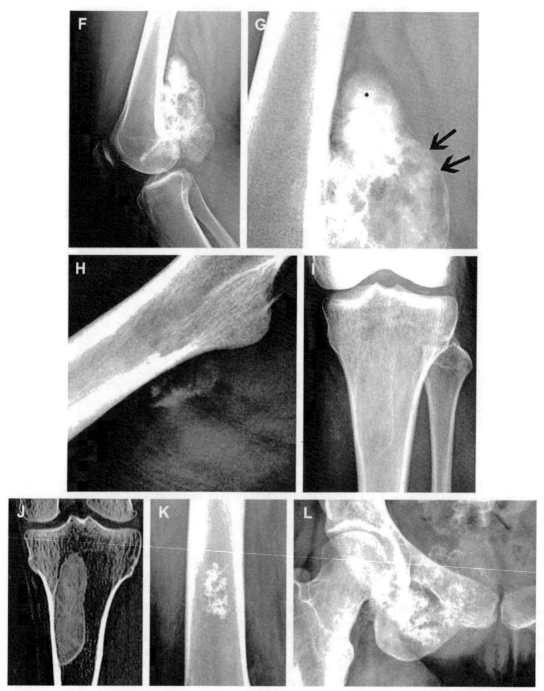

Fig. 3. Two types of mineralization are seen in a patient with a dedifferentiated parosteal osteosarcoma on a lateral radiograph (*F*), as well as a magnified view of the area of higher-grade tumor (*G*), showing mature ossification in the low-grade parosteal osteosarcoma (*arrows*) and less well defined "cumulus cloud" mineralization in the higher-grade dedifferentiated osteosarcoma (*asterisk*). Amorphous mineralization is seen in calcium hydroxyapatite deposition disease on radiography (*H*), the "ground-glass" matrix of fibrous dysplasia is seen on radiography (*I*) and CT (*J*), and the "rings and arcs" of a chondroid matrix neoplasm are seen radiographically in an enchondroma (*K*) and in a chondrosarcoma (*L*).

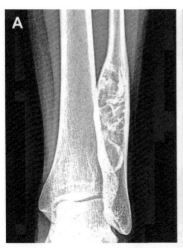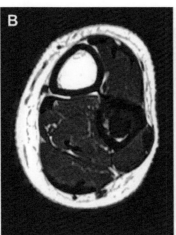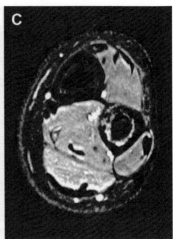

Fig. 4. Radiography (*A*) and T1-weighted (*B*) and T2-weighted (*C*) MR images of a fibrous cortical defect of the left distal fibula in a 15-year-old girl. Note the low signal intensity of the lucent lesion on both T1 and T2 MR images.

that are geographic, but the faster growth of this tumor does not usually allow for reactive bone formation (Fig. 5). Aggressive bone lesions often have poorly defined margins on radiographs, which can have a moth-eaten or permeative appearance. This is typified by osteomyelitis (Fig. 6), as well as primary lymphoma of bone.

The reaction of the host bone is another clue to the behavior of a bone tumor. Slow-growing lesions cannot only cause the adjacent trabecular bone to produce a zone of reactive bone about them, but such lesions can also stimulate periosteal new bone formation as they erode cortex. In contrast, rapidly growing lesions expand faster than the ability of the periosteum to form a shell of new-containing bone about the tumor.

The major drawback of conventional radiography in the evaluation of bone tumors is its 2-dimensional portrayal of a dynamic 3-dimensional relationship. For example, it has been estimated that up to 40% of a vertebral body can be destroyed by a metastatic lesion without definite visualization on radiography. This is why the introduction of CT has been such a revolutionary advance in the staging of bone tumors (Fig. 7).

Computed Tomography of Bone

The introduction of CT in 1974 marked a major milestone in diagnostic imaging. Today, despite the widespread use of MRI, CT still has an important role in the evaluation of bone tumors. CT is usually less expensive than MRI, examination times can be 10 or more times faster than the latter, and CT can be the only suitable cross-sectional imaging modality for staging a bone

mass in severely obese or claustrophobic patients or those with pacemakers. For both calcifications and gas within bone and soft tissue, as well as in the demonstration of subtle cortical alteration by aggressive masses, CT is actually superior to MRI. Modern helical CT scanners, by virtue of their capability to obtain submillimeter section thicknesses, are able to reformat image data in any desired plane.

CT is superb in the demonstration of subtle density differences in tissues, as well as in spatial resolution. Density of tissues on CT is expressed by Hounsfield units (HU), with the density of pure water having a value of zero. HU measurements are variable, dependent on both the manufacturer of the CT scanner and the technical parameters used to obtain the CT scan. Cortical bone has a density of 1000 to 4000 HU, fat has a density of about −100 HU, muscle has a density of 40 to 50 HU, and tendon has a density of 90 to 100 HU. Because of the characteristic negative attenuation values of fat, CT can be diagnostic in the case of intraosseous lipomas (Fig. 8). Similarly, CT is often superior to MRI in depicting mineralization in tumors as areas of high attenuation, and usually demonstrates the distinguishing features of the mineralization in superior fashion compared with conventional radiography. Examples of the various types of mineralization encountered radiographically and by CT are summarized in Fig. 3.

MAGNETIC RESONANCE IMAGING OF BONE

With the exceptions outlined in the preceding section, the single best tool for evaluating and

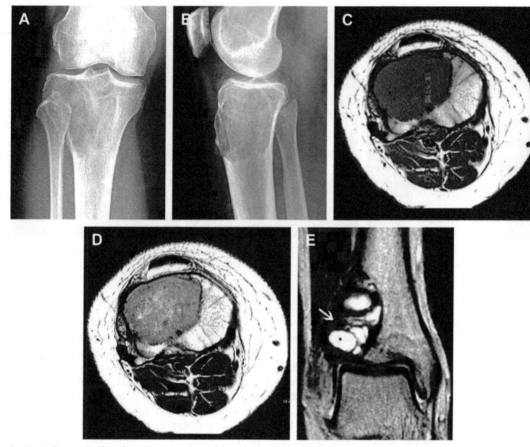

Fig. 5. Radiography (*A, B*) and T1-weighted (*C*) and T2-weighted MR images (*D*) of a giant-cell tumor of the prox-imal tibia show a lucent lesion extending to the articular cortex of the lateral tibial plateau. Note the margins of the lesion by radiography are geographic, but do not show any surrounding reactive bone. Another giant-cell tumor of the distal tibia in a different patient (*E*) shows a prominent component of high-signal fluid from secondary aneurysmal bone cyst formation by T2 MRI (*asterisk*), as well as very low signal hemosiderin in the tumor (*arrow*).

staging bone tumors is MRI. The basic principles of MRI are summarized in several excellent review articles.[9–12] MRI maximizes contrast between normal tissues and tumors and, unlike CT, it permits direct visualization of the abnormality in any desired plane. The multiplanar capability of MRI helps the surgeon to better visualize the tumor, allowing better understanding of the anatomy and easier surgical planning. MRI is also superior to CT in demonstrating the relation-ship of the tumor to adjacent uninvolved bone marrow, as well as being superior in defining the relation of soft tissue components of aggressive bone lesions to adjacent neurovascular structures.

Unlike CT, in which the images are a display of the difference in x-ray attenuation caused by the various densities of different tissues, MRI exploits the differences in proton relaxation between tissues to produce image contrast. The nearly universal presence of hydrogen in biomolecules makes MRI of living systems possible. Almost all hydrogen in nature consists of its lightest isotope, H-1, whose nucleus, a lone proton, possesses a net magnetic moment or dipole moment. When the proton in a hydrogen nucleus is placed in an external magnetic field, the magnetic moment of the proton will tend to align with the applied magnetic field, in which case those protons are termed as being in their ground state. If these protons are subjected to an electromagnetic ra-diofrequency pulse of the proper energy, a number of the tissue protons will alter the alignment of their dipole moment to opposite that of the applied magnetic field, a higher energy or excited state. When that radiofrequency pulse ends, those excited tissue protons will tend to return to their

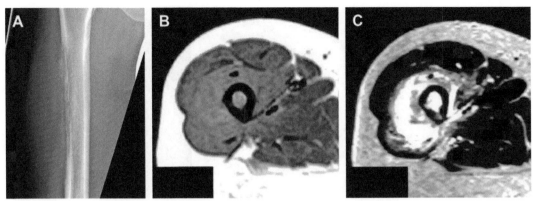

Fig. 6. Radiography (*A*) and T1-weighted (*B*) and T2-weighted (*C*) MR images show a typical permeative radiographic pattern in staphylococcal osteomyelitis. Note the extensively abnormal juxtacortical soft tissue signal in (*C*). The margin of the soft tissue component of most primary bone sarcomas is usually better defined (contrast with the Ewing sarcoma in Fig. 9).

ground state by giving off radiofrequency energy, which can be measured. The methods used to spatially encode the location of tissue protons are beyond the purposes of this article, but these methods allow production of an MR image.

Another difference from CT is the ability to change the way in which the image is produced, termed the *pulse sequence*. A useful simplification to understanding tissue contrast in MRI is to describe pulse sequences by their weighting. Image weighting in MRI is of primary importance in manipulating contrast between bone and soft tissue tumors and normal tissues. The commonly encountered MR images are classified as Tl-weighted, proton density–weighted, and T2-weighted images. T1-weighted images provide excellent spatial resolution, but contrast between many tumors and normal tissue is often minimal.

T2-weighted images usually provide good contrast between tumors and normal tissue (Fig. 9), and these sequences are sensitive in the depiction of fluid and edema, which appear of high signal intensity relative to normal tissues. Another pulse sequence commonly encountered in musculoskeletal imaging is the STIR (short tau inversion recovery) sequence, in which contrast between high-signal edema, fluid, and water-rich tumors and low-signal muscle and bone is maximized.

The common operator-specific variables found as an annotation on MRI are TR (repetition time) and TE (echo time), both measured in milliseconds. For Tl-weighted images, TR is usually in the range of 400 to 600 ms, whereas TE varies from 20 to 30 ms. T2-weighted images have a much longer TR (usually >2000 ms) and longer TE (usually >60). STIR images carry an additional parameter,

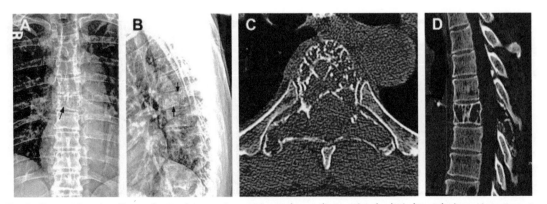

Fig. 7. Conventional radiographs can be very insensitive to bone destruction by lytic bone lesions. Anteroposterior (AP) (*A*) and lateral (*B*) radiographs of a T6 plasmacytoma show only subtle endplate irregularity at the affected level (*arrows*). Axial (*C*) and reformatted coronal CT images (*D*) clearly show the extent of bone destruction by the lesion.

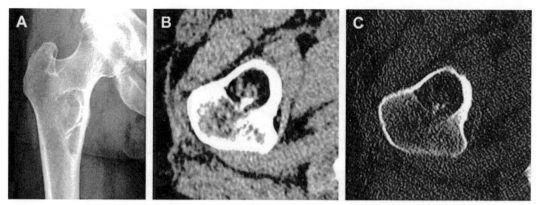

Fig. 8. A 37-year-old woman found incidentally to have a lesion of the right proximal tibia. An AP radiograph of the right hip (*A*) shows a lucent, intramedullary lesion of the right proximal femur. Soft tissue (*B*) and bone window (*C*) CT images through the lesion show it is mostly composed of tissue of fat attenuation.

the inversion time, TI, usually about 140 ms at 1.5 T. The inversion time is designed to null the signal from fat, thus usually optimizing the conspicuity of pathology. Intravascular paramagnetic contrast agents, typically chelates of the strongly paramagnetic rare earth element gadolinium, are often used in imaging of bone tumors to provide additional information concerning the vascularity of the lesion. Such contrast agents shorten T1 relaxation in target tissues, causing them to show increased signal on T1-weighted images (see **Figs. 9** and **10**).

In most bone tumors, MRI excels in staging the lesion, but does not provide any additional information toward a particular diagnosis. One notable exception is fibrous tumors. Most nonlipomatous bone tumors are of low signal on T1-weighted images, usually appearing of similar signal intensity to muscle, but such tumors usually appear at least partly of higher signal intensity than muscle on T2-weighted images. Fibrous tumors of bone are often the exception to this general rule. Many benign and some malignant fibrous tumors appear of low signal relative to muscle on *both* T1-weighted *and* T2-weighted images (see **Fig. 4**). Under certain conditions, biomolecules containing paramagnetic iron can profoundly influence the signal observed with some bone tumors. Deoxyhemoglobin, methemoglobin, and hemosiderin can all profoundly alter the signal observed from some tumors on MRI, with these hemoglobin breakdown products altering the observed signal in different ways. This can be seen in both an aneurysmal bone cyst and a giant cell tumor (see **Fig. 5**). An additional feature encountered in some bone tumors can provide diagnostic information on MRI: signal voids from feeding vessels in some hypervascular tumors. One more specific imaging feature of some less common bone tumors should

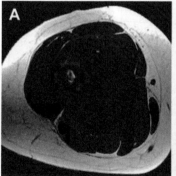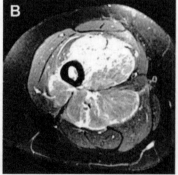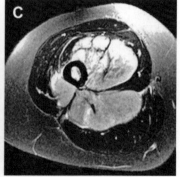

Fig. 9. T1-weighted (*A*), T2-weighted (*B*), and T1-weighted postcontrast (*C*) MR images from a patient with a Ewing sarcoma of the right femur. A gadolinium chelate contrast agent was administered intravenously at a dose of 1 mmol/kg before obtaining image (*C*). Note the greater contrast between the tumor and adjacent muscle on the T2 and T1 postcontrast images.

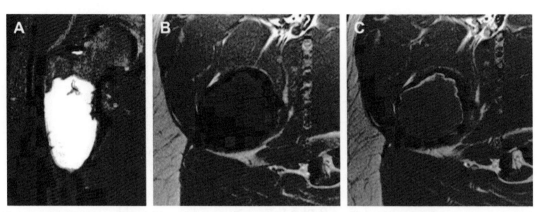

Fig. 10. STIR (*A*), T1-weighted (*B*), and T1 postcontrast (*C*) MR images of a unicameral bone cyst of the right femur. Note the extremely thin, uniform zone of contrast enhancement about the cyst in *C*.

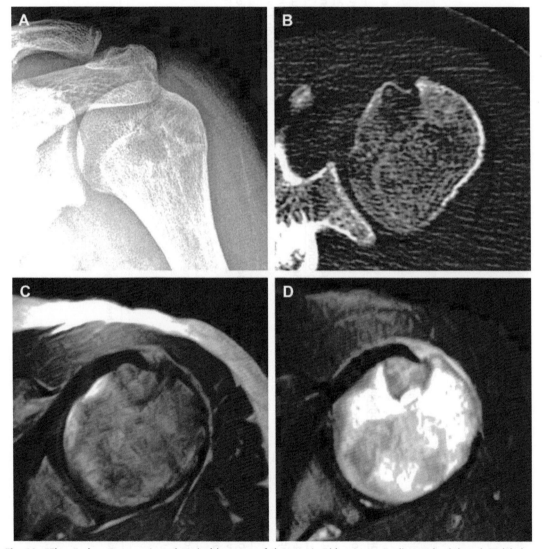

Fig. 11. "Flare" phenomenon in a chondroblastoma of the proximal humerus. Radiography (*A*) and CT (*B*) show a lucent lesion of the humeral head. T1-weighted (*C*) and T2-weighted (*D*) axial MR images show extensive, poorly defined altered marrow signal surrounding the lesion.

Table 1
Imaging features of some bone tumors that suggest specific histologies

Tumor	Demographics	Radiography	Computed Tomography	Magnetic Resonance Imaging	Specific Pathologic Feature
Intraosseous lipoma	Adults		Intramedullary, fat attenuation	Lesion isointense to fat on all sequences	Adipocytes
Fibrous cortical defect	Adolescents	Eccentric, metaphyseal lesion of long bones	Soft tissue attenuation, no matrix mineralization	Lesion parenchyma low signal on T1WI and T2WI	Fibrocytes
Giant-cell tumor of epiphysis	Adults	Ends of long bones, spine	Soft tissue attenuation, no matrix mineralization	Lesion frequently much lower in signal relative to fat on T2WI. Fluid-fluid levels.	Hemosiderin, hemorrhage
Enchondroma, low-grade chondrosarcoma	Adults	Metaphyses of long bones, pelvis	Soft tissue attenuation; density ≤ muscle, chondroid matrix mineralization	Portion of lesion very high signal on T2WI	Hydrogen bonded water in cartilage ground substance
Chondroblastoma	Children and adolescents	Epiphyses of long bones	Soft tissue attenuation, matrix mineralization in some tumors	Perilesional edema ("flare")	Chondroblasts with associated reticular mineralization. Surrounding marrow edema

Abbreviations: T1WI, T1-weighted image; T2WI, T2-weighted image.

be mentioned: perilesional edema or flare. This is seen as an ill-defined region of increased marrow signal outside of the margin of the lesion on T2-weighted or STIR images, and can be seen with chondroblastoma, osteoblastoma, and osteoid osteoma (**Fig. 11**).

SUMMARY

The role of the radiographic characterization of mineralization within a bone lesion in aiding its identification has already been mentioned. Other imaging features of some bone lesions that suggest a specific histology are listed in **Table 1**.

In this brief review, we have attempted to show how some imaging features of bone tumors can give valuable clues as to their histology. The clinical presentation of the patient, however, helped by close cooperation among the radiologist, pathologist, and orthopedic surgeon remain paramount in both achieving an accurate diagnosis of bone tumors and optimizing their management.

REFERENCES

1. Jaffe HL. Tumors and tumorous conditions of the bones and joints. Philadelphia: Lea & Febiger; 1958. p. 12.
2. Miller TT. Bone tumors and tumorlike conditions: analysis with conventional radiography. Radiology 2008;246:662–74.
3. Madewell JE, Ragsdale BD, Sweet DE. Radiologic and pathologic analysis of solitary bone lesions. I. Internal margins. Radiol Clin North Am 1981;19: 715–48.
4. Ragsdale BD, Madewell JE, Sweet DE. Radiologic and pathologic analysis of solitary bone lesions. II. Periosteal reactions. Radiol Clin North Am 1981;19: 749–83.
5. Sweet DE, Madewell JE, Ragsdale BD. Radiologic and pathologic analysis of solitary bone lesions. III. Matrix patterns. Radiol Clin North Am 1981;19: 785–814.
6. Lodwick GS. The bones and joints. Chicago: Year Book Medical Publishers; 1971.
7. Lodwick GS, Wilson AJ, Farrell C, et al. Determining growth rates of focal lesions of bone from radiographs. Radiology 1980;134:577–83.
8. Lodwick GS, Wilson AJ, Farrell C, et al. Estimating rate of growth in bone lesions: observer performance and error. Radiology 1980;134:585–90.
9. Partain CL, Price RR, Patton JAP, et al. Nuclear magnetic resonance imaging. Radiographics 1984; 4:5–25.
10. Elliott DO. Magnetic resonance imaging fundamentals and system performance. Radiol Clin North Am 1987;25:409–17.
11. Pooley RA. AAPM/RSNA physics tutorial for residents. Fundamental physics of MR imaging. Radiographics 2005;25:1087–99.
12. Armstrong P, Keevil SF. Magnetic resonance imaging-1: basic principles of image production. BMJ 1991;303:35–40.

ARTHRITIS PATHOLOGY

Edward F. DiCarlo, MD[a,b], Michael J. Klein, MD[a,b,c],*

KEYWORDS

- Degenerative joint disease • Osteoarthritis • Subchondral insufficiency fracture
- Inflammatory disease • Avascular necrosis • Septic/infectious arthritis • Joint replacement
- Gout • Iron overload • Ochronosis

ABSTRACT

The pathologic examination of failed joints, whether natural or artificial, is an indispensable part of the understanding of arthritis, as it is the last, and still best opportunity to determine or verify the correct diagnosis. Accuracy in pathologic diagnosis, based on a firm understanding of the various disease processes, provides reliable data for use in clinical registries, provides an opportunity to explain the "unusual" clinical presentation, and ultimately gives the "best evidence" for basing further treatments and prognosis for the individual patient.

OVERVIEW: BASIC CONCEPT OF ARTHRITIS

The 2 most common types of joint affected by arthritis of any kind are either diarthrodial (synovial) or amphiarthrodial (intervertebral discs). Most of the conditions affecting these joints are centered on diarthrodial joints, which is the focus of this article.

A functioning diarthrodial joint depends on the normal function of all of its components; an abnormality centered in one component eventually affects the others. The components of a diarthrodial joint are the articular cartilage; bones; menisci, if present; ligaments, tendons, capsular tissues; and neuromuscular elements. Some form of arthropathy develops when inflammation, degeneration, deformation, or abnormal deposits affect any of these components. In practice, the term "arthritis" is usually considered synonymous with "arthropathy," because most cases of disease in fact have either a primary or secondary inflammatory component. This in turn reduces the uncertainty about when to use such terms as "arthritis" and the somewhat awkward terms "arthrosis" and "arthritidies."

DISEASE CLASSIFICATION

The classification of arthritic diseases is based on the putative site of initiation or concentration of the disease process. Disease arising from degenerative changes, such as osteoarthritis, affects the cartilage initially. Inflammatory diseases, such as rheumatoid arthritis, the seronegative spondyloarthropathies, and infection begin in the synovium or bone. Diseases characterized by acute or chronic deformity of the joint, which is maintained primarily by the bone, include trauma, the dysplasias, collapse, and Paget disease. Depositional diseases such as gout and ochronosis result when deposits of crystals or aberrant chemical components accumulate in the soft tissues and bones of the joint, respectively.

In this classification scheme, most conditions are arbitrarily considered primary – arbitrary, in that many cases of osteoarthritis, for example, lack an identifiable specific inciting or precipitating event. Likewise, the inflammatory diseases such as rheumatoid arthritis and ankylosing spondylitis are considered primary because they have early joint involvement. On the other hand, so-called secondary inflammatory joint disease may occur much later in cases of the seronegative

---

[a] Department of Pathology and Laboratory Medicine, Hospital for Special Surgery, 535 East 70th Street, New York, NY 10021, USA
[b] Joan and Sanford Weill College of Medicine of Cornell University, 1300 York Avenue, New York, NY 10065, USA
[c] Memorial Sloan-Kettering Cancer Center and Memorial Hospital for Cancer and Allied Diseases, 1275 York Avenue, New York, NY 10065, USA
* Corresponding author. Department of Pathology and Laboratory Medicine, Hospital for Special Surgery, 535 East 70th Street, New York, NY 10021.
E-mail address: KleinM@HSS.EDU

Surgical Pathology 5 (2012) 15–65
doi:10.1016/j.path.2011.07.009

Table 1
Diagnosis distribution of large joints, 1997 versus 2007

| | Hip | | | | Knee | | | | Shoulder | | | |
| | 1997 | | 2007 | | 1997 | | 2007 | | 1997 | | 2007 | |
	No	%	No	%	No	%	No	%	No	%	No	%
Diagnoses:												
DJD	491	83	597	75	569	93	898	93	29	67	33	69
AVN	62	10	43	5	13	2	1	0	5	12	4	8
Neck Fx.	22	4	21	3	0	0	0	0	5	12	8	17
Inflamm.	11	2	14	2	32	5	17	2	4	9	2	4
Subchon. Fx.	2	0.3	90	11	0	0	51	5	0	0	1	2
Rapid	2	0.3	25	3	0	0	2	0.2	0	0	0	0
Septic	1	0.2	2	0.3	0	0	1	0.1	0	0	0	0
Total Count:	591		792		614		970		43		48	

Abbreviations: AVN, avascular necrosis; DJD, degenerative joint disease; Fx, fracture; Inflamm, inflammation; Subchon, subchondral.

spondyloarthropathies and arthropathies associated with other diseases, such as inflammatory bowel disease and reactive arthritis (Reiter syndrome).

Although the pathologic classification of the various joint diseases has remained fairly constant, several conditions have been added to the list of distinct entities over the past decade. The conditions that are presented in this article and their relative frequencies as they were encountered by the authors from 1997 to 2007 are listed in Table 1. These years were chosen because they span a period from before the reporting of more recently appreciated conditions to well into the first decade of this millennium—a period designated as the "The Bone and Joint Decade for the Prevention and Treatment of Musculoskeletal Disorders."[1] The condition-specific experience by the authors is presented in Table 2, with summary information covering 2005 through 2009, a period when all of the conditions listed in Table 1 were included in the diagnostic acumen of the authors.

DISEASE FEATURES

DEGENERATIVE JOINT DISEASE

Degenerative joint disease (DJD) or osteoarthritis (OA) is the most common form of arthritis encountered in clinical and pathologic practice (see Table 1). The causes of this form of arthritis are

Table 2
Anatomic distribution by diagnosis, 2005 through 2009

| Joint | Osteoarthritis | | Subchondral Fracture | | Rapidly Destructive | | Inflammatory Disease | | Avascular Necrosis | | Septic Arthritis | | Implant Failure | |
	No	%	No	%	No	%	No	%	No	%	No	%	No	%
Hip	3109	36.7	502	57.0	118	95.2	59	29.8	210	90.1	9	17.0	502	52.2
Knee	4426	52.2	360	40.9	6	4.8	71	35.9	4	1.7	30	56.6	411	42.8
Shoulder	280	3.3	12	1.4	0	0.0	13	6.6	16	6.9	6	11.3	31	3.2
Elbow	39	0.5	2	0.2	0	0.0	11	5.6	1	0.4	1	1.9	10	1.0
Ankle	49	0.6	4	0.5	0	0.0	3	1.5	1	0.4	2	3.8	5	0.5
Small, Upper	143	1.7	0	0.0	0	0.0	22	11.1	1	0.4	1	1.9	0	0.0
Small, Lower	429	5.1	1	0.1	0	0.0	19	9.6	0	0.4	4	7.5	2	0.2
	8475	—	881	—	124	—	198	—	233	—	53	—	961	—

many, but are usually related to a lifelong accumulation of traumatic insults to the joint components in the absence of rare familial syndromes.

Age and Skeletal Distribution

Degenerative disease of the joints, not related to developmental abnormalities or associated with specific incidences of trauma, is usually encountered in mature individuals because degenerative disease occurs over a lifetime of activity. With the exception of posttraumatic osteoarthropathy, the incidence of DJD/OA increases with age and has an average age in the upper 60s for both men and women; 60% of surgical specimens are from women. Both large and small joints are affected. As seen in **Table 2**, the hips and knees are the 2 most commonly affected large joints, the metatarsophalangeal joint of the great toe and the interphalangeal joints of the toes are the most common small joints affected, and the carpometacarpal joint (the basal joint) of the thumb is the most commonly affected small joint of the hand.

Gross Pathology

DJD/OA is characterized grossly by a set of morphologic features beginning with fibrillation and disruption, followed by loss of the articular cartilage in the weight-bearing region of the joint, and then dense sclerosis of the exposed bone, with osteochondral proliferations, known as marginal osteophytes, developing nearly simultaneously at the periphery of the joint surfaces (**Figs. 1** and **2**). Osteophytosis, the development of marginal osteophytes, is a nearly obligatory hallmark of DJD/OA and is a proliferative feature that occurs simultaneously with the loss of the cartilage as long as the degenerative process occurs at a rate that permits the growth of osteophytes. It should also be emphasized that osteophytes commonly develop in compartments of the knee that do not show loss of the compartmental cartilage.

The cut surface of the bone beneath the exposed surface shows sclerosis that extends to variable depths into the underlying bone. Varying degrees of mucocystic degeneration, occasionally referred to as "subchondral cysts," and more correctly as "subarticular cysts," or pseudocystic degeneration, may be apparent in the superficial bone as well (**Fig. 3**).

The gross appearance of synovial tissue is highly variable and ranges from smooth and glistening through variable degrees of granular, nodular, and papillary hyperplasia and hypertrophy with or without brown coloration caused by hemosiderosis. The absence of synovial infiltrates permits the delicate vessels to be seen through the transparent lining layer (**Fig. 4**).

Microscopic Pathology

Histologically, the classic case of DJD/OA shows loss of the cartilage centrally, sclerosis of the exposed bone, and marginal osteophytosis (**Fig. 5**). The degenerating cartilage shows variable

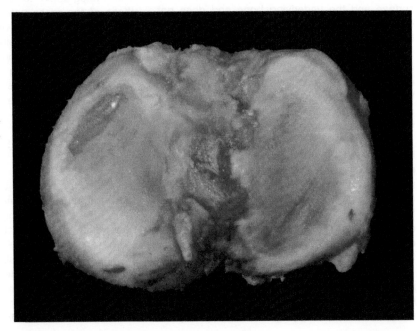

Fig. 1. This photograph of a right knee joint affected by DJD/OA shows loss of a small region of cartilage and exposure of sclerotic bone at the anteromedial border with early local osteophytes and a small osteophyte at the anterior border of the otherwise well-maintained lateral compartment.

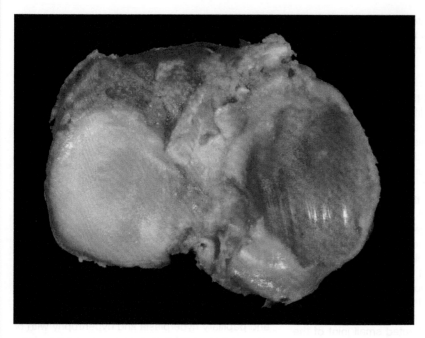

Fig. 2. This photograph of a left knee joint affected by DJD/OA shows extensive loss of the cartilage of the medial compartment with sclerosis and ridging of the exposed bone and moderate marginal osteophytosis. Slight marginal osteophytosis is apparent in the otherwise well-maintained lateral compartment as well.

degrees of fibrillation, focal loss of the chondrocytes, and variable degrees of chondrocytic proliferation ("cloning") (**Fig. 6**). With thinning of the cartilage, the calcified zone thickens, the tide mark becomes reduplicated, and the bony end plate becomes thickened as well, leading to dense bony sclerosis composed mostly of lamellar matrix (**Fig. 7**). As can also be appreciated in **Fig. 5**, the sclerosis tends to be limited to the exposed bony surface and the underlying bone and does not extend very far beneath the surfaces still covered by cartilage, even if the cartilage is not intact.

Pseudocysts are rounded defects in the superficial bone containing fibromyxoid tissue, fibrovascular tissue, or mucoid fluid. Bone overlying these pseudocysts may be necrotic or fractured and is composed of reactive osteochondral tissue, including woven bone (**Fig. 8**).

Osteophytes begin as progressive growth of bone through the marginal bony end plate with progressive growth of the overlying cartilage and may reach a very large size. This cartilage has a cursory resemblance to normal articular cartilage, but it is somewhat more fibrous and less organized (**Fig. 9**). Hematopoietic marrow is frequently present in the intertrabecular spaces of the osteophyte.

The synovium shows various degrees of hyperplasia of the lining layer (**Fig. 10**). Inflammation is nearly universally present, most commonly as small perivascular aggregates of lymphocytes, but may be focally intense and contain a higher proportion of plasma cells with or without Russell bodies and occasionally even isolated perivascular germinal centers (**Fig. 11**). Evidence indicates that this inflammation, even at low levels, may be pathogenetic in the disease process.[2–4]

Radiographic Features

The radiographic features of DJD/OA parallel those of the gross pathologic features. Loss of the cartilage correlates with loss of the joint space in the center of the joint. Sclerosis and cystic degeneration in the bone correlate with similar features in the opposing surfaces of the narrowed joint space. Osteophytes are seen as bony excrescences arising from the edges of the joint lines (**Fig. 12**).

INSUFFICIENCY DISEASE/SUBCHONDRAL FRACTURE

Insufficiency fracture in the subchondral location (subchondral insufficiency fracture [SIF]) was rarely reported before the end of the 1990s but is now a fairly frequent diagnosis in the experience of the authors (see **Table 1**). SIF is a fracture occurring beneath the subchondral bony end plate that rapidly leads to degeneration of the joint. Because the fracture is often subtle and not usually identified radiographically, nearly all cases are regarded as DJD/OA clinically; however,

Fig. 3. (*A*) This photograph of a femoral head affected by DJD/OA shows loss of the cartilage at the superior surface with a prominent medial osteophyte filled with hematopoietic marrow (*left*) and well-defined subarticular fibromyxoid pseudocysts beneath the exposed surface. (*B*) The corresponding specimen radiograph emphasizes the medial osteophyte and the pseudocysts but also shows the sclerosis in the superficial bone.

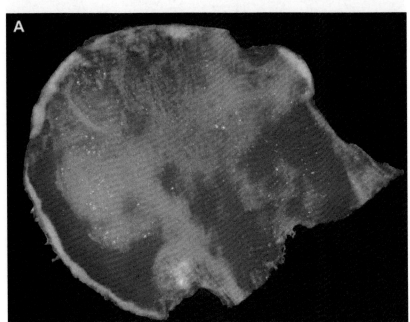

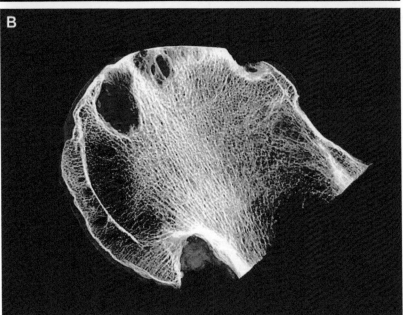

a hallmark clinical feature of this condition is intense pain and disability grossly out of proportion to the degree of radiographically apparent deformity of the affected joint.

Age and Skeletal Distribution

Subchondral insufficiency fracture is a disease of elderly adults. Nearly 50% of the patients are older than 70. Slightly more than 60% of the cases occur in women. It has been speculated that SIF represents either a consequence or a potential harbinger of systemic osteoporosis. Because insufficiency is a relative term, however, it is possible that the condition can also develop in overweight adults in their 50s and 60s who do not appear to be osteoporotic. As can be seen in **Table 2**, the femoral head/hip joint is the most

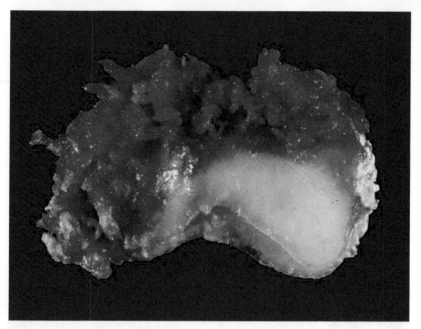

Fig. 4. This photograph of the synovium from the supra-patellar pouch of a knee affected by DJD/OA shows delicate fibrillation with delicate blood vessels just visible through the transparent superficial lining layer.

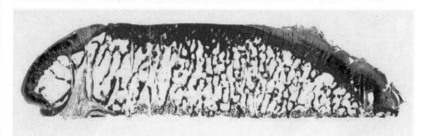

Fig. 5. This photomicrograph of a femoral condyle affected by DJD/OA shows the central loss of the cartilage with sclerosis of the bone, thinning and degeneration of the residual cartilage, and a prominent marginal osteophyte (*left*) (hematoxylin and eosin [H&E], original magnification ×0.5).

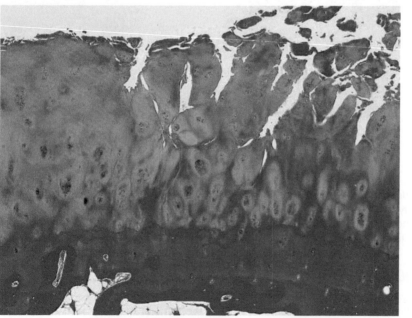

Fig. 6. This photomicrograph of degenerate cartilage shows the surface disruption with fibrillation, patchy loss of the chondrocytes and proliferation or "cloning" of the surviving chondrocytes. Note also the duplication of the tidemark over an otherwise minimally affected bony end plate (H&E, original magnification ×10).

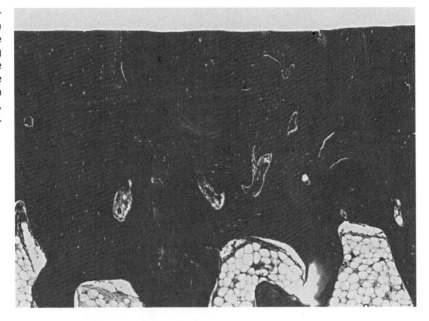

Fig. 7. This photomicrograph of exposed bone in DJD/OA shows the dense sclerosis owing to filling of the space between the original trabeculae (pale staining) by the addition of lamellar bone (H&E, original magnification ×10).

common site affected, followed by the knee and the humeral head/shoulder. Many of the cases affecting the knee were previously diagnosed as spontaneous osteonecrosis, known as SPONK (SPontaneous OsteoNecrosis of the Knee), thought to be a form of osteonecrosis/avascular necrosis (AVN) without any of the usual associations for that condition.[5,6]

Gross Pathology

The gross appearance of SIF is variable and occasionally resembles that of Stage 3 AVN (see later in this article), which explains much of the difficulty in distinguishing between these 2 conditions.

In general, the cartilage is thinned and may even be absent, and a small, shallow excavation or region of collapse may be apparent. A flap of

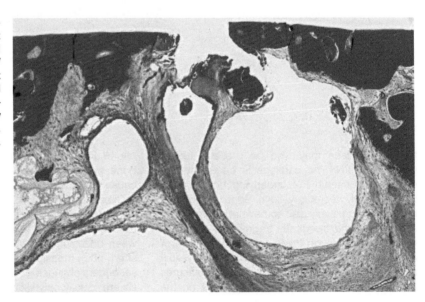

Fig. 8. This photomicrograph of a pseudocyst just beneath the exposed articular surface in DJD/OA shows a small defect in the overlying bone and empty, previously fluid-filled spaces defined by fibromyxoid septa (H&E, original magnification ×2.5).

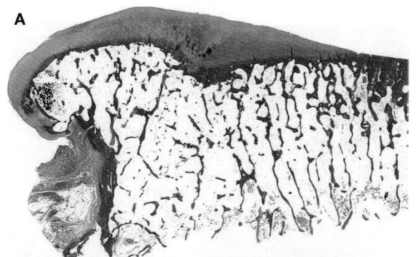

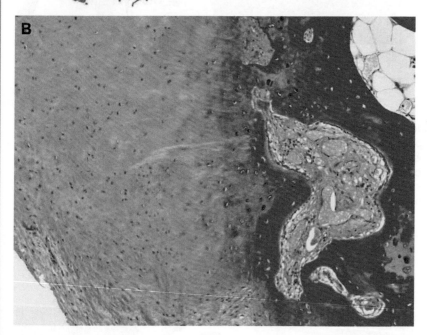

Fig. 9. These photomicrographs of an osteophyte show (*A*) extension beyond the original joint margin resulting from osteochondral growth at the periphery of the joint (H&E, magnification ×1) and (*B*) remodeling endochondral ossification at the base of the layer of mostly fibrochondral tissue (H&E, original magnification ×10).

thinned cartilage may also be present, further mimicking AVN. The cartilage is frequently thin enough to observe the underlying bone that is usually focally necrotic (yellow). Bone not covered by cartilage is usually also somewhat sclerotic, but also yellow and frequently fragmented (**Fig. 13**). Cut sections through these regions show thin or absent cartilage overlying a narrow zone of yellow necrosis or tan sclerosis that usually measures less than 8 mm in thickness and abuts on the

undersurface of the bony end plate (**Fig. 14**). The bone beneath this zone may be hyperemic because of hematoma.

Cystic degeneration is not usually present unless secondary degeneration has supervened. Likewise, because the duration of symptoms between onset and surgical replacement is usually short, often measured in months instead of years, secondary changes, such as marginal osteophytosis are usually only slight or not present.

Fig. 10. These photomicrographs of synovium in DJD/OA show (*A*) the normally thin synovial lining layer as well as interstitial mucoid degeneration and a focus of perivascular chronic inflammation, and (*B*) micropapillary hyperplasia of the lining layer in this region (*A* and *B,* H&E, original magnification ×20).

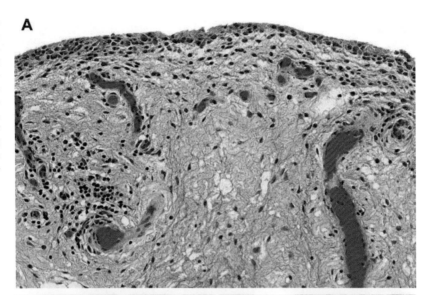

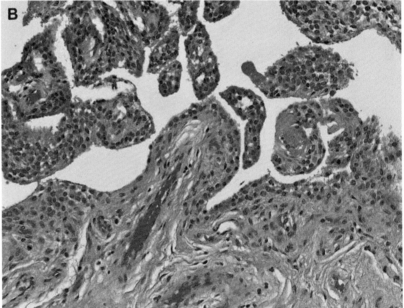

Microscopic Pathology

In general, the articular cartilage is thin and somewhat fibrillated, in contrast to the generally well-maintained cartilage in AVN. The bone beneath this thinned cartilage shows a linear zone of fracturing, frequently with superficial necrosis, and other reactive changes in the marrow that run parallel to and immediately beneath the bony end plate (Fig. 15). In some cases, well-developed fracture callus without necrosis is present in this location, representing a chronic, remodeling, healed fracture (Fig. 16).

Radiographic Features

The radiographic features of SIF are often subtle and not easily recognized (Fig. 17). The primary feature of subchondral fracture at the time of radiographic evaluation is narrowing of the joint space up to a moderate degree with little or no subchondral bony sclerosis and with small or no osteophytes at all. Only occasionally, and usually only after very careful examination, can a discontinuity or flattening of the convex articular surface be identified. Likewise, only rarely is a fracture line with or without sclerosis apparent on routine

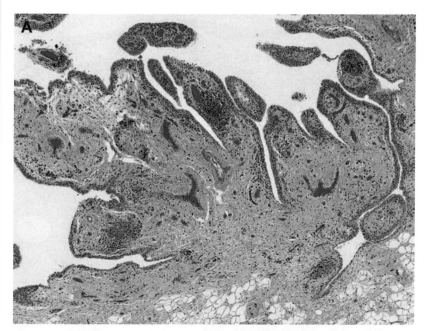

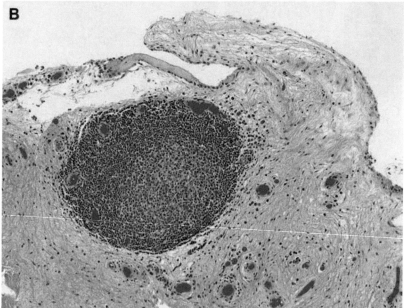

Fig. 11. These photomicrographs of synovium in DJD/OA show (*A*) papillary hypertrophy with a moderate degree of perivascular and interstitial chronic inflammation (H&E, magnification ×5), and (*B*) a single germinal center (H&E, original magnification ×10).

radiographs. Because of a greater degree of overlap of the bones, the diagnostic features are less likely to be identified in the hip joint than in the knee or shoulder joints. Magnetic resonance imaging (MRI) may show signs of fracture with hematoma and diffuse "edema pattern," but MRI is not often used in radiographic analysis.[7]

RAPIDLY DESTRUCTIVE OSTEOARTHRITIS

Rapidly destructive OA (RDOA), like SIF, was only rarely diagnosed before the end of the 1990s (see Table 1). The diagnosis of RDOA is suggested by the radiographic progression of a case of relatively mild OA progressing to destruction of the joint over a relatively short period, usually measured

Fig. 12. This plain radiograph of the case presented in **Fig. 3** shows the corresponding loss of the radiographic joint space, the sclerosis and "cystic" degeneration of the head and acetabulum, and the large medial osteophyte.

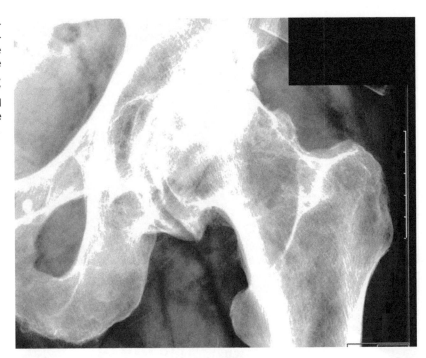

in months.[8] It has been suggested that RDOA is a more rapidly developing form of subarticular insufficiency fracture, which may account for its concurrent recognition along with SIF.[9–11]

Age and Skeletal Distribution

RDOA is generally a condition of the mature or elderly adult with nearly 80% of the cases occurring in those older than 60. Nearly 70% of the

Fig. 13. This photograph of the surface of a femoral head affected by SIF shows cartilage that is thin enough to see patchy yellow necrosis in the underlying bone. Note also the small osteophytes.

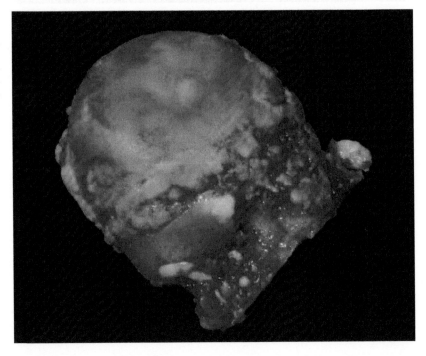

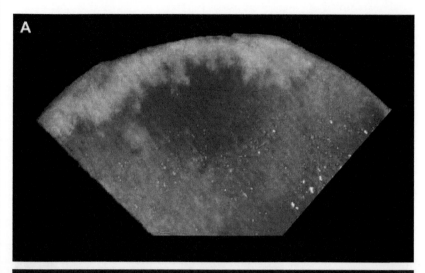

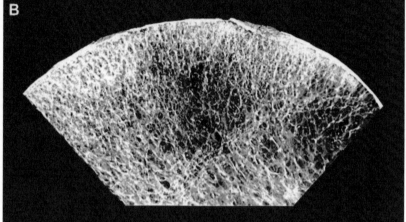

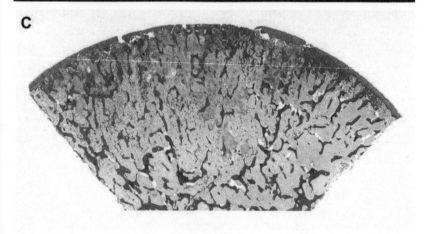

Fig. 14. These images are of the same case as presented in **Fig. 13.** (*A*) The cut surface shows focal loss and thinning of the cartilage with a narrow superficial zone of necrosis with a thin zone of sclerosis (*top right*). (*B*) The specimen radiograph of the same sample that shows the superficial sclerosis to the right as well as superficial rarefaction owing to the necrosis and fractured bone. (*C*) The histologic section that shows corresponding features of necrosis, fragmentation, and collapse of the cartilage and the sclerosis owing to callus near the right edge of the section (H&E, original magnification ×1).

Fig. 15. These photomicrographs of an acute case of SIF show (*A*) a thin layer of cartilage overlying a superficial zone of fracture with necrosis and osteochondral callus, and (*B*) a surface devoid of cartilage with a superficial zone of sclerotic and fractured trabeculae and associated fracture callus, much of which is secondarily necrotic (H&E, original magnification ×5).

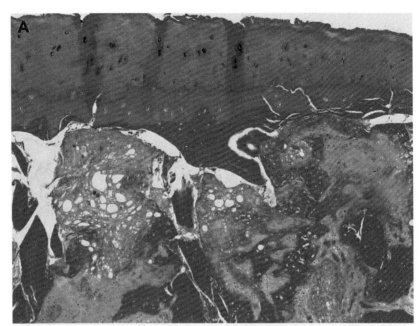

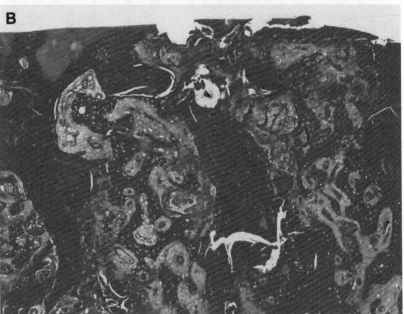

cases occur in women. As can be seen in **Table 2**, the hip is affected in approximately 95% of the cases and the authors have identified the remaining cases only in the knee. None of the patients were known to have a neuropathic illness or a known reason to suspect such an illness, either before or after diagnosis.

Gross Pathology

Grossly, a joint affected by RDOA shows dramatic deformity owing to destruction of the cartilage and variable amounts of the bone resulting in flattening of the articular surface or even a deep saddle-shaped deformity (**Fig. 18**A). The surface is usually devoid of cartilage except for at the extreme

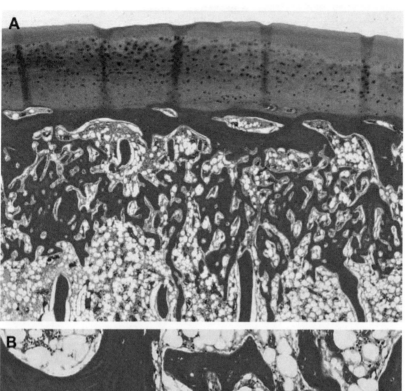

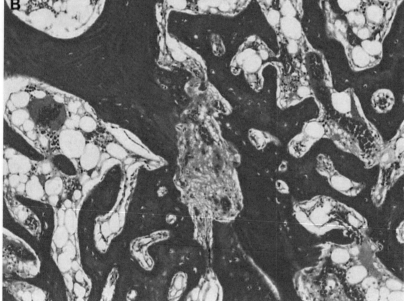

Fig. 16. These photomicrographs of a case of chronic SIF show (*A*) a band of remodeling trabecular fracture callus beneath the bony end plate (H&E, original magnification ×2.5) and (*B*) the same region at higher magnification with a broken trabecula encased in trabecular callus composed of woven and lamellar matrix (H&E, original magnification ×10).

periphery of the joint, which usually does not show significant osteophytosis. The exposed bone is fragmented and necrotic. The synovium is often thickened and gritty owing to the accumulation of articular detritus.

Sectioning into the bone shows patchy sclerosis and focal rarefaction with patchy necrosis extending to variable depths into the underlying cancellous bone (see **Fig. 18**B, C).

Microscopic Pathology

The histologic features of RDOA reflect the accelerated destructive changes occurring in the joint. The articular surface mostly consists of exposed, fragmented bone that is necrotic and fragmented with scattered foci of callus within the necrotic region (**Fig. 19**). A small amount of residual cartilage, usually present at the margin of the articular surface, shows variable degrees of degeneration

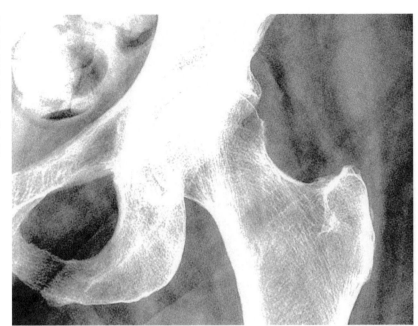

Fig. 17. This plain radiograph of the case of SIF illustrated in **Figs.** 13 and 14 shows the subtle flattening of the femoral head and only a slight degree of osteophytosis despite a report of excruciating pain. A subtle zone of superficial sclerosis was not appreciated preoperatively.

with or without a slight degree of osteophytosis. Bone at the periphery of the necrotic zone may show various degrees of fracture callus (**Fig. 20**). The large amount of cartilaginous and bony detritus produced by the rapidly destructive process induces a substantial cellular reaction composed of mononuclear macrophages and giant cells, resulting in a noninflammatory, nonnecrotizing, loose granulomatous reaction within the bone (**Fig. 21**) and the synovium (**Fig. 22**).

Radiographic Features

Before the onset of the rapidly progressive component, RDOA presents radiographically as early or moderate OA that progresses over a fairly brief period to extreme destruction of the affected joint in a manner mimicking a Charcot (neuropathic) joint, except that the condition is symptomatically painful. Marginal osteophytosis is usually minimal, or not changed from its appearance before the destructive phase of the disease, and is markedly reduced for the degree of deformity of the joint (**Fig. 23**).

INFLAMMATORY DISEASE

The inflammatory arthropathies, most notably rheumatoid arthritis, and to a lesser degree, ankylosing spondylitis and psoriatic arthritis, have maintained clinical prevalence over the years.[12–15] Nonsurgical treatment, however, has improved to

the point where cases of these conditions are much less common in a surgical pathology practice than they once were (see **Table 1**). When these conditions are encountered, the findings reflect either very active joint disease that has failed treatment or late, end-stage, clinically "burned-out" disease.

Age and Skeletal Distribution

The surgically treated inflammatory diseases have a wide range of age and skeletal distributions and therefore can be seen in any joint and at any age. The more active cases are usually seen in children and young adults, whereas the less active or end-stage cases are usually seen in older adults. In contrast to degenerative diseases, inflammatory diseases usually affect the smaller joints, especially of the hands and wrist, with the elbow being the most commonly affected large joint (see **Table 2**). When the large joints are affected, especially the mature knee, degenerative disease of one compartment may be superimposed; this is a separate condition that does not represent end-stage arthritis.

Gross Pathology

The earliest manifestations of inflammatory disease arise in the synovium, which shows thickening and variable papillary hypertrophy, with a variable amount of surface fibrin overlying reddish-brown and tan synovial tissue (**Fig. 24**).

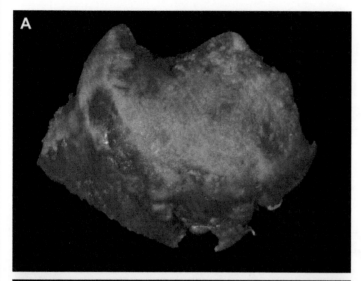

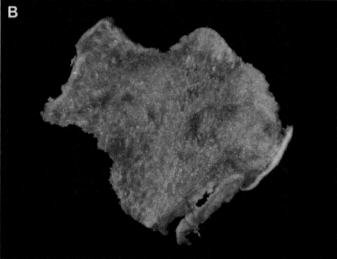

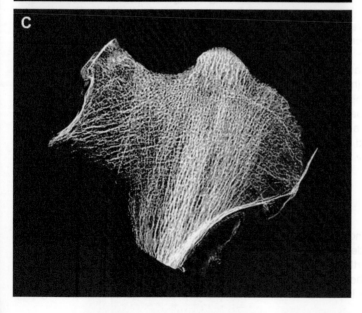

Fig. 18. (A) This photograph of a formalin-fixed femoral head shows the necrosis and fragmentation of the bone representing the markedly deformed, exposed articular surface after rapid destruction of the over-lying cartilage and bone. Notice the absence of osteophytes. (B) This photograph of the cut surface from the same femoral head shows a varia-bly thick superficial zone of necrosis with mottling and loss of the fatty yellow marrow. (C) This specimen radiograph of the same femoral head shows the sclerosis associated with collapse and fracturing of the superfi-cial bone without the typical bony sclerosis of DJD. Small osteophytes are visible at the articular margins.

Fig. 19. This photomicrograph of the superficial bone exposed after rapid destruction shows fragmentation of the trabeculae with detritus and necrosis of the marrow fat (H&E, original magnification ×5).

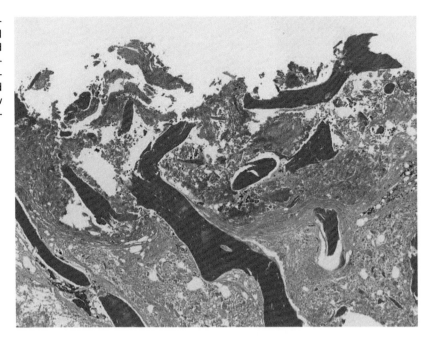

As the disease progresses, the synovial tissue produces a pannus (covering) that causes erosive destruction of the soft tissues of the joint beginning at the joint periphery. The soft tissues, including the cartilage, intracapsular ligaments, and menisci, are progressively destroyed, resulting in the appearance of erosions without osteophytes at the margins of the articular surfaces (**Fig. 25**). These erosions involve the cartilage as well as the subchondral bone, occasionally leading to collapse of the undermined articular surface. The bone usually has some degree of osteoporosis.

The synovial hypertrophy and the destructive features often persist until all of the cartilage has

Fig. 20. This photomicrograph of the peripheral exposed surface shows fracture callus adjacent to the small amount of residual cartilage at the medial border of the articular surface (H&E, original magnification ×5).

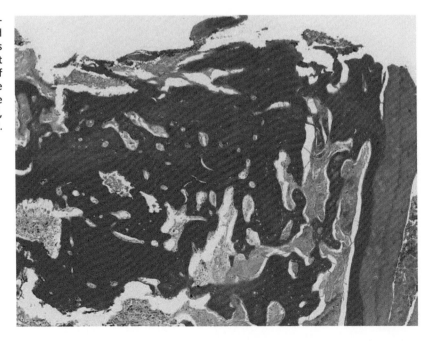

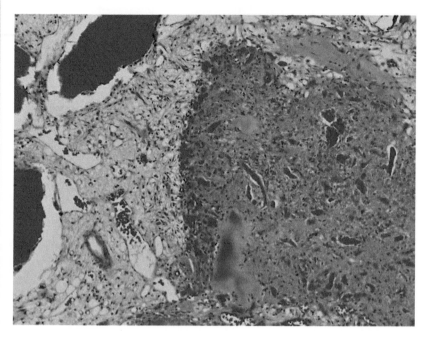

Fig. 21. This photomicrograph from the bone at the periphery of the necrotic region shows accumulated articular detritus with an associated granulomatous reaction and granular degeneration of the marrow fat (H&E, original magnification ×10).

been destroyed in the late stage of the disease. By that time, the articular surfaces show variable degrees of patchy excavation and patchy sclerosis of the exposed bone. Fibrosis of the synovial tissue and focal or widespread fibrous ankylosis occur mostly in the small joints.

Microscopic Pathology

The inflammatory features are most readily seen in the synovium. The synovial lining layer is usually markedly thickened and frequently contains multinucleate synovial giant cells (**Fig. 26**). The hallmark feature of RA synovium is the inflammation, which

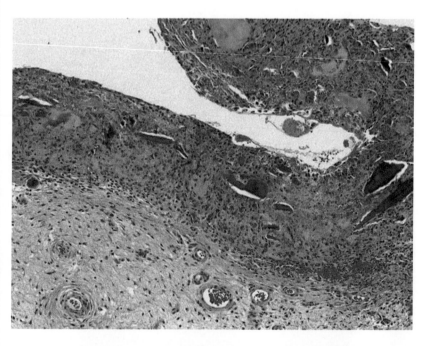

Fig. 22. This photomicrograph from the synovium in a hip joint affected by RDOA shows accumulated articular detritus with an associated granulomatous reaction (H&E, original magnification ×10).

Fig. 23. (*A*) This plain radiograph of a hip joint shows moderate deformity of the femoral head in a case of recent-onset hip pain. Notice the degree of deformity without appreciable osteophytes. (*B*) This plain radiograph of the same hip taken 2 months later shows the hallmark marked deformity occurring over a short period, still with the absence of osteophytes.

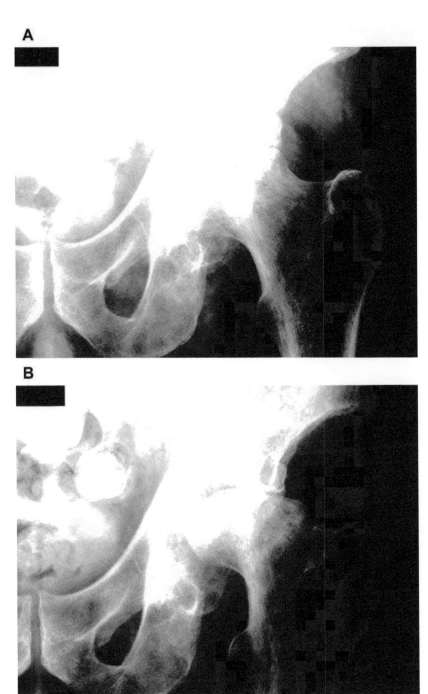

consists of an extensive infiltrate of chronic inflammation composed of a mixture of lymphocytes and plasma cells with variable amounts of Russell bodies, multinucleate plasma cells, and germinal centers (**Fig. 27**). Neutrophils may be seen in the superficial tissue, as they are caught while in transit through the tissue into the joint fluid; they are not accompanied by necrosis, do not represent infection, and account for the high neutrophil count in rheumatoid synovial fluid (**Fig. 28**). The

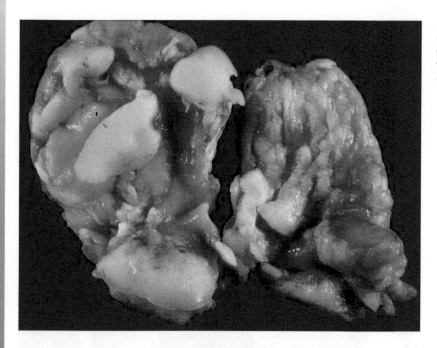

Fig. 24. This photograph of rheumatoid synovium shows the thickening and tan appearance with globules of coagulated fibrin.

deeper tissues show variable degrees of interstitial mucoid degeneration and perivascular chronic inflammation.

The joint surfaces in active inflammatory disease frequently show destruction of the cartilage by inflammatory pannus as well as undermining the articular surface with a distinctive variety of degeneration of the cartilage that produces Weichselbaum lacunae, which represents invasion into the territorial zones of the superficial chondrocytes (**Fig. 29**). The cartilage is eventually completely destroyed and the exposed bone shows variable degrees of rarefaction and patchy sclerosis. In some cases, pseudocysts containing

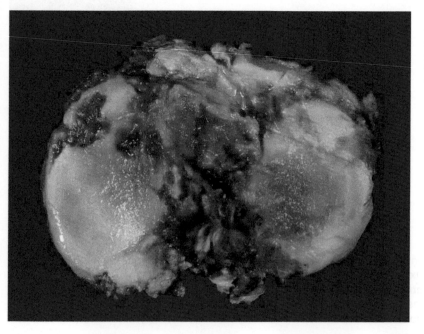

Fig. 25. This photograph of a right tibial plateau affected by RA shows peripheral erosions of the cartilage without osteophytes.

Fig. 26. This photomicrograph of the synovial lining layer shows hyperplasia as well as numerous scattered multinucleate synovial giant cells (H&E, original magnification ×40).

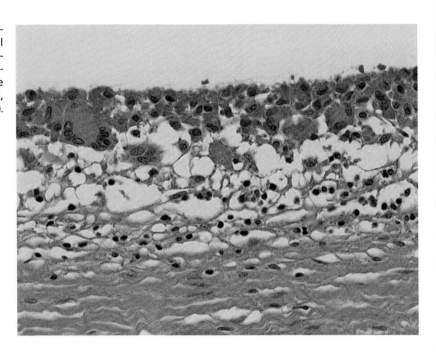

numerous neutrophils intermixed with macrophages may also be present in the superficial exposed bone (**Fig. 30**).[16] Inflammatory infiltrates composed of a mixture of lymphocytes and plasma cells are also frequently present in the bone marrow.

In cases of end-stage disease, degenerative changes including osteosclerosis and noninflammatory cystic degeneration with telltale marginal erosions but without marginal osteophytes constitute the typical findings. When degenerative joint disease is superimposed on inflammatory disease,

Fig. 27. This photomicrograph of RA synovium shows papillary hypertrophy with hyperplasia of the lining and intense inflammation including germinal centers (H&E, magnification ×10).

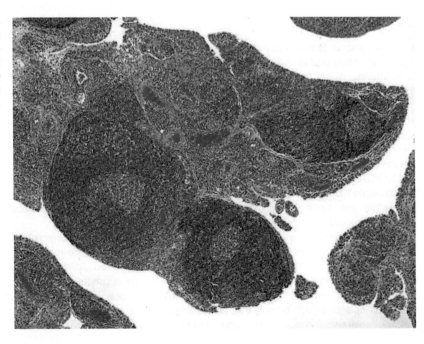

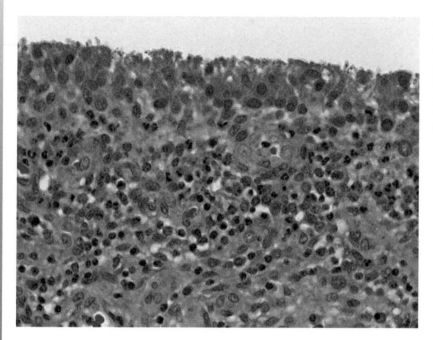

Fig. 28. This photomicrograph of RA synovium shows numerous neutrophils in transit through the tissue and into the lining layer, through which they gain access to the synovial fluid (H&E, magnification ×40).

such as happens in the knee, it usually involves only one compartment and then it has the typical features of DJD/OA, including central loss of the cartilage with eburnation of the exposed bone and marginal osteophytosis, although these features may be somewhat blunted (**Fig. 31**).

Radiographic Features

The radiographic features of inflammatory disease reflect the stage and activity of the disease. In the early stages, usually best seen in the small joints of the hand, hypertrophy of the synovium appears as soft tissue swelling. Destruction of the joint begins at the edges of the articular surfaces, with relative sparing of the joint space until the destruction of the cartilage is nearly complete, at which point the joint space is also significantly narrow. Unlike in DJD/OA, the loss of the joint space is not accompanied by sclerosis of the exposed bone, but rather the bone is porotic, typical of the juxta-articular osteoporosis of RA. The destruction of the joint from the periphery generates marginal erosions, which persist throughout the clinical course. In cases of psoriatic arthritis, osteophytes may be present and even overshadow the otherwise erosive changes. With later stages of RA, the joint space is narrowed; the bone shows patchy sclerosis, rarefaction, and structural derangement; and the alignment of the joint is markedly abnormal.

INFARCTION/OSTEONECROSIS DISEASE

Avascular necrosis (AVN) is the term applied to the special case of bone infarction (osteonecrosis) arising in the end of a bone leading to potential consequences to the adjacent joint. Before the use of steroids in the treatment of various forms of inflammatory disease, infarction in bone was seldom encountered in any significant numbers independent of such conditions as sickle cell disease, caisson-workers' disease (decompression sickness), Gaucher disease, and various infections and fractures.[17] As seen in **Table 1**, however, the incidence of AVN as encountered in surgical pathologic practice has declined since more widespread use of nonsteroidal anti-inflammatory agents has developed over the past several decades.

Unlike osteonecrosis ("bone infarction"), which occurs in the medullary regions elsewhere in the skeleton, AVN leads to joint disease because the mechanical forces applied to the infarcted subarticular cancellous bone cause the accumulation of nonhealing trabecular fractures that result in ultimate collapse of the joint surface. The resulting

Fig. 29. These photomicrographs of RA articular surfaces show (*A*) erosive synovial pannus covering the cartilage, and (*B*) inflammatory pannus undermining the cartilage and bone with associated destruction of the these components and invasion of the chondrocytic territorial zones producing Weichselbaum lacunae (H&E, original magnification ×10).

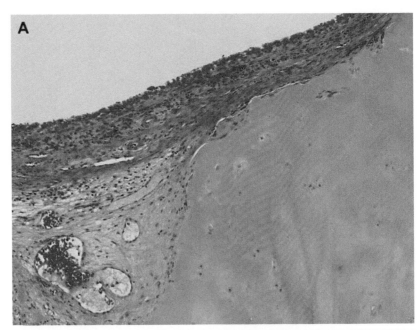

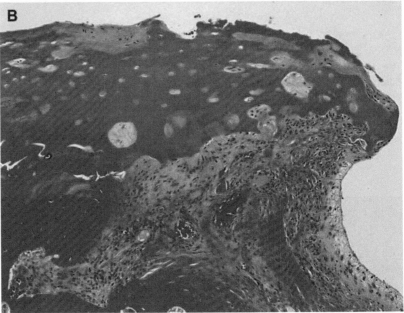

incongruity of the opposing collapsed convex and intact concave surfaces results in secondary degenerative disease.

Age and Skeletal Distribution

AVN is known to occur in any age group, but is generally a disease of the young adult skeleton, because it is most commonly associated with the use of steroids for the treatment of various inflammatory conditions that develop in the younger skeleton. AVN is most commonly encountered in the elderly adult skeleton after fracture, frequently of the femoral neck. Table 2 shows the skeletal distribution of AVN with special note that it is nearly always centered on the convex side of the joint, eg, the femoral head of the hip, the humeral head of the shoulder, the dome of the talus of the ankle, or a femoral condyle of the knee.

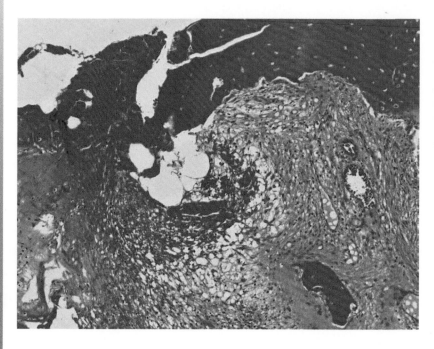

Fig. 30. This photomicrograph of a superficial pseudocyst in RA shows fibrin and a mixture of inflammatory cells including neutrophils representing an inflammatory pseudoabscess and mimicking infection (H&E, original magnification ×10).

Gross Pathology

The gross appearance of a joint affected by AVN differs somewhat depending on the stage of the disease, as defined by Ficat and Arlet[18]; the differences are summarized in Table 3. In most cases of surgically excised specimens, the articular surface shows a segment of fairly well maintained articular cartilage that is depressed (collapsed) into the underlying bone (Fig. 32). The periphery of the collapsed segment is usually buckled and at least focally torn, and the resulting flap of cartilage may lift from the underlying bone. In late-stage AVN, the load usually supported by the collapsed necrotic region is transferred to the surrounding

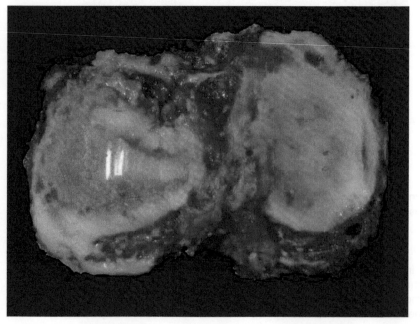

Fig. 31. This photograph of a left tibial plateau in a patient with RA shows loss of the cartilage centrally in the lateral compartment with sclerosis of the exposed bone and associated marginal osteophytes, features typical of DJD/OA occurring without preceding RA.

Table 3
Stages of avascular necrosis

	Pathology (Feature/% Cases)	X-rays	MRI
Stage 1	Osteonecrosis without reparative activity (2%)	No signs	Subchondral signal increase
Stage 2	Osteonecrosis with marginal sclerosis (4%)	Curvilinear sclerosis in bone	Marginal reduction in signal
Stage 3	Osteonecrosis with collapse (43%)	Crescent sign	Fragmentation and collapse
Stage 4	Secondary Degenerative Joint Disease (34%)	Collapse and OA	Superimposed degeneration

Abbreviations: MRI, magnetic resonance imaging; OA, osteoarthritis.

noncollapsed region and causes loss of the cartilage with eburnation of a rim of exposed bone, thinning of the surrounding residual cartilage, and variable degrees of marginal osteophytosis, all features of secondary osteoarthritis.

The cut surface of the collapsed joint shows a usually well-defined zone of bright yellow necrosis beneath the articular end plate and extending into the subarticular bone usually for a distance of greater than 1.5 cm. A fracture line is usually visible within this necrotic zone immediately beneath the end plate and less commonly at

the base of the necrotic zone on the necrotic side of the reparative tissue, which is usually sclerotic, tan, fibrous, and hyperemic (**Fig. 33**).

Microscopic Pathology

The microscopic features of interest in AVN occur both within the necrotic zone and at the periphery of the necrotic zone. Within the necrotic zone, which involves the bony end plate and extends into the underlying cancellous bone, all of the marrow contents and all of the bony trabeculae

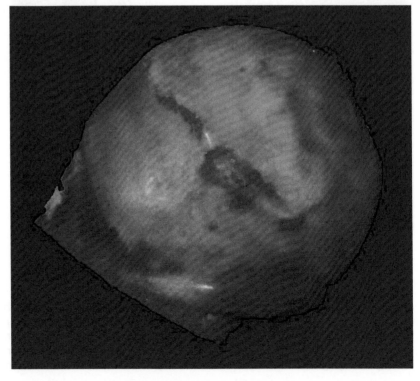

Fig. 32. This photograph of a femoral head affected by AVN shows curvilinear buckling of the cartilage and loss of sphericity owing to collapse of the underlying necrotic bone.

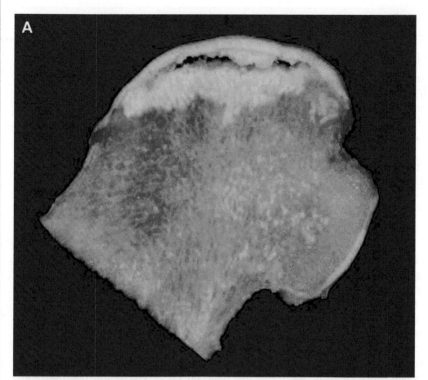

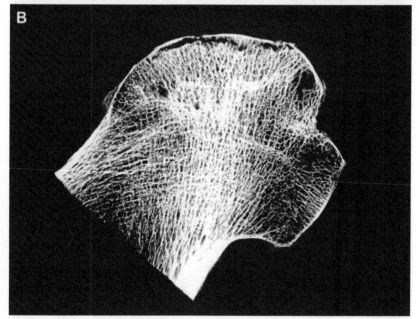

Fig. 33. These images of the same case of AVN of a femoral head show (*A*) the cut surface with the subchondral region of necrosis, and (*B*) the specimen radiograph with a fracture line representing the "crescent sign" beneath the bony end plate and with a hazy zone of sclerosis representing the peripheral reparative activity.

are necrotic. In cases of AVN of Stage 3 or higher, there is also a nonhealing fracture within the necrotic zone (Fig. 34).

In all stages of AVN, except Stage 4, the articular cartilage overlying the necrotic zone is structurally well maintained. Inside the bone, the viable tissue at the periphery of the necrotic zone begins the reparative process described as "creeping substitution." Repair in this manner is necessary to maintain the mechanical competence of the bone

Fig. 34. This photomicrograph of AVN of the femoral head shows a nonhealing fracture line beneath the bony end plate and bony sclerosis and marrow calcification at the periphery of the necrotic zone (H&E, original magnification ×1).

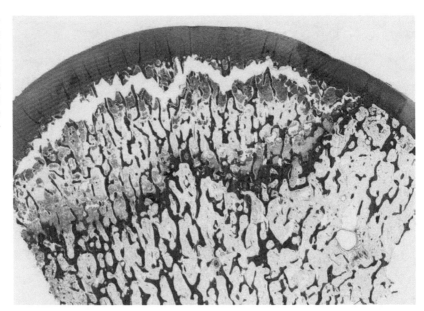

throughout the healing process. In the early phase of repair, macrophages accumulate at the periphery of the infarct and remove the necrotic marrow contents (**Fig. 35**A). Stromal and bone-competent elements follow closely behind and begin to lay down new bone using the necrotic trabeculae as templates (see **Fig. 35**B). It is this second phase, in which bone is deposited, that defines Stage 2 AVN radiographically. Over time, this reparative activity can either reach completion, or, as in most cases, fail to progress, leaving a boundary of dense bone and calcified, fibrotic marrow that for all intents and purposes poses a boundary to any further healing (**Fig. 36**).

Radiographic Features

The radiographic features of AVN also depend on the stage of the disease and are also summarized in **Table 3**. The degree of radiographic deformity defines the stage of the condition in an affected joint. In Stage 1 disease, the plain radiograph frequently demonstrates no abnormality, whereas the presence of radiographically visible sclerosis in a "serpiginous" or curvilinear manner indicates Stage 2 disease. Stage 3 disease is characterized by collapse of the articular surface owing to the fracture that occurs superficially in the necrotic zone with or without extension to the periphery of the necrotic zone. The presence of this fracture beneath the end plate is responsible for the "crescent sign" regarded as a hallmark radiographic

sign of AVN with collapse (see **Fig. 33**B; **Fig. 37**).[19] Finally, after the collapse, Stage 4 disease is characterized by the presence of secondary degenerative changes, such as loss of the joint space, bony sclerosis, cystic degeneration, and marginal osteophytosis.

SEPTIC/INFECTIOUS DISEASE

Infection in a joint constitutes one of the true medical/surgical emergencies in orthopedic practice aside from catastrophic fracture. Infection in a joint frequently follows infection in the bone ("osteomyelitis"), but may occur de novo. Although osteomyelitis is clinically more common in the young patient, a surgical pathologist is more likely to encounter it in adult specimens. The most common organisms are staphylococcal species (*Staphylococcus aureus*, *Staphylococcus epidermidis*, methicillin-resistant *Staphylococcus aureus*), but other organisms, such as beta hemolytic *Streptococcus,* and Enterococcal species comprise most of the remaining gram-positive organisms. Gram-negative organisms commonly include *Klebsiella*, *Proprionobacterium acnes*, especially after prior joint surgery,[20] and *Escherichia coli,* especially in the spine. Rarely, mycobacteria and even fungi are isolated.

During infection, irreversible inflammatory destruction of the cartilage occurs early and can be well established by the time the infection is

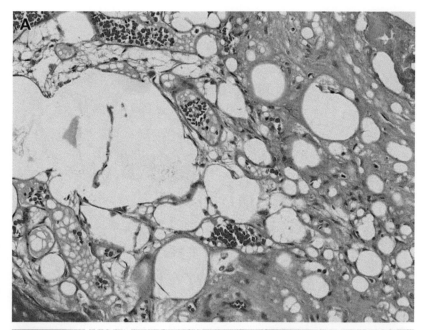

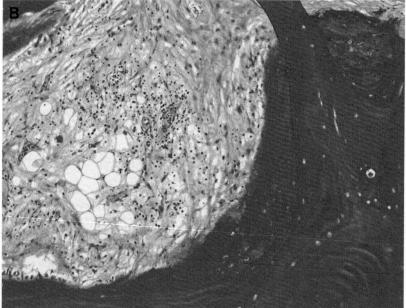

Fig. 35. These photomicrographs from the periphery of the infarct in AVN show (*A*) macrophages and vascular elements in the process of replacing the necrotic marrow contents and (*B*) new bone being deposited on the surfaces of the necrotic bone as part of "creeping substitution" (H&E, *A*: original magnification ×20, *B*: original magnification ×10).

documented. Therefore, it is crucial that suspected infection be treated early, even before proof of the infection can be established. In surgical pathology practice, the disease has been well established and has progressed to a point requiring surgical intervention, which may even include eventual joint replacement. Fortunately, as seen in **Table 1**, this has remained a rare occurrence.

Age and Skeletal Distribution

Infection can occur at any age, and usually starts in the bone (osteomyelitis), with joint involvement occurring as a less common, but significant

Fig. 36. This photomicrograph from the border of the necrotic region in AVN shows the substantial zone of bony and marrow sclerosis that acts as a barrier to any further reparative activity (H&E, original magnification ×5).

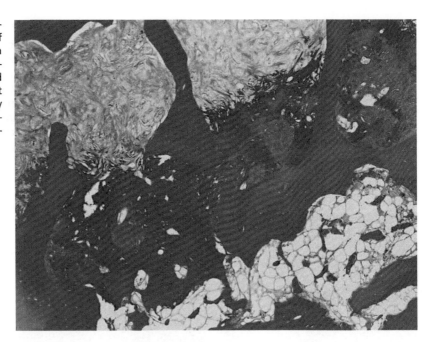

complication. Infection in children is usually of the metaphyses of the long bones, but in adults it is more common in the spine. The nearest joints can be affected, but in de novo cases, any joint can be affected. The knee is the most commonly affected nonspinal joint, followed by the hip and shoulder, with or without prior infection in the adjacent bones (see **Table 2**).

Gross Pathology

Grossly, an infected joint shows destruction of the cartilage in a patchy manner with variable degrees

Fig. 37. This plain radiograph of the case in **Fig. 32** shows the irregular loss of sphericity corresponding to the fracture-associated depression of the articular surface of the femoral head. A crescent sign can be discerned beneath the collapsed surface.

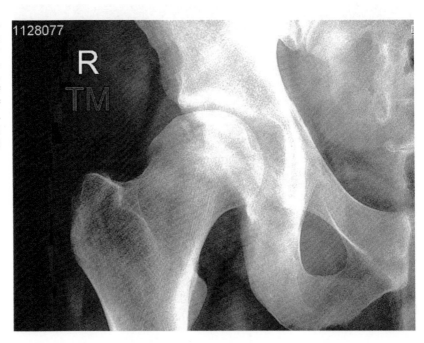

of surface hematoma as well as focal hemorrhagic necrosis in the cancellous bone (Fig. 38). Because the features are destructive and tend to be fairly rapid, compensatory changes, such as osteosclerosis and marginal osteophytosis, are not usually present, but sclerosis is a feature of chronic infection. Cystic degeneration may also present as a feature of the destruction. The synovial tissue is also variably exudative and hemorrhagic.

Microscopic Pathology

The overall appearance is that of necrotizing inflammation that consists of a mixture of all types of inflammatory cells, although neutrophils are the main element in early disease in the joint, synovium, and bone. The surfaces of the cartilage are usually focally covered and invaded by neutrophils (Fig. 39). Mixed inflammation with patchy necrosis of the bone and marrow, as well as inflammatory

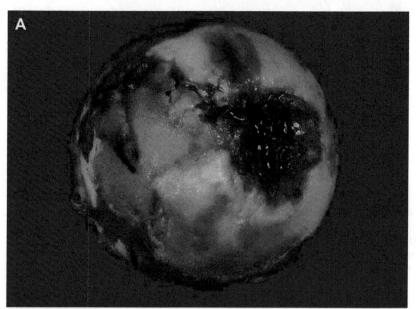

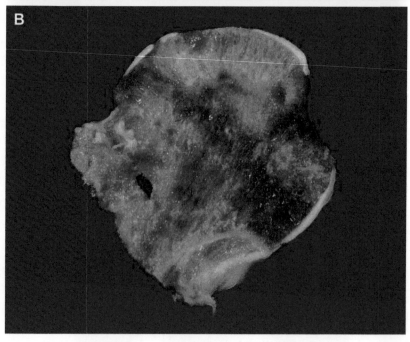

Fig. 38. These images of the same septic femoral head show (A) irregular erosion and thinning of the articular cartilage on the surface with hematoma in the fovea, and (B) patchy necrosis and hemorrhage in the cancellous bone visible on the cut surface.

Fig. 39. This photomicrograph of septic arthritis shows destruction of the cartilaginous matrix by adherent neutrophils and associated necrosis of the superficial chondrocytes (H&E, original magnification ×20).

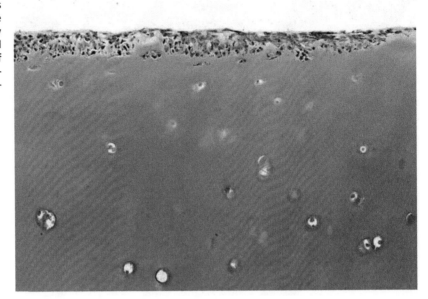

destruction of the necrotic bone is also present (**Fig. 40**). In chronic infection, plasma cells and lymphocytes predominate. The features of septic arthritis are consistent and uniform for the nonmycobacterial bacterial organisms.

As in other tissues, mycobacterial infection in the joints and affected bone are granulomatous and necrotizing. Likewise, fungal infections are necrotizing and occasionally produce a somewhat distinctive variety of loose granuloma (**Fig. 41**).

Radiographic Features

The radiographic features of infection in the joint reflect the destructive effects of the inflammation on the soft and bony tissues. The soft tissues usually show swelling, best visible in MRI studies, especially early in the disease process. When joint disease becomes clinically apparent, the joint space becomes irregularly narrow and the bone undergoes rarefaction with residual bone appearing somewhat sclerotic. In the chronic state, the bone shows patchy sclerosis involving cortical and cancellous bone and the soft tissues remain swollen.

JOINT REPLACEMENT

Joint replacement is widely regarded as one of the most successful surgical procedures that modern medicine has developed, with hundreds of thousands of large and small joint replacement procedures performed every year in the United States alone.[21] The prevalence of implanted artificial joints, combined with a small but definite failure rate,[22] makes the examination of tissues from failed implants the second most common joint-related procedure in surgical pathology practice (see **Table 1**). Over the years, the major challenges in pathologic assessment of failed artificial joints result from the increasing diversity in the various cements, plastics, ceramics, and metals used in ever-more complex components.[23] The variety of these components has presented the pathologist with a variety of tissue reactions that, fortunately, are distinctive.

Reactions to the implanted materials are grouped into foreign-body reactions, superimposed infections, and the increasingly encountered immunologically mediated reactions.

Gross Pathology

The gross appearance of the pseudocapsule and membranes from the joint and at the implant interface is similar for accumulation of cement and polyethylene debris. The surface ranges from smooth to polypoid and the color ranges from tan through yellow to orange (**Fig. 42**). When metallic debris is present, the tissue can be gray to black as well (**Fig. 43**). When cement is present, the tissue is usually gritty.

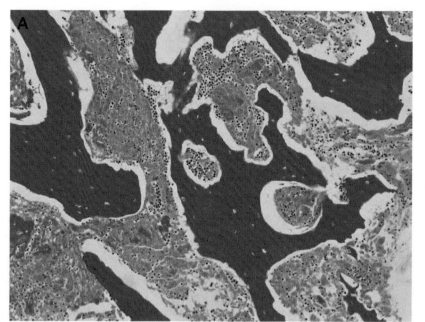

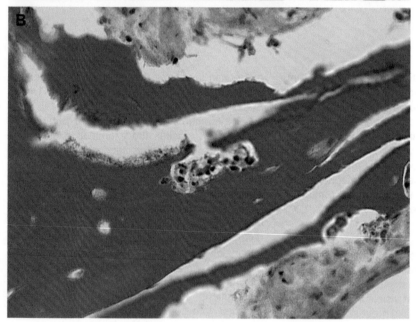

Fig. 40. These photomicrographs of the bone in septic arthritis show (*A*) the necrotizing and inflammatory quality of the marrow components (H&E, original magnification ×10) and (*B*) erosion of necrotic fragments of bone directly by neutrophils, perhaps the only instance in which bone is removed by a cell other than an osteoclast (H&E, original magnification ×40).

Microscopic Pathology

The microscopic features of the foreign body reaction consist of macrophages present focally or in large sheets. The macrophages are accompanied by multinucleate giant cells of various sizes depending on the size of the particulate debris. More than one kind of particle may be present in a single giant cell. A variable but usually slight degree of perivascular lymphocytic inflammation is also present within the reaction tissue. Frequently, there is also hyaline sclerosis and focal infarction.

Cement debris

The "cement" is produced from a mixture of polymethyl methacrylate (PMM) beads and liquid methyl methacrylate with an incorporated contrast

Fig. 41. This photomicrograph of fungal infection shows a fairly distinctive loose and vascular form of granulomatous inflammation of that class of infection. (H&E, original magnification ×10).

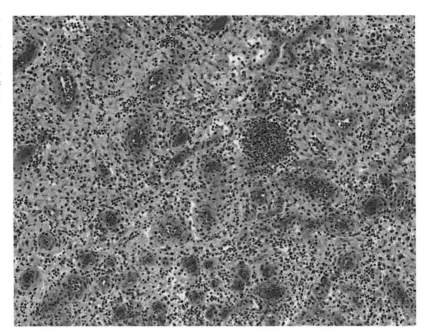

agent that makes the cement mantle visible radiographically. The tissue reaction is to the methacrylate and to the contrast agent (**Fig. 44**A). The PMM is dissolved during routine histologic processing so it does not remain in paraffin sections. The reaction to the "cement" debris varies from sheets of mononuclear macrophages with pale blue, granular cytoplasm, to single giant cells containing single clear beads of PMM, to masses of giant cells surrounding larger particles composed of aggregates of beads with intermixed contrast agent. When the contrast agent is barium sulfate, it is seen as fine granules within the cells and cement interstices (see **Fig. 44**B). When the contrast agent is powdered zirconium oxide, its particles are round and refractile and have a central

Fig. 42. This photograph of the pseudo-capsule from a failed, cemented polyethylene implant shows the sometimes striking nodular and papillary, variably colored features associated with these materials and their associated secondary reactions of necrosis, fibrin, and sclerosis.

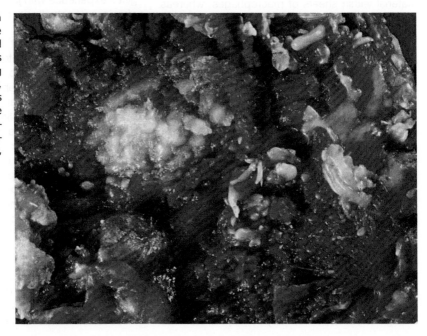

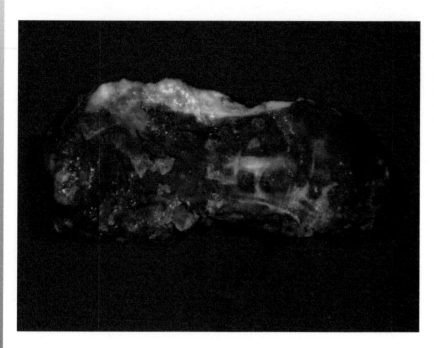

Fig. 43. This photograph of the pseudo-capsule containing debris from a failed titanium implant is particularly heavy, but shows the typical gray to black tissue-staining common to all metals.

pale zone creating a resemblance to tiny donuts (Fig. 45).

Polyethylene debris

The tissue reaction to polyethylene debris depends strongly on the size of the particles, which are brightly visible, and best seen, in polarized light (Fig. 46). Fine particles appear as small shards of material within sheets of macrophages, whereas ever-larger particles are associated with giant cells and masses of giant cells.

Metallic debris

Metallic debris is usually present as black (optically opaque) irregular particles in the tissues or in macrophages (Fig. 47). The particles are too small to generate large giant cells, although they may be present in giant cells that also contain other types of debris. Occasional particles of corrosion products (rustlike) are present and may then induce a giant-cell reaction. Chronic inflammation composed of lymphocytes and plasma cells is not uncommon in reactions to metallic debris.

Ceramic debris

Debris from ceramic implants, whether aluminum oxide (alumina) or zirconium oxide (zirconia), bears similarities to that seen in the ceramic contrast agent in cement. However, debris usually consists of larger particles, which may or may not have an associated macrophage or giant cell reaction (Fig. 48).

Infection in Artificial Joints

The assessment of infection in the tissues around an artificial joint is likely the most problematic and most important part of the surgical pathologist's experience with joint implants. The pathologist is not actually identifying the presence of infection, however, but rather is identifying the histologic features that are usually associated with infection and therefore may be indicative of infection in any specific case. The result of the frozen section assessment for infection is another piece of information that must be interpreted by the surgeon within the clinical context.

An infected membrane grossly has a somewhat fibrinous and granular surface with variable degrees of hyperemia or hematoma. Rarely is there evidence of frank purulence.

In the microscopic examination of an implant membrane for the presence of infection, it is widely agreed that the presence of neutrophils to some extent is the main predictor of infection in frozen sections. Tissues having more than 2 to 5 neutrophils per high-power field, in at least 5 fields, are usually regarded as being infected and are reported as such.[24] The importance of the touch preparation prepared from blotted cut surfaces cannot be overstated in the microscopic

Fig. 44. These photomicrographs of cement debris show (*A*) the sheetlike mononuclear and giant cell reaction to the "beaded" particles of cement debris cleared from the tissue during routine embedding (H&E, original magnification ×10) and (*B*) the granular barium sulfate that is used as a radiographic contrast agent in many methyl methacrylate cement formulations (H&E, original magnification ×40).

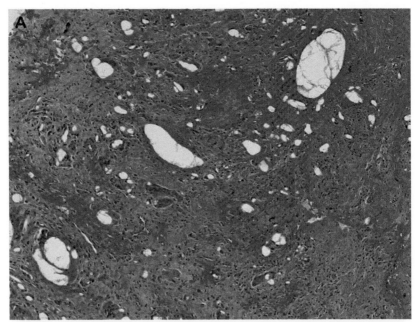

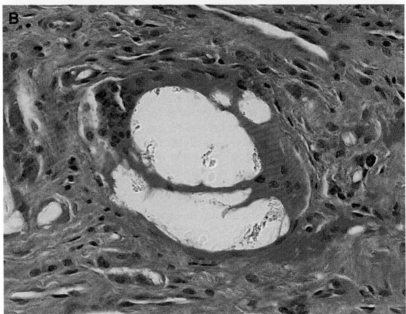

assessment of infection in joint tissues. Noninfected membranes have only rare neutrophils, appropriate for the amount of blood on the slide, whereas infected membranes nearly always have an increased proportion of neutrophils. **Table 4** shows a summary of the interpretations provided by the authors from frozen-section assessment. Features that are consistent with infection or cannot exclude infection are illustrated in **Fig. 49**. It may not be possible to support or exclude the possibility of infection in every case. This problem is usually a result of the presence of persistent inflammation from the primary disease, the presence of fibrin without tissue, or the presence of intense electrocautery effect. Examining additional tissue may be helpful in these situations.

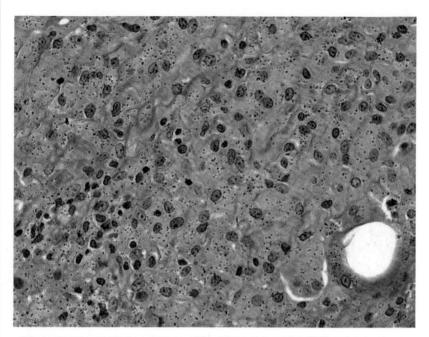

Fig. 45. This photomicrograph of zirconium oxide contrast agent shows the typical tiny "donut" appearance of the particles owing to their refractile qualities (H&E, original magnification ×40).

Immunologic Reactions in Artificial Joints

Sensitivity to metals has been a known, if rare, condition, since the use of metallic implants for joint replacement and appears to be undergoing a resurgence.[25] An unusual inflammatory reaction, however, perhaps representing some type of delayed hypersensitivity reaction, is increasingly being observed in the capsules and bones around implants composed of metal components articulating with other metal components, so-called metal-on-metal (MoM) implants.[26–28] A scheme for grading this reaction, given the unfortunate term "ALVAL" for atypical lymphocytic vasculitis-associated lesion, has been proposed.[29]

The excised interface membrane grossly is covered by loose or coagulated fibrin and may be granular and red or smooth and somewhat yellow-tan. The membrane is variably thick and rubbery owing to fibrin and fibrous tissue.

Microscopically, the membrane has a layered appearance, with the inner surface covered by fibrin or synovial cells, a central layer of denser compacted fibrin or fibrous tissue with a variable amount of scattered inflammatory cells, including macrophages and lymphocytes, and an outer layer composed of vascular loose connective tissue. A variable degree of lymphocytic inflammation occurs around small arteries in this outer layer (Fig. 50). The fibrin and the fibrous layers may also show infarction without significant inflammation.

Occasionally, a layer of macrophages may border regions of infarction in the fibrous layer, but frequently only noninflammatory granulation tissue or a transition to viable fibrous tissue without inflammation is present. The perivascular inflammation is composed of a mixture of small lymphocytes with an increased proportion of T-lymphocytes, with variable numbers of plasma cells and occasional eosinophils. Macrophages containing distinctive globular inclusions are frequently present in the tissues (Fig. 51).

Although the proposed scoring system attempts to quantify the severity of the reaction based on the degree of inflammation and architectural effacement, the clinical significance and validity of this type of reaction are not well understood and not universally accepted.[30,31]

MISCELLANEOUS METABOLIC DISEASES

Certain well-recognized, morphologically definable metabolic conditions illustrate the concept of arthritis presented earlier in this article.

The most commonly encountered metabolic conditions involving the joints are associated with deposition of various crystalline and noncrystalline materials in the tissues of the joints. The deposition of these materials ultimately compromises the mechanical performance of these tissues.

Fig. 46. These photomicrographs of the polyethylene debris show (*A*) a sheet of mononuclear and scattered giant cells containing shards of polyethylene of various sizes and (*B*) the same field demonstrating the strong birefringence of the debris as seen in polarized light (H&E, original magnification ×10).

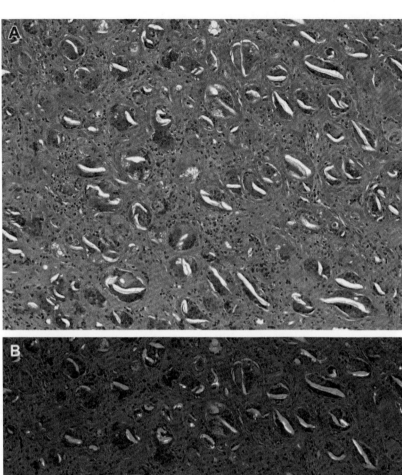

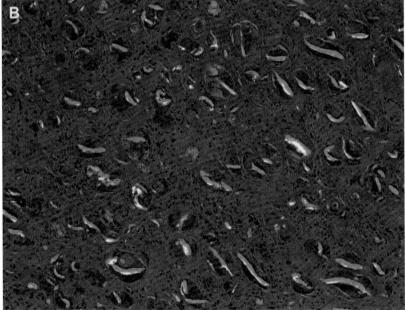

Gout/Calcium Pyrophosphate Deposition Disease

The 2 most common crystalline deposits in the joints are monosodium urate (MSU) and calcium pyrophosphate (CPP), deposits in gout and pseudogout, respectively. Whereas deposits of MSU certainly have clinical consequences, the same is not always true with deposits of CPP. Gout manifests clinically as remarkably painful firm swellings or masses in and around joints. Pseudogout is so named because of the occasional case that overlaps with gout in signs and symptoms.

The radiographic features of each disease easily distinguish between them, as MSU deposits are

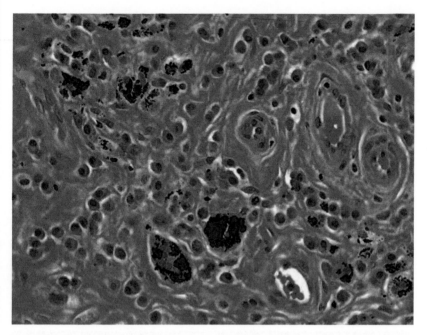

Fig. 47. This photomicrograph of metallic debris shows small irregular particles of black (optically opaque) metallic debris within macrophages and small giant cells. The plasma cells in the background are unique to this case, although inflammation is typical (H&E, original magnification ×40).

not radiodense and appear only as space-occupying and erosive masses around affected joints, whereas deposits of CPP are visible radiographically, usually as finely punctate or linear deposits that are not usually massive or destructive in the affected joint (Figs. 52 and 53A).

The gross pathologic features of these conditions reflect their radiographic features. Deposits of MSU are bulky and white, occasionally hemorrhagic, and are usually found in the soft tissues of the joint and in the superficial bone at the periphery of the joint surface (see Fig. 52B).

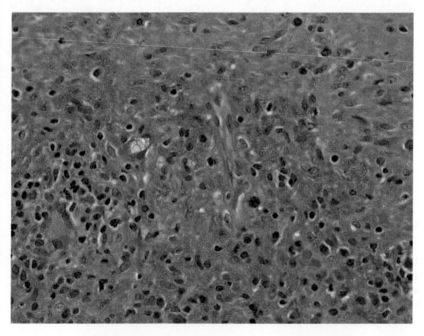

Fig. 48. This photomicrograph of ceramic debris shows irregular particles of refractile debris within small giant cells and macrophages (H&E, original magnification ×20).

Table 4
Frozen section diagnoses for infection of implants (2005 through 2009)

Diagnosis	Cases (no)	% Cases
No evidence of infection	223	85
Consistent with infection	18	7
Infection cannot be ruled out	20	8
All diagnoses	261	100

Deposits of CPP are finely punctate and linear and occasionally more massive and are present within the substance of the menisci, which are frequently torn, the capsular and ligamentous tissues, the articular cartilage, and the synovium when a large amount of material is deposited (see **Fig. 53**B). The presence of CPP deposits within the chondral and fibrochondral tissues of the joint gives rise to the radiographic and gross morphologic term of "chondrocalcinosis."

The microscopic features of each condition depend on the characteristics of the crystalline

Fig. 49. (*A*) This photomicrograph of an infected implant membrane shows cellular fibrinous exudate overlying edematous granulation tissue showing scattered neutrophils (H&E, original magnification ×20). (*B*) This photomicrograph of an implant membrane in which infection cannot be ruled out shows an intact lining with sclerosis and band-like chronic inflammation consistent with persistence of a rheumatoid infiltrate, but the neutrophils prevent a definitive statement regarding infection (H&E, original magnification ×20).

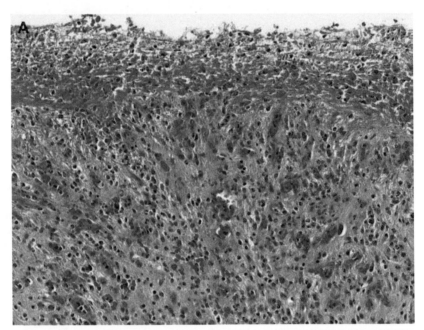

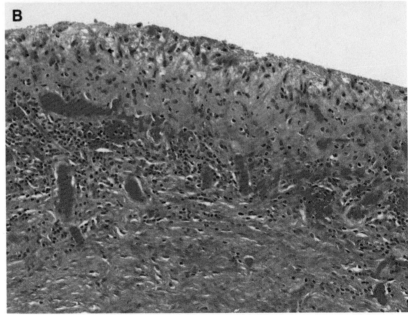

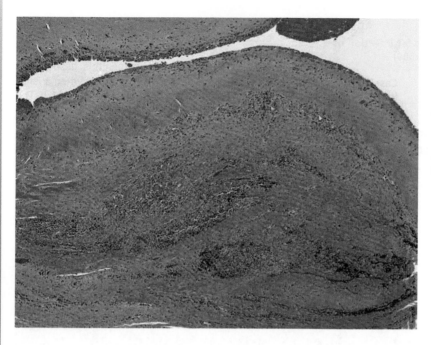

Fig. 50. This photomicrograph of a suspected immune-based reaction shows the layered appearance of the implant membrane with granular material at the surface, variably cellular fibrotic layers, and basilar, band-like perivascular chronic inflammation (H&E, original magnification ×2.5).

material and on the tissue in which the deposit develops. In gout, the crystals are needle-shaped and negatively birefringent (yellow in properly aligned compensated polarized light microscopy), are present in bulky masses within the soft tissues as brown crystals or crystal-bearing pink matrix, and are associated with a prominent mononuclear and giant cell reaction at the periphery of the deposit (**Fig. 54**). In deposits of CPP, the crystals are rhomboidal and positively birefringent (blue in properly aligned compensated polarized light microscopy), are present as delicate, deep-blue condensations displacing the stroma of the chondral tissue, and do not have an associated cellular

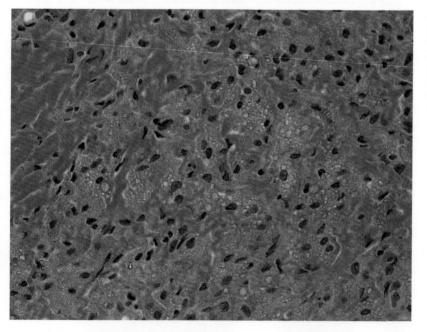

Fig. 51. This photomicrograph of a suspected immune-based reaction in a metal-on-metal implant shows sheets of macrophages containing globular inclusions (H&E, original magnification ×20).

Fig. 52. (*A*) This plain radiograph shows destruction of the proximal side of the first metacarpo-phalangeal joint with soft tissue swelling but without calcification in a case of gout. (*B*) This photograph of fragments of a gouty deposit shows multiple aggregates of chalky white material (bar = 1 cm).

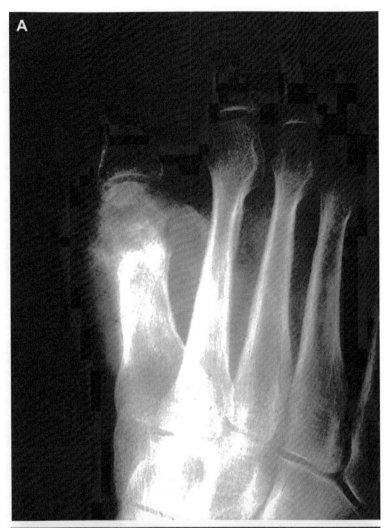

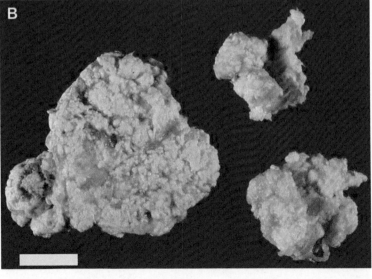

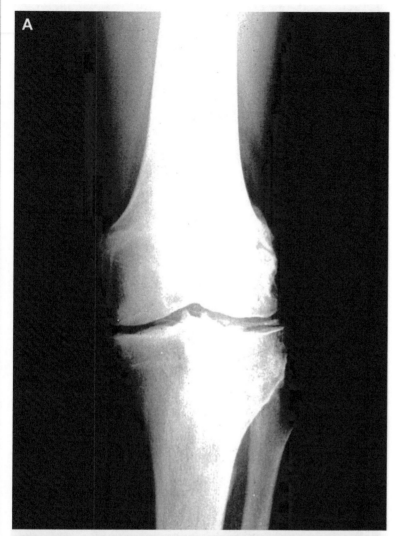

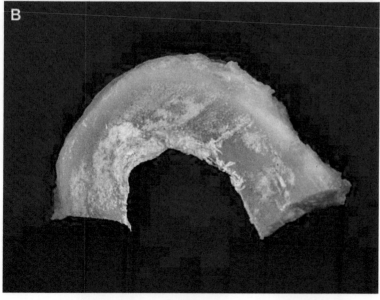

Fig. 53. (A) This plain radiograph shows delicate, flecklike radiodensities in the lateral meniscus indicative of chondrocalcinosis associated with deposits of calcium pyrophosphate. (B) This photograph of a meniscal segment shows the chalky white, smudged, punctate and streaklike deposits of calcium pyrophosphate.

Fig. 54. (*A*) This photomicrograph of a gouty deposit shows the crystals and associated peripheral cellular reaction typical of gout (H&E, original magnification ×20). (*B*) This photomicrograph of the same field shows the brightly birefringent needle-shaped crystals of gout in polarized light (polarized, original magnification ×20).

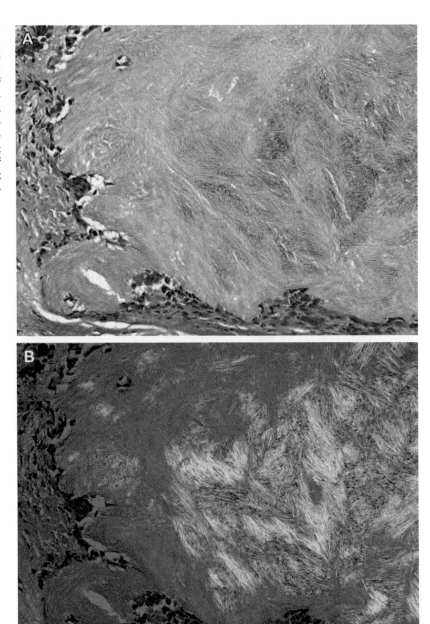

reaction at the periphery of the deposits in these tissues (**Fig. 55**). However, when CPP deposits are in the synovium, such deposits usually do have a somewhat subdued peripheral granulomatous reaction.

In tissue sections that have been stained with hematoxylin and eosin, it sometimes is not possible to see the crystals. This is because the pH of the hematoxylin, and sometimes even the eosin, is acidic, causing dissolution of the crystals during the staining process. This process affects both crystals, but MSU crystals are more susceptible. Simply recutting a tissue section without staining, or staining only in the eosin, may permit visualization of the crystals in the tissues. If even this fails, an accurate diagnosis can still be suggested by the presence of "ghosts" of the crystals left behind within the matrix in which they develop (**Fig. 56**).

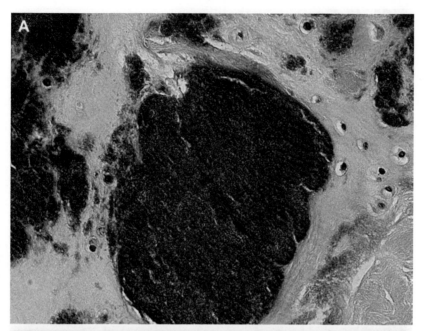

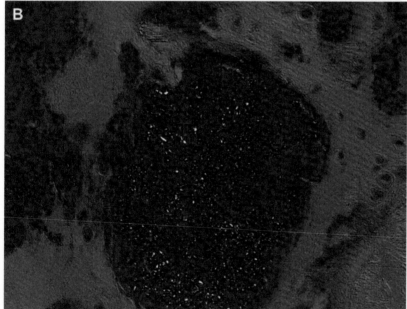

Fig. 55. (A) This photomicrograph of a globular CPP deposit shows the chondroid quality of the surrounding tissue without a significant peripheral cellular reaction (H&E, original magnification ×20). (B) This photomicrograph of the same field shows the somewhat birefringent rhomboidal crystals of CPP in polarized light (polarized, original magnification ×20).

The effect of gout on the function of an affected joint is fairly apparent, as the destructive nature of the deposits is radiographically and grossly evident. Gouty deposits undermine the joint structure and expand the soft tissues, further comprising the mechanics of the joint. The effect of CPP deposits on the joint is much less clear and there is still a lack of consensus in this regard. Individuals who suffer from pseudogout clearly have an arthritic condition; however, the overwhelming number of examples of CPP deposition occurs in individuals who otherwise have degenerative joint disease. The increase in both the incidence of CPP deposition and the age of the patients appears to support the notion that CPP deposition is likely secondary to the degenerative state, the incidence of which is also known to increase with age.

Fig. 56. (*A*) This photomicrograph of a gouty deposit shows the needle-shaped ghosts of dissolved crystals (H&E, original magnification ×40). (*B*) This photomicrograph of a CPP deposit shows the typical rhomboidal ghosts of dissolved crystals (H&E, original magnification ×40).

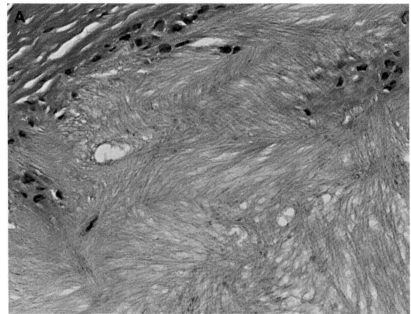

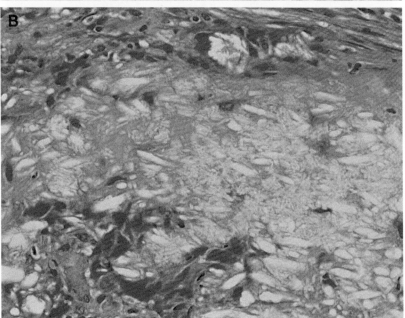

Iron Overload: Intra-articular Bleeding, Systemic Iron Overload

Iron may accumulate in a joint by 1 of 2 mechanisms: intra-articular and systemic. The most common intra-articular source of iron deposition in a joint is trauma usually associated with an unstable degenerate joint that results in the accumulation of iron in the synovium, and occasionally in the articular cartilage to some widely variable degree. Hemophilia is a historically significant and devastating cause of intra-articular bleeding, with iron overload usually in a large joint.[32] Pigmented villonodular synovitis is an uncommon cause of intra-articular bleeding as

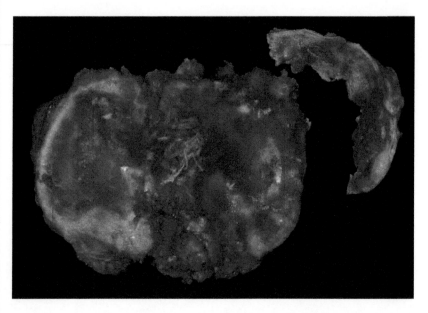

Fig. 57. This photograph of a knee affected by extensive iron overload caused by bleeding shows intense synovial hemosiderosis as well as staining and degeneration of the cartilage with focal eburnation of exposed bone resulting in degenerative joint disease.

well. Secondary hemosiderosis and primary hemochromatosis are uncommon systemic causes of iron-associated joint disease.[33,34] Regardless of the cause, the common feature of iron overload is the accumulation of iron in the soft tissues and chondrocytes.

Grossly, local intra-articular bleeding causes accumulation of iron pigment in the superficial cells and tissues, whereas systemic causes of iron overload, usually without frank bleeding into the joint, cause accumulation of the iron in the deeper cells and tissues first (Fig. 57).

Regardless of the mechanism, the findings in the tissues and cells are similar. Many of the chondrocytes and stromal fibroblasts appear hypereosinophilic, with shrunken cytoplasm and a nucleus that is either absent or undergoing degeneration, features indicative of cell death (Fig. 58). Prussian

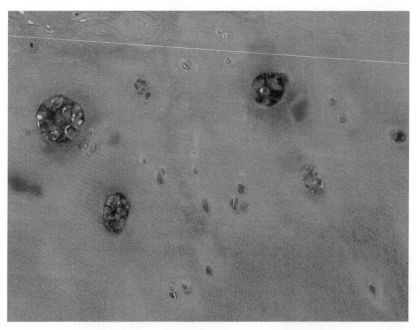

Fig. 58. This photomicrograph of hemosiderotic arthropathy associated with hemochromatosis shows granular eosinophilic necrosis of chondrocytes with cloning of surviving chondrocytes (H&E, original magnification ×20).

blue staining of the tissues demonstrates iron deposits in chondrocytes and other stromal cells, including synovial lining cells and meniscal fibroblasts (Fig. 59). When the stromal cells die because of this form of metabolic toxicity, their custodial function supporting the matrix is eliminated. Without correctly functioning cellular components, the matrices begin to break down at a greater rate, leading to failure of the joint, a form of degenerative arthritis.

Although the specific abnormalities resulting in hemophilia and hemochromatosis are recognizably different, the mechanism of arthritis in these 2 conditions is similar, even if occurring at different rates. In hemophilia, the repeated episodes of hemarthrosis results in greater and more rapid destruction of the affected joint, whereas the slower processes involved in hemochromatosis lead to a more widespread variety of degenerative disease that manifests in later adult life.

Ochronosis

Ochronosis is the pathologic manifestation in the tissues of alkaptonuria, which is the disease associated with deficiency of the enzyme homogentisic acid oxidase. The clinical manifestations stem from accumulation of homogentisic acid (homogentisate) in cartilage and other dense connective tissues with the resulting darkening caused by

nonenzymatic oxidative polymerization that produces first a yellow and then brownish pigmentation in the tissue over the duration of the disease. Ochronotic pigmentation in the joints leads to a disseminated degenerative arthritis involving diarthrodial joints and also the amphiarthrodial joints of the spine. Ochronotic pigmentation occurs in other dense connective tissues in the body and leads to darkening of the ears and nose, as well as to dysfunction in the cardiac valves. Interestingly, many of the patients having joint surgery have already had cardiac-valve surgery.

In contrast to cases of iron overload, where the iron interferes with the metabolic functions of the cells, the ochronotic pigment appears to alter the mechanical properties of the chondroid matrices, making them less malleable and more brittle, contributing to their destruction.[35] The gross pathologic features of the arthritis of ochronosis consist of dark brown to black discoloration of the cartilage, meniscus, and capsular tissues (Fig. 60A). Cross sections of the cartilage and menisci show pigmentation that is more intense deep in the tissues than at the surfaces (see Fig. 60B). In contrast, newer chondroid tissues, such as that seen over the osteophytes and in any reparative regions, are not pigmented, indicating that the process of pigmentation takes long-term exposure to the homogentisate. The pigmented cartilage has a more brittle consistency, leading to focal loss of

Fig. 59. This photomicrograph of the same case as in Fig. 58 shows iron pigment in the individual necrotic chondrocytes as well as in the surviving chondrocytic clones (Prussian Blue, original magnification ×20).

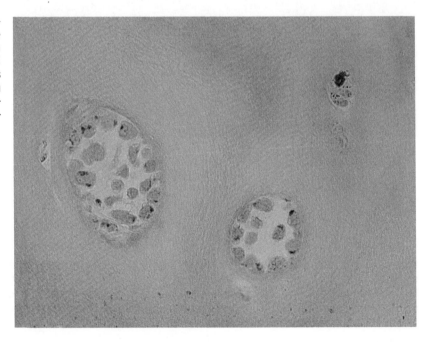

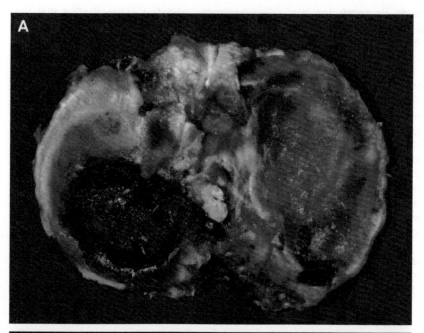

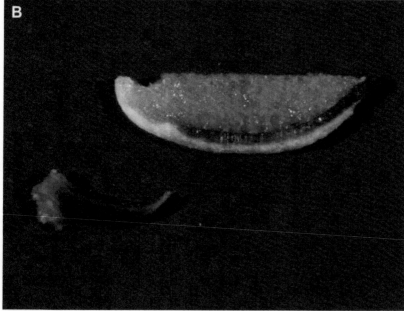

Fig. 60. These photographs of the same knee affected by ochronosis show (A) the disruption and focal loss of the darkly pigmented degenerate cartilage with pale osteophytes and (B) the coloration of the deep region of the cartilage and meniscus on cut section, whereas the osteophyte, being newer tissue, is not discolored.

the cartilage because of degeneration and shearing at the cartilage-bone interface (Fig. 61). Fragmentation and tearing of the cartilage, menisci, and capsular tissues cause granular pigmentation of the synovium owing to accumulation of the pigmented articular detritus (Fig. 62). The finding of such pigmented detritus in the synovium is a clear-cut indication of the brittleness of the affected matrices and is a hallmark of the disease in diarthrodial joints.

Fig. 61. This photomicrograph of the cartilage-bone interface shows delicate splits resulting from shearing owing to stiffness of the cartilage resulting from the altered mechanical properties of ochronotic cartilage (H&E, original magnification ×10).

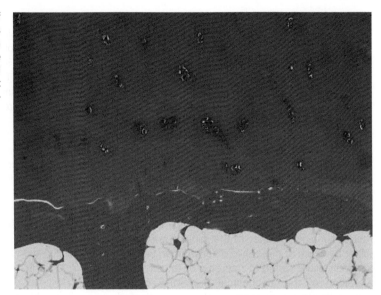

Fig. 62. These photomicrographs from the same case of ochronotic arthropathy show (*A*) accumulation of pigmented cartilage fragments in the capsular tissue that also show chondroid degeneration (H&E, original magnification ×5) and (*B*) delicate particles of pigmented cartilaginous detritus in the slightly hyperplastic and slight inflamed synovium (H&E, original magnification ×10).

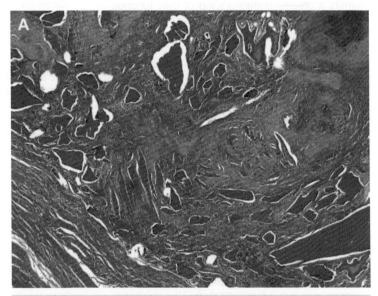

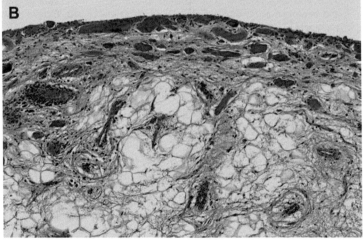

SUMMARY

The modern concepts of arthritis arose from an ever-more sophisticated appreciation of the ways that all of the components of the joints contribute to the painless, smooth, and stable movement of the joints throughout appropriate ranges of motion. Therefore, it follows logically that abnormality or malfunction, either intrinsic or imposed, in any one of the joint's components can be expected to lead to malfunction in the other components and thus lead to failure of the joint as an anatomic/functional unit. Joints can be affected by overuse; inflammation, including infection; mechanical insufficiency of the joint components, either because of metabolic disease or an inability to repair injury owing to necrosis or toxicity; and alteration of the mechanical properties of the various tissue components. Such a sophisticated approach to the health and diseases of the joints permits a greater understanding of their function and how they experience dysfunction and allow for the recognition of newer modes of failure as they occur.

The pathologic examination of failed joints, whether natural or artificial, is an indispensable part of this approach to the understanding of arthritis, as it is the last, and still best opportunity to determine or verify the correct diagnosis. Accuracy in pathologic diagnosis, based on a firm understanding of the various disease processes, provides reliable data for use in clinical registries, provides an opportunity to explain the "unusual" clinical presentation, and ultimately gives the "best evidence" for basing further treatments and prognosis for the individual patient.

REFERENCES

1. Garfin SR, Andersson G, Gronblad M, et al. The bone and joint decade 2000-2010 for prevention and treatment of musculoskeletal disorders. Spine 1999;24(11):1055.

2. Pearle AD, Scanzello CR, George S, et al. Elevated high-sensitivity C-reactive protein levels are associated with local inflammatory findings in patients with osteoarthritis. Osteoarthritis Cartilage 2007; 15(5):516–23.

3. Scanzello CR, Umoh E, Pessler F, et al. Local cytokine profiles in knee osteoarthritis: elevated synovial fluid interleukin-15 differentiates early from end-stage disease. Osteoarthritis Cartilage 2009;17(8):1040–8.

4. Scanzello CR, McKeon B, Swaim BH, et al. Synovial inflammation in patients undergoing arthroscopic meniscectomy: molecular characterization and relationship with symptoms. Arthritis Rheum 2011;63(2): 391–400.

5. Ahuja SC, Bullough PG. Osteonecrosis of the knee, a clinicopathological study in twenty-eight patients. J Bone Joint Surg Am 1978;60(2):191–7.

6. Yamamoto T, Bullough PG. Spontaneous osteonecrosis of the knee: the result of subchondral insufficiency fracture. J Bone Joint Surg Am 2000;82(6): 858–66.

7. Yamamoto T, Schneider R, Bullough PG. Subchondral insufficiency fracture of the femoral head: histopathologic correlation with MRI. Skeletal Radiol 2001;30(5):247–54.

8. Yamamoto T, Schneider R, Iwamoto Y, et al. Rapid destruction of the hip joint in osteoarthritis. Ann Rheum Dis 2008;67(12):1783–4.

9. Yamamoto T, Schneider R, Iwamoto Y, et al. Bilateral rapidly destructive arthrosis of the hip joint resulting from subchondral fracture with superimposed secondary osteonecrosis. J Bone Joint Surg Am 2000;82(6):858–66.

10. Yamamoto T, Schneider R, Iwamoto Y, et al. Rapid destruction of the femoral head after a single intra-articular injection of corticosteroid into the hip joint [Erratum in J Rheumatol 2006;33(10):2101]. J Rheumatol 2006;33(8):1701–4.

11. Yamamoto T, Bullough PG. The role of subchondral insufficiency fracture in rapid destruction of the hip joint: a preliminary report. Arthritis Rheum 2000; 43(11):2423–7.

12. Walberger JM, Firestein GS. Rheumatoid arthritis, B-epidemiology, pathology and pathologenesis. Chapter 6. In: Klipple JH, editor. Primer on the rheumatic diseases. 13th edition. New York: Springer; 2008. p. 122.

13. Gladman DD. Psoriatic arthritis, A–clinical features. Chapter 8. In: Klipple JH, editor. Primer on the rheumatic diseases. 13th edition. New York: Springer; 2008. p. 170.

14. Van der Heijde D. Ankylosing spondylitis, A–clinical features. Chapter 9. In: Klipple JH, editor. Primer on the rheumatic diseases. 13th edition. New York: Springer; 2008. p. 193.

15. Cantini F, Niccoli L, Nannini C, et al. Psoriatic arthritis: a systematic review. Int J Rheum Dis 2010;13(4):300–17.

16. O'Connell JX, Nielsen GP, Rosenberg AE. Subchondral acute inflammation in severe arthritis: a sterile osteomyelitis? Am J Surg Pathol 1999;23(2): 192–7.

17. Bullough PG, DiCarlo ED. Subchondral avascular necrosis, a common cause of arthritis. Ann Rheum Dis 1990;49:412–20.

18. Ficat RP, Arlet J. Functional investigation of bone under normal conditions. In: Hungerford DS, editor. Ischemia and necrosis of bone. Baltimore (MD): Williams and Wilkins; 1980. p. 29–52.

19. Norman A, Bullough PG. The radiolucent crescent sign—an early diagnostic sign of avascular necrosis

of the femoral head. Bull Hosp Joint Dis 1963;24:
99–104.

20. Dodson CC, Craig EV, Cordasco FA, et al. Propiono-
bacterium acnes infection after shoulder arthros-
copy: a diagnostic challenge. J Shoulder Elbow
Surg 2010;19(2):303–7.

21. Kurtz S, Ong K, Lau E, et al. Projections of primary
and revision hip and knee arthroplasty in the United
States from 2005 to 2030. J Bone Joint Surg Am
2007;89(4):780–5.

22. Kurtz S, Mowat F, Ong K, et al. Prevalence of
primary and revision total hip and knee arthroplasty
in the United States from 1990 through 2002. J Bone
Joint Surg Am 2005;87(7):1487–97.

23. Sargent A, Goswami T. Pathophysiologic aspects of
hip implants. J Surg Orthop Adv 2006;15(2):111–2.

24. Della Valle C, Parvizi J, Bauer TW, et al. Diagnosis of
periprosthetic joint infections of the hip and knee.
J Am Acad Orthop Surg 2010;18(12):760–70.

25. Campbell P, Shimmin A, Walter L, et al. Metal sensitivity as a cause of groin pain in metal-on-metal hip
resurfacing. J Arthroplasty 2008;23(7):1080–5.

26. Willert H-G, Buchhorn GH, Fayyazi A, et al. Metal-
on-metal bearings and hypersensitivity in patients
with artificial hip joints: a clinical and histomorpho-
logical study. J Bone Joint Surg Am 2005;87:28–36.

27. Mahendra G, Pandit H, Kliskey K, et al. Necrotic and
inflammatory changes in metal-on-metal resurfacing
hip arthroplasties. Acta Orthop 2009;80(6):653–9.

28. Pandit H, Vlychou M, Whitwell D, et al. Necrotic
granulomatous pseudotumors in bilateral resurfacing hip arthroplasties: evidence for a type IV immune
response. Virchows Arch 2008;453(5):529–34.

29. Campbell P, Ebramzadeh E, Nelson S, et al. Histologic features of pseudotumor-like tissues from
metal-on-metal hips. Clin Orthop Relat Res 2010;
468(9):2321–7.

30. Fujishiro T, Moojen DJ, Kobayashi N, et al. Perivascular and diffuse lymphocytic inflammation are not
specific for failed metal-on-metal hip implants. Clin
Orthop Relat Res 2010;469(4):1127–33.

31. Kwon YM, Thomas P, Summer B, et al. Lymphocyte
proliferation responses in patients with pseudotumors following metal-on-metal hip resurfacing arthroplasty. J Orthop Res 2010;28(4):444–50.

32. Lafeber FP, Miossec P, Valentino LS. Physiopa-
thology of hemophilic arthropathy. Haemophilia
2008;14(Suppl 4):3–9.

33. Richette P, Ottaviani S, Vicaut E, et al. Musculoskeletal complications of hereditary hemochromatosis:
a case-control study. J Rheumatol 2010;37(10):
2145–50. [Epub 2010 Aug 3].

34. Sahinbegovic E, Dallos T, Aigner E, et al. Musculoskeletal disease burden of hereditary hemochromatosis. Arthritis Rheum 2010;62(12):3792–8.

35. Lagier R. Ochronotic arthropathy, an approach to
osteoarthritis bone remodelling. Rheumatol Int 2006;
26(6):561–4.

THE ROLE OF THE PATHOLOGIST IN DIAGNOSING PERIPROSTHETIC INFECTION

Thomas W. Bauer, MD, PhD[a],*, Riku Hayashi, MD, PhD[b]

KEYWORDS

• Periprosthetic infection • Arthroplasty infection • Serologic testing

ABSTRACT

Most patients who undergo total joint arthroplasty experience dramatic relief of pain and improved ambulation for many years, but some eventually develop pain, often accompanied by radiographic evidence of bone resorption around their implants. The most frequent cause of device failure is osteolysis, but infection is another important cause of pain and arthroplasty failure. The distinction between infection and aseptic loosening is important because the 2 conditions are treated very differently. The purpose of this article is to summarize the role of the anatomic and clinical pathologist in helping distinguish aseptic loosening from infection.

Key Points
DIAGNOSING PERIPROSTHETIC INFECTION

Distinction between infection and aseptic loosening is important because the 2 conditions are treated very differently.

The results of microbiologic cultures of periprosthetic tissue samples or joint fluid collected during a revision arthroplasty operation are often considered the "gold standard" for the diagnosis of periprosthetic infection.

The most frequently used intraoperative test for infection is the interpretation of frozen sections of tissue obtained from the joint capsule or periprosthetic membrane.

The authors support American Academy of Orthopaedic Surgeons Practice Guidelines that strongly recommend against Gram stains for the intraoperative diagnosis of periprosthetic infection because of the high percentage of false positives.

The challenge for new molecular tests will be to distinguish clinically important infections from trace levels of necrotic bacteria or contaminants, and to provide that information quickly enough to be of practical help in guiding patient care.

OVERVIEW

Most patients who undergo total joint arthroplasty experience dramatic relief of pain and improved ambulation for many years, but a small proportion of patients eventually develop pain, often accompanied by radiographic evidence of bone resorption around their implants. The most frequent cause of device failure has been osteolysis indirectly induced by an inflammatory reaction to particles of wear debris, but infection is another

[a] Departments of Pathology, Orthopaedic Surgery and the Spine Center, The Cleveland Clinic, 9500 Euclid, Cleveland, OH 44195, USA
[b] Department of Orthopaedic Surgery, Yokohama City University School of Medicine, Yokohama, Japan
* Corresponding author. Department of Pathology, The Cleveland Clinic, 9500 Euclid, Cleveland, OH 44195.
E-mail address: bauert@ccf.org

Surgical Pathology 5 (2012) 67–77
doi:10.1016/j.path.2011.10.001
1875-9181/12/$ – see front matter © 2012 Elsevier Inc. All rights reserved.

important cause of pain and arthroplasty failure. The distinction between infection and aseptic loosening is important because the 2 conditions are treated very differently. A device that has failed because of aseptic loosening is removed and replaced in one operation, whereas an infected implant may require the additional morbidity of a 2-stage procedure along with the use of local and systemic antibiotics. If a periprosthetic infection is not recognized at the time of revision arthroplasty, then the infection is likely to persist, leading to continued pain, bone loss, and additional operations. Surgeons use a combination of physical examination, imaging studies, and laboratory tests to help diagnose infection,[1–3] but many of those tests are nonspecific and the results are often equivocal. The purpose of this article is to summarize the role of the anatomic and clinical pathologist in helping distinguish aseptic loosening from infection.

> **Pathologic Key Features**
> PERIPROSTHETIC INFECTION
>
> *Periprosthetic Infection:*
> - Neutrophils infiltrating the joint capsule or peri-implant membrane at a maximum tissue concentration of at least 5 polymorphonuclear leukocytes per high-power field in at least 5 fields.
>
> *Particle-Induced Aseptic Loosening*
> - "Foamy" macrophages
> - Foreign-body–type granulomas
> - Birefringent particles (polyethylene)
> - Opaque particles (metal, barium sulfate, and/or zirconium dioxide)

OVERVIEW OF TESTING ALGORITHM

An algorithm commonly used by surgeons to distinguish between aseptic loosening and periprosthetic infection is summarized in **Fig. 1**. If the outcome of that algorithm suggests infection, then many surgeons will abort the planned revision arthroplasty operation and instead proceed with a 2-stage procedure, in which the infected devices are removed and replaced with a "spacer" composed in part of bone cement that has been permeated with antibiotics. The patient is then

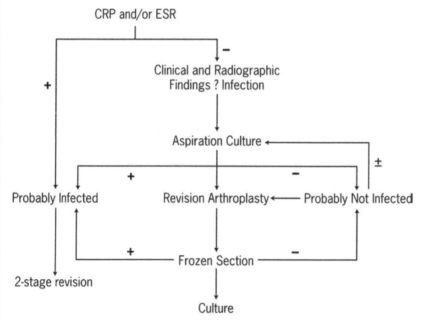

Fig. 1. Among the first tests used to diagnose infection are the serum CRP and ESR. If these are elevated in the appropriate clinical context, then the implant is probably infected. If both are negative but other clinical factors still suggest the possibility of infection, then joint fluid is commonly aspirated and submitted for microbiologic culture. If the results are equivocal, the aspiration can be repeated, but negative aspiration culture usually rules out infection. If during the course of a revision arthroplasty operation the surgeon becomes suspicious of infection, then a frozen section of the joint capsule or peri-implant membrane is often requested. Acute inflammation in the frozen section usually indicates infection, whereas the absence of acute inflammation suggests aseptic loosening and can safely be followed by revision arthroplasty. (*Adapted from* Journal of Bone and Joint Surgery American, December, 2006, 88, S4, Periprosthetic infection: what are the diagnostic challenges? Parvizi, 138–47.)

treated with additional antibiotics, and if subsequent clinical and serologic features suggest that the infection has been resolved, the patient returns to the operating room about 6 weeks later, at which time the cement spacer is removed and replaced with a new total joint prosthesis. In part because of the serious consequences of missing a periprosthetic infection, surgeons often use a combination of tests to help guide treatment of painful joints that might be infected.

DIAGNOSTIC TESTS FOR ARTHROPLASTY INFECTION

SEROLOGIC TESTS

The most important preoperative serologic tests include the Westergren erythrocyte sedimentation rate (ESR), a measure of the rate at which red blood cells sediment from whole blood, and the C-reactive protein (CRP), a protein produced in the liver. ESR and CRP levels normally increase rapidly after joint arthroplasty, reaching peak levels several days after the operation. In the absence of an infection (or underlying inflammatory arthropathy), the serum CRP level usually returns to normal about 3 weeks after arthroplasty. ESR decreases more slowly than the CRP, and may remain slightly elevated for 6 weeks after arthroplasty. In the absence of an underlying systemic inflammatory condition, increased levels of the ESR, and especially CRP, longer than 3 months after arthroplasty suggest the possibility of infection.[4]

Many studies have evaluated the use of these serologic tests for diagnosing a periprosthetic infection. For example, Spangehl and coworkers[5] prospectively tested the specificity and sensitivity of several tests to diagnose infection in a series of 202 revision arthroplasty operations. After excluding cases with underlying inflammatory arthropathies, the ESR had sensitivity and specificity values of 82% and 85% respectively. The CRP was a slightly better test, with sensitivity of 86% and specificity of 92%. Neither of these tests is diagnostic of infection in isolation, but values that increase or fail to decrease 3 months after an arthroplasty operation suggest the strong possibility of infection. Although the subject of relatively few studies so far, the level of serum interleukin-6 (IL-6) is another serologic test that may be useful in diagnosing infection. In one recent study, serum IL-6 was reported to have a higher predictive value than many other serologic markers when used to diagnose periprosthetic infections.[6] One advantage of this test is that the IL-6 level returns to normal within 48 hours after the operation and does not appear to be elevated in patients with aseptic loosening.

INTRAOPERATIVE TESTS

Although the serologic tests described previously can provide surgeons with information before a revision arthroplasty operation, sometimes it is not until the middle of an operation that a surgeon's suspicion of infection is increased. Unfortunately, few tests are available with turnaround time short enough to provide "real-time" intraoperative results.

GRAM STAINS OF ASPIRATED JOINT FLUID

One of those tests is a Gram stain of aspirated joint fluid or tissue. This is a very poor test. Many studies have documented poor predictive value of negative Gram stains, primarily because of the high frequency of false negative results.[3,7] Although some surgeons recognize the relatively poor value of a negative intraoperative Gram stain, the perception persists that a positive stain is diagnostic of infection. Several studies have documented false positive results, however, and we have recently discovered necrotic bacterial "corpses" in commercially purchased reagents that were used to dilute tissue samples between biopsy and staining.[8] Those necrotic bacteria were found to adhere to cells on a smear, developed gram-positive staining, and were interpreted as positive test results. The use of Millipore filtering of all reagents used in specimen transportation and staining procedure greatly reduced these false positive results, but we still agree with the Practice Guidelines of the American Academy of Orthopaedic Surgeons

---

△△ *Differential Diagnosis*
PERIPROSTHETIC INFECTION

- Tissue around an implant with a periprosthetic infection is characterized by acute inflammation (neutrophils).

- Another common cause of implant failure is bone resorption induced by particles of wear debris. These partially necrotic tissue samples are characterized by foreign-body granulomatous inflammation, especially foamy macrophages. Birefringent particles of polyethylene and opaque particles of metal, barium sulfate, or zirconium are often visible, but there is minimal acute inflammation.

- Tissue around implants that are painful because they failed to achieve adequate initial fixation usually lacks inflammation.

(AAOS), which strongly recommend against the use of this test for the intraoperative diagnosis of peri-prosthetic infection.[3]

JOINT FLUID LEUKOCYTE COUNTS

A second test available during the course of an operation is the joint fluid leukocyte count. Both the absolute number of cells per fluid volume and the fractional proportion of neutrophils can be helpful to diagnose infection, but defining cutoff values has been confusing, in part because of inconsistent (and sometimes incorrect) published units for volumes.[2] The investigators of one recent study used receiver operator characteristic curves to calculate that in their hospital, the optimum cutoff value for total joint fluid leukocytes is 1100 cells/μL.[9] They similarly found that a cutoff of 63% or more neutrophils provided independent diagnostic information with respect to the presence of infection.

INTERPRETATION OF FROZEN SECTIONS OF PERI-IMPLANT TISSUES

Probably the most frequently used intraoperative test for infection at most hospitals in the United States is the interpretation of frozen sections of tissue obtained from the joint capsule or periprosthetic membrane.

Pyogenic bacteria induce acute inflammation characterized by neutrophils (polymorphonuclear leukocytes). Some implant membranes show marked acute inflammation in which the high concentration of neutrophils is essentially diagnostic of ongoing infection (**Figs. 2** and **3**).

On the other hand, tissues around implants that have failed because of aseptic, particle-induced osteolysis commonly show necrosis and an inflammatory infiltrate composed of mostly macrophages ("foamy" macrophages), giant cells, and occasional lymphocytes, but essentially no neutrophils (**Fig. 4**). In cases of aseptic loosening, the absence of neutrophils on a frozen section can help support the clinical impression of aseptic loosening.

Biopsies that are often more difficult to interpret are those from cases that are clinically equivocal, and that contain a low concentration of neutrophils. Many studies have attempted to define optimum cutoff criteria for the tissue concentration of neutrophils to support the diagnosis of infection,[10–23] and have been recently reviewed in detail.[2] In general, requiring a high concentration of neutrophils to diagnose infection will yield high specificity (few false positive diagnoses), but relatively low sensitivity (a higher proportion of false negative diagnoses). Alternatively, interpreting a low concentration of neutrophils as suggestive of infection increases sensitivity, but decreases specificity. A meta-analysis by the AAOS Clinical Practice Guidelines committee[3] used raw data contained in 4 studies that used a cutoff value of 10 neutrophils in each of 5, ×400 high-power fields,[18–21] and another 4 studies that used 5 neutrophils in each of 5 high-power fields as

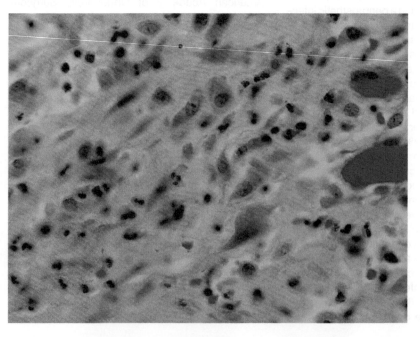

Fig. 2. Typical appearance of tissue adjacent to an infected total hip or knee prosthesis. The concentration of neutrophils exceeds 5 per ×400 high-power field (hematoxylin-eosin [H&E], original magnification ×400).

Fig. 3. Another example of a joint capsule around an infected total knee prosthesis. Neutrophils within capillaries (marginating) are not predictive of infection, but those that involve the extravascular fibrous membrane suggest infection (H&E, original magnification ×200).

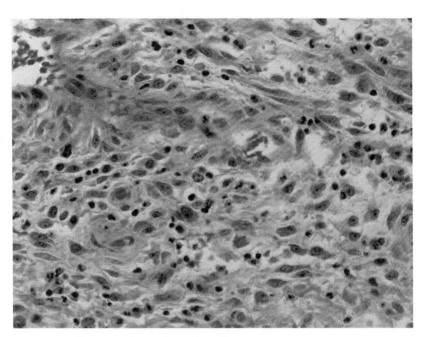

a cutoff for diagnosing infection.[3,15,22,23] Both cutoff levels were interpreted as good diagnostic tests, but as expected, requiring fewer neutrophils per unit area slightly reduced specificity but increased sensitivity.

There are several caveats to interpreting frozen sections to diagnose infection at revision arthroplasty:

- Joint capsules as well as peri-implant membranes of patients with an underlying inflammatory arthropathy (such as rheumatoid arthritis) often contain inflammation, so criteria for diagnosing infection in those patients have not been established.
- Inflammatory cells can be difficult to identify in tissue samples that have been cauterized (Fig. 5), so we encourage surgeons to use as little cautery as possible when submitting these samples for frozen section.
- Surgeons often ream the femoral or tibial canal to obtain a sample, so pathologists need to recognize that neutrophils within hematopoietic bone marrow do not necessarily reflect an infection (Fig. 6).
- Lymphocytes and plasma cells are commonly present in biopsies of patients who have been treated with antibiotics for infection, but these cells are nonspecific and are not predictive of active infection.
- Some specimens obtained at the second stage of a 2-stage revision arthroplasty for known infection contain extensive surface necrosis, thick fibrous membranes, sheets of lymphocytes and plasma cells, and marked perivascular lymphocytes (Fig. 7). These morphologic features are similar to those described as an "inflammatory pseudotumor" and are attributed to metal ions from failed metal-metal total hip prostheses.[24] When this inflammatory reaction develops around an antibiotic-containing cement spacer, however, the inflammatory reaction is unlikely to reflect an immune reaction to metal ions ("pseudo-inflammatory pseudotumor").
- Inflammation is not uniformly distributed around the arthroplasty, so evaluation of biopsies from several different sites increases sensitivity over a single biopsy. It is also important for the tissue submitted for frozen section to adequately represent the implant membrane or joint capsule, and not contain only superficial fibrin. Neutrophils often become entrapped in superficial fibrin and are not predictive of infection (Fig. 8).

Although we use the same histologic criteria for diagnosing active infection when a bone cement spacer is being removed during the second stage of a 2-stage revision arthroplasty for infection, as we do for frozen sections obtained at revision arthroplasty, to our knowledge, the predictive value of these observations after the use of local and systemic antibiotics requires further study.

Communication between surgeon and pathologist is key to help both physicians determine the

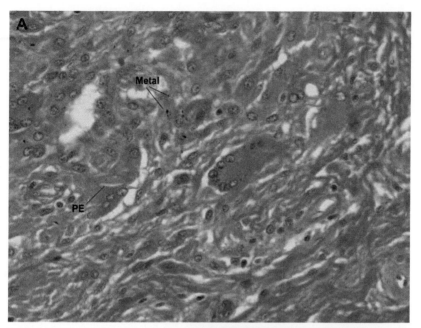

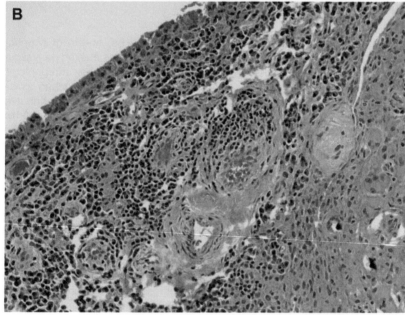

Fig. 4. (*A*) Typical appearance of tissue adjacent to an implant that has developed aseptic loosening because of bone resorption indirectly stimulated by the macrophage and giant cell reaction to particles of orthopedic wear debris. An arcuate "space" contains a shard of polyethylene (PE) wear-debris (better visualized with the use of polarized light). Small opaque particles of metal are also present in macrophages and giant cells. There is no acute inflammation (H&E, original magnification ×400). (*B*) Membranes around implants that develop aseptic loosening sometimes contain lymphocytes, plasma cells, and perivascular inflammation, but these features are not predictive of infection (H&E, original magnification ×200).

clinical importance of inflammation in any given case.

IMPROVING SENSITIVITY OF MICROBIOLOGIC CULTURES

The results of microbiologic cultures of periprosthetic tissue samples or joint fluid collected during a revision arthroplasty operation are often considered the "gold standard" for the diagnosis of periprosthetic infection. Intraoperative cultures are undoubtedly important to both document the presence of infection and to identify the organism to determine susceptibility, but false positive intraoperative cultures, presumably caused by contamination, are relatively common. There are also well-recognized cases with negative intraoperative cultures in which the histology of peri-implant membranes showed acute inflammation, and subsequent clinical course confirmed

Fig. 5. Neutrophils can be difficult to distinguish from lymphocytes and eosinophils if the peri-implant tissue contains artifacts related to the use of intraoperative cautery (H&E, original magnification ×200).

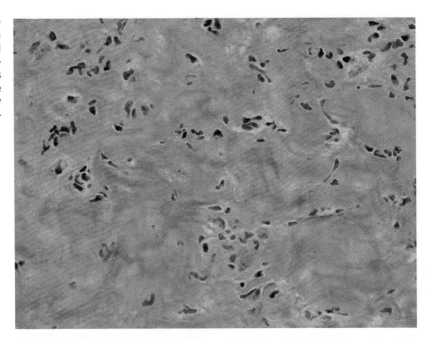

infection. For example, Atkins and colleagues[25] described a prospective series of 297 patients, 41 of whom had clinically evident infections. In that study, only 65% of samples from the infected patients grew organisms thought to be responsible for the infection. For this reason, some investigators recommended that 5 or 6 different samples be submitted, and a cutoff of 3 or more positive cultures be used to diagnose infection. The AAOS Clinical Practice Guidelines do not specify an optimum number of cultures to be submitted during revision arthroplasty, but recommend the surgeon submit at least 2.[3]

Although false negative results are most commonly the consequence of recent antibiotics, other factors that can yield false negative cultures

Fig. 6. Hematopoietic bone marrow is often present in frozen sections of specimens obtained from the femoral or tibial canal. Neutrophils within bone marrow are not predictive of infection (H&E, original magnification ×200).

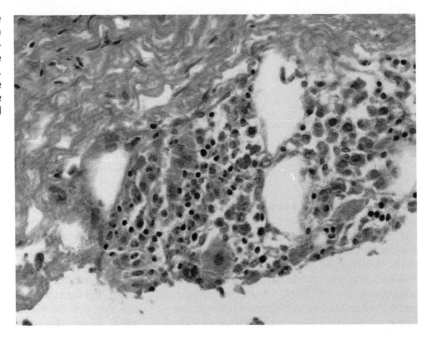

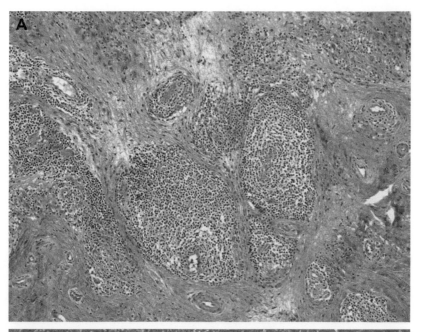

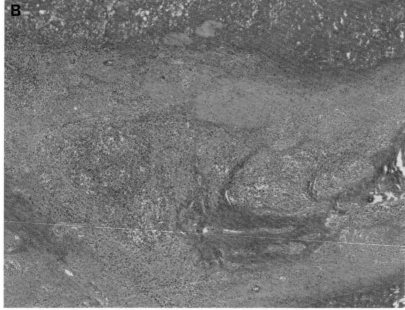

Fig. 7. (*A*) A prominent infiltrate of lymphocytes and plasma cells, in both diffuse and perivascular distribution is sometimes present at the second stage of a 2-stage revision for an infected prosthesis (in this case, a previously infected total knee prosthesis). This chronic inflammatory reaction is not predictive of persistent infection (H&E, original magnification ×40). (*B*) Areas of extensive necrosis along with diffuse and perivascular chronic inflammation have been associated with failed metal-metal hip prostheses ("inflammatory pseudotumor"), but a similar appearance can be seen around other types of failed implants, especially at the second-stage reconstruction for infection (H&E, original magnification ×40).

include cauterization of tissues before culture, and infections with low virulent, fastidious organisms that, sometimes protected by biofilm, may exist in a dormant state on the implant. Several studies have documented the efficacy of sonicating retrieved implants to increase culture yield,[26–28] presumably by disrupting the biofilm. Based in part on in vitro studies to determine optimum sonication conditions,[29] we add approximately 500 mL of Ringer lactate solution to the clean, sterile container with the retrieved implant, sonicate for 5 minutes, and then culture aliquots of the sonicate fluid. Comparisons with tissue and aspirated fluid cultures obtained at the same time have shown good correlation in many cases and, in a few cases, the sonicate fluid has yielded the only positive cultures. Sonication appears to be of most value when used to evaluate implants from

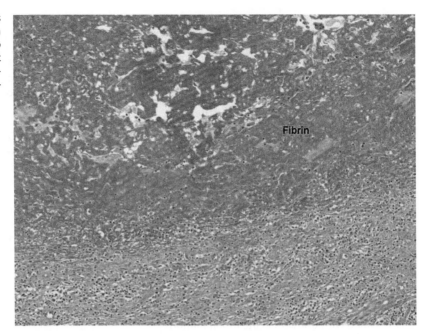

Fibrin

Fig. 8. Inflammatory cells entrapped in the fibrin that is often adherent to the surface of the implant membrane are not predictive of infection (H&E, original magnification ×200).

patients who received antibiotics shortly before implant removal.[27]

MOLECULAR TECHNIQUES TO DIAGNOSE INFECTIONS

It is widely believed that the incidence of periprosthetic infections is underdiagnosed, but the true magnitude of that underdiagnosis is unknown. Several studies have used the polymerase chain reaction (PCR) to seek evidence of periprosthetic infections, usually targeting the 16S rRNA gene that is highly conserved in nearly all bacteria. For example, Tunney and colleagues[30] reported PCR evidence of bacteria in fluid sonicated from 72% of 120 hip implants retrieved at revision arthroplasty. Other investigators have also reported cases of PCR-positive, culture-negative cases.[31,32] Some of those PCR-positive cases were probably culture-negative cases because of the use of perioperative antibiotics, but other cases could be culture negative because the bacteria were in a dormant state encased in biofilm, or because the organisms simply did not grow using standard microbiologic methods. Alternatively, some of those cases could represent clinically false positive PCR results owing to either contamination during specimen handling, contamination of PCR reagents with bacterial DNA,[33] or the detection of DNA from dead bacteria. Recent studies are under way to minimize the detection of DNA from dead bacteria, either through the use of reverse transcription PCR to localize mRNA,[34] or by using a DNA cross-linking agent, such as propidium monoazide.[35]

Conventional PCR has the advantage of high sensitivity, but does not provide information about the species of bacteria, information needed to select antibiotic therapy. Recent advances in molecular testing, such as the use of postamplification pyrosequencing[32] or multiplex PCR,[36] may help overcome that limitation of conventional PCR. Another way to improve the specificity of PCR is to use primers and probes directed against a specific organism, or the group of organisms most likely to be involved with clinically important orthopedic infections. For example, Sakai and colleagues[37] have developed a PCR assay for staphylococci in which postamplification melting curve analysis allows distinction between *Staphylococcus aureus* and coagulase-negative staphylococci. Kobayashi and colleagues[32] have used a combination of a modified universal PCR and sequencing technology to identify bacteria based on the DNA sequences that determine gram-positive versus gram-negative staining, whereas Moojen and colleagues[38] used a "reverse line blot" method in which oligonucleotide probes of organisms commonly involved in orthopedic infections were bound to membranes and reacted with PCR amplicons to provide bacterial species information. Thus, combinations of specific PCR

Pitfalls
PERIPROSTHETIC INFECTION

! Acute inflammation in periprosthetic tissue of a patient with an underlying noninfectious inflammatory arthropathy (such as rheumatoid arthritis) is not necessarily predictive of infection.

! Neutrophils entrapped in superficial fibrin are not predictive of infection.

! Neutrophils in capillaries (marginating) are not predictive of infection.

! Neutrophils in bone marrow may not be predictive of infection.

! Lymphocytes and plasma cells alone are not predictive of infection.

! In rare cases, tissue necrosis induced by impingement or implant dislocation can be associated with transient acute inflammation in the absence of infection.

! A very recent periprosthetic fracture can also be associated with transient acute inflammation in the absence of infection.

assays may ultimately prove to be more useful than broad-spectrum, so-called "universal" bacterial assays.

Other new techniques that may have a role in diagnosing infection include the use of microarray and proteomics technologies. The challenge for all of the new molecular tests will be to distinguish clinically important infections from trace levels of necrotic bacteria or contaminants, and to provide that information quickly enough to be of practical help in guiding patient care.

The role of the pathologist is to work with the orthopedic surgeon to help optimize the predictive value of serologic, microbiologic, morphologic, and molecular diagnostic tests to improve the recognition of clinically important periprosthetic infections.

REFERENCES

1. Love C, Tomas MB, Marwin SE, et al. Role of nuclear medicine in diagnosis of the infected joint replacement. Radiographics 2001;21:1229–38.

2. Bauer TW, Parvizi J, Kobayashi N, et al. Diagnosis of periprosthetic infection. J Bone Joint Surg Am 2006; 88:869–82.

3. Della Valle C, Parvizi J, Bauer TW, et al. AAOS Clinical Practice Guideline Summary: The diagnosis of periprosthetic joint infections of the hip and knee. J Am Acad Orthop Surg 2010;18:760–70.

4. Ghanem E, Antoci V Jr, Pulido L. The use of receiver operating characteristics analysis in determining erythrocyte sedimentation rate and C-reactive protein levels in diagnosing periprosthetic infection prior to revision total hip arthroplasty. Int J Infect Dis 2009;13:e444–9.

5. Spangehl M, Masri B, O'Connell J, et al. Prospective analysis of preoperative and intraoperative investigations for the diagnosis of infection at the sites of two hundred and two revision total hip arthroplasties. J Bone Joint Surg Am 1999;81:672–83.

6. Di Cesare P, Chang E, Preston C, et al. Serum interleukin-6 as a marker of periprosthetic infection following total hip and knee arthroplasty. J Bone Joint Surg Am 2005;87:1921–7.

7. Ghanem E, Ketonis C, Restrepo C, et al. Periprosthetic infection: where do we stand with regard to Gram stain? Acta Orthop 2009;80:37–40.

8. Oethinger M, Warner DK, Schindler SA, et al. Diagnosing periprosthetic infection false-positive intraoperative gram stains. Clin Orthop Relat Res 2011;469:954–60.

9. Ghanem E, Parvizi J, Burnett RS, et al. Cell count and differential of aspirated fluid in the diagnosis of infection at the site of total knee arthroplasty. J Bone Joint Surg Am 2008;90:1637–43.

10. Feldman D, Lonner J, Desai P, et al. The role of intraoperative frozen sections in revision total joint arthroplasty. J Bone Joint Surg Am 1995;77:1807–13.

11. Charosky C, Bullough P, Wilson P. Total hip replacement failures: a histologic evaluation. J Bone Joint Surg Am 1973;55:49–58.

12. Mirra J, Amstutz H, Matos M, et al. The pathology of the joint tissues and its clinical relevance in prosthesis failure. Clin Orthop Relat Res 1976;117: 221–40.

13. Mirra J, Marder R, Amstutz H. The pathology of failed total joint arthroplasty. Clin Orthop 1982;170: 175–83.

14. Fehring T, McAlister J. Frozen histologic section as a guide to sepsis in revision joint arthroplasty. Clin Orthop Relat Res 1994;304:229–37.

15. Lonner J, Desai P, Dicesare P, et al. The reliability of analysis of intraoperative frozen sections for identifying active infection during revision hip or knee arthroplasty. J Bone Joint Surg Am 1996;78:1553–8.

16. Athanasou N, Pandey R, de Steiger R, et al. Diagnosis of infection by frozen section during revision arthroplasty. J Bone Joint Surg Br 1995;77:28–33.

17. Pandey R, Berendt A, Athanasou N. Histological and microbiological findings in non-infected and infected revision arthroplasty tissues. Arch Orthop Trauma Surg 2000;120:570–4.

18. Della Valle C, Bogner E, Desai P. Analysis of frozen sections of intraoperative specimens obtained at

the time of reoperation after hip or knee resection arthroplasty for the treatment of infection. J Bone Joint Surg Am 1999;81:684–9.

19. Banit DM, Kaufer H, Hartford JM. Intraoperative frozen section analysis in revision total joint arthroplasty. Clin Orthop Relat Res 2002;401:230–8.

20. Ko PS, Ip D, Chow KP, et al. The role of intraoperative frozen section in decision making in revision hip and knee arthroplasties in a local community hospital. J Arthroplasty 2005;20:189–95.

21. Nunez LV, Buttaro MA, Morandi A, et al. Frozen sections of samples taken intraoperatively for diagnosis of infection in revision hip surgery. Acta Orthop 2007;78:226–30.

22. Frances BA, Martinez FM, Cebrian Parra JL. Diagnosis of infection in hip and knee revision surgery: intraoperative frozen section analysis. Int Orthop 2007;31:33–7.

23. Schinksy MF, Della Valle CJ, Sporer SM. Perioperative testing for joint infection in patients undergoing revision total hip arthroplasty. J Bone Joint Surg Am 2008;90:1869–75.

24. Campbell P, Ebramzadeh E, Nelson S. Histological features of pseudotumor-like tissues from metal-on-metal hips. Clin Orthop Relat Res 2010;468:2321–7.

25. Atkins BL, Athanasou N, Deeks JJ, et al. Prospective evaluation of criteria for microbiological diagnosis of prosthetic-joint infection at revision arthroplasty. J Clin Microbiol 1998;36:2932–9.

26. Sampedro MF, Huddleston PM, Piper KE, et al. A biofilm approach to detect bacteria on removed spinal implants. Spine 2010;35:1218–24.

27. Trampuz A, Piper KE, Jacobson MJ, et al. Sonication of removed hip and knee prostheses for diagnosis of infection. N Engl J Med 2007;357:654–63.

28. Kobayashi H, Oethinger M, Tuohy MJ, et al. Improved detection of biofilm-formative bacteria by vortexing and sonication: a pilot study. Clin Orthop Relat Res 2008;466:1360–4.

29. Kobayashi N, Bauer TW, Tuohy MJ, et al. Brief ultrasonication improves detection of biofilm-formative bacteria around a metal implant. Clin Orthop Relat Res 2007;457:210–3.

30. Tunney MM, Patrick S, Gorman SP. Improved detection of infection in hip replacements. A currently underestimated problem. J Bone Joint Surg Br 1998;80:568–72.

31. Mariani BD, Martin DS, Levine MJ. Polymerase chain reaction detection of bacterial infection in total knee arthroplasty. Clin Orthop Relat Res 1996;331:11–22.

32. Kobayashi N, Procop GW, Krebs V. Molecular identification of bacteria from aseptically loose implants. Clin Orthop Relat Res 2008;466:1716–25.

33. Newsome T, Li B, Zou N, et al. Presence of bacterial phage-like DNA sequences in commercial Taq DNA polymerase reagents. J Clin Microbiol 2004;42:2264–7.

34. Bergin PF, Doppelt JD, Hamilton WG, et al. Detection of periprosthetic infections with use of ribosomal RNA-based polymerase chain reaction. J Bone Joint Surg Am 2010;92:654–63.

35. Kobayashi H, Oethinger M, Tuohy MJ. Distinction between intact and antibiotic-inactivated bacteria by real-time PCR after treatment with propidium monoazide. J Orthop Res 2010;28:1245–51.

36. Achermann Y, Vogt M, Leung M. Improved diagnosis of periprosthetic joint infection by multiplex PCR of sonicated fluid from removed implants. J Clin Microbiol 2010;48:1208–14.

37. Sakai H, Procop W, Kobayashi N, et al. Simultaneous detection of Staphylococcus aureus and coagulase-negative staphylococci in positive blood cultures by real-time PCR with fluorescence resonance energy transfer probe sets. J Clin Microbiol 2004;42:5739–44.

38. Moojen DJ, van Hellemondt G, Vogely HC, et al. Incidence of low-grade infection in aseptic loosening of total hip arthroplasty. Acta Orthop 2010;81:667–73.

BONE CYTOLOGY: A REALISTIC APPROACH FOR CLINICAL USE

Diana M. Cardona, MD*, Leslie G. Dodd, MD

KEYWORDS

• Bone • Benign • Malignant • Cytology • FNA

ABSTRACT

This article presents the use of bone cytology for diagnosis of bone tumors. It discusses critical factors and considerations of fine-needle aspiration and bone cytology and presents diagnostic options and differential diagnosis for benign and malignant bone lesions. Osteomyelitis, chrondroblastoma, Langerhans cell histiocytosis, chondromyxoid fibromas, enchondromas, giant cell tumor of bone, osteosarcoma, chondrosarcoma and variants, Ewing sarcoma, chordoma, plasmacytoma, multiple myeloma, lymphoma, and metastatic bone disease are presented.

OVERVIEW: CRITICAL PREANALYTICAL FACTORS AND CONSIDERATIONS

Although open biopsy is the widely accepted procedure of choice for the diagnosis of bone tumors, there are some disadvantages that could potentially be avoided through the use of fine-needle aspiration (FNA) and cytologic analysis. The associated medical costs and risks of infection, hematoma, patient discomfort, pathologic fracture, and contamination of surrounding tissues are dramatically reduced through the use of FNA.[1–5] Outside the setting of a few large orthopedic centers, however, this methodology has not gained wide acceptance, likely due to unease of pathologists and presumed difficulties in obtaining adequate or diagnostic material.

The use of FNA for the diagnosis of bone lesions was first introduced by Coley and colleagues[6] in 1931 and further simplified and promoted in 1970 with the introduction of fluoroscopy.[7] Since its inception, the reported sensitivity and specificity ranges for FNA of bone lesions have been 93% to 100% and 86% to 100%, respectively.[8,9] Accuracy rates have varied tremendously, ranging from 53.8% to 100%.[5,10–13] When assessing for secondary malignant disease, the accuracy rates tend to be higher than when looking at primary bone tumors alone.[11,14] In most instances, skeletal metastatic disease and lymphoproliferative disease can be reliably and safely diagnosed by

Key Points
BONE CYTOLOGY AND FINE-NEEDLE ASPIRATION

- FNA is especially appropriate for some of the more commonly encountered bone lesions, including metastases, plasmacytoma, lymphoma, EWS, giant cell tumor, and benign and malignant matrix-forming neoplasms.

- Clinical and radiographic correlation is crucial to triaging appropriate cases for FNA and for the diagnostic interpretation of aspirated material.

- The advantage of FNA over other diagnostic techniques is the ability to determine specimen adequacy in real time, which should help diminish the number of inadequate or nondiagnostic biopsies.

- Other potential benefits of FNA, particularly when compared with open biopsy, include cost savings and decreased patient morbidity and inconvenience as well as faster turnaround time for diagnosis.

Department of Pathology, Duke University Medical Center, Box 3712, Durham, NC 27710, USA
* Corresponding author.
E-mail address: Diana.cardona@duke.edu

Surgical Pathology 5 (2012) 79–100
doi:10.1016/j.path.2011.07.008
1875-9181/12/$ – see front matter © 2012 Elsevier Inc. All rights reserved.

surgpath.theclinics.com

FNA. When only categorizing primary bone lesions as either benign versus malignant, however, accuracy rates also increase (94%).[11] Furthermore, this distinction alone often provides the needed information for further management decisions. Often of concern are the insufficiency/inadequacy rates for FNA, which vary from 0 to 33%[9,12] and are highly dependent on the availability of on site assessment of sample adequacy.

The authors agree that, in certain clinical settings, the usefulness of FNA is of limited benefit. For example, lesions in which the cortical surface remains intact or appears thickened, tumors with extensive sclerotic matrix production, and/or largely cystic lesions should be avoided (ie, fibrous dysplasia, aneurysmal bone cyst [ABC], and so forth), because the sampling or diagnostic yield likely is low.[10,15] Therefore, analysis of the radiographic appearance should provide the needed gross information to triage a case to the most appropriate sampling technique, aspiration versus open biopsy. Once the decision for FNA is made, the use of image guidance (fluoroscopy or CT guidance), targeting the periphery of the lesion to avoid potential central necrosis and the use of immediate adequacy assessment aid in increasing the diagnostic yield.[10,11] But what must be stressed is that there should be no hesitation in requesting further sampling by either repeat FNA or open biopsy if there is a discrepancy or doubt as to sample adequacy. In the current cost-saving environment and with desire for less-invasive techniques, FNA remains an attractive option provided clinicians, radiologists, and pathologists approach the diagnosis as a collaborative effort.

BENIGN LESIONS

By no means is this an exhaustive list, because lesions with a high radiographic suspicion of being a unicameral or bone cyst ABC, fibrous dysplasia, nonossifying fibroma, or osteoid osteoma should be avoided due to the high risk of nondiagnostic sampling.[10,15] Understanding the radiographic findings and differential diagnosis is critical before any FNA procedure and specimen assessment.

OSTEOMYELITIS

The development of acute osteomyelitis can occur via hematogenous dissemination or direct inoculation, such as with skin ulceration or direct trauma. In cases of contiguous extension, the diagnosis is often not in question because radiographic findings or gross observation of underlying bony change is seen. In cases of acute hematogenous spread, the patient population tends to be children

under the age of 15 years.[16] Correlation with radiographic findings, which can vary from unapparent to aggressive and destructive, and clinical laboratory studies, such as an elevated erythrocyte sedimentation rate and left shifted white blood cell count, support the diagnosis. The clinical course tends to be relapsing and remitting with patients presenting with fever, local swelling, and bone pain that primarily affects the metaphysis of long tubular bones, clavicles, spine, and pelvis.[17]

FNA Cytology for Osteomyelitis

Aspiration cytology is usually performed in cases with significant bone destruction and/or soft tissue extension.[18] The typically cellular smears contain a mixture of acute and chronic inflammatory cells, with a predominance of neutrophils, cellular debris, and necrosis (Fig. 1).[19] Foci of histiocytic inflammation can be seen.[17] Although these findings are supportive of the diagnosis, Gram staining and cultures of the aspirated material often provide a definitive answer and the identity of the specific infectious agent.[18,19] The most commonly implicated microbes include *Staphylococcus aureus*, *Streptococcus pyogenes*, and *Haemophilus influenza*.[16]

Differential Diagnosis for Osteomyelitis

The differential diagnosis for osteomyelitis or Brodie abscess typically includes eosinophilic granuloma (Langerhans cell histiocytosis) and, if aggressive-appearing on imaging studies, a primary bone tumor, such as Ewing sarcoma (EWS).[17] Although histiocytes can be seen in the setting of osteomyelitis, they should not be the predominant cell type, demonstrate the characteristic morphology (longitudinal nuclear grooves), or have a marked associated eosinophilic infiltrate. Additionally, cell types other than inflammatory cells and osteoblasts/osteoclasts, frank cytologic atypia, or mitotic activity should not be identified in the setting of osteomyelitis. Chronic recurrent multifocal osteomyelitis is a rare, noninfectious, systemic inflammatory disorder that affects children and young adults and that radiographically and histologically can mimic osteomyelitis.[16,17]

LANGERHANS CELL HISTIOCYTOSIS

Langerhans cell histiocytosis is a clonal and, therefore, neoplastic condition that most commonly affects children younger than age 5 years but is a disease that can affect any age group. There is a slight male predominance and the craniofacial bones, followed by the femur, humerus, pelvis, ribs, and spine, are the sites of most frequent involvement.[16,17] When present as a solitary

Fig. 1. This image illustrates a mixture of neutrophils and histiocytes from a focus of acute osteomyleitis. The histiocytic cytoplasm contains several phagocytized neutrophils.

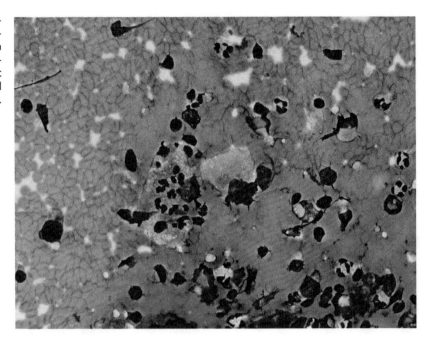

bone lesion, the term, *eosinophilic granuloma (EG)*, is often used. When multifocal, a few distinct clinical syndromes exist, such as Hand-Schüller-Christian syndrome and Letterer-Siwe disease, which share the same histologic findings but are prognostically and biologically distinct. Although technically a misnomer, EG is still the most widely recognized term for the solitary bone lesion of the histiocytoses family of disease. Radiographically, EG tends to be intramedullary, well defined, and lytic but typically lacks a reactive sclerotic rim. When EG involves the vertebral bodies, bone destruction can lead to flattening (vertebra plana).

FNA Cytology for Langerhans Cell Histiocytosis

FNA smears of EG are usually hypercellular and comprised of the distinctive plump, round to ovoid histiocytes with large, pale nuclei. The nuclei are frequently characterized as having a kidney shape with longitudinal grooves or folded contours and inconspicuous to prominent nucleoli (**Fig. 2**A). Binucleated cells and/or multinucleated cells are often noted. These nuclear features are best highlighted on the Papanicolaou stain. The background infiltrate is composed of scattered inflammatory cells, most notably many eosinophils.[17,20,21] The cytologic picture is characteristic, but if a cell block or additional smears are available, immunohistochemistry for S-100 protein and CD1a can help confirm the diagnosis, because the histiocytes

should be positive (see **Fig. 2**B).[20] Although not needed, electron microscopic examination reveals the pathognomonic Birbeck granules.[22]

Differential Diagnosis for Langerhans Cell Histiocytosis

The radiographic and cytologic differential diagnosis potentially include osteomyelitis, chondroblastoma, and, in the adult population, metastatic disease (ie, melanoma). Recognition of the characteristic histiocyte morphology, associated inflammatory milieu, lack of matrix production, absence of cytologic atypia, and immunohistochemical analysis should aid in this distinction.[17,20,23]

CHONDROBLASTOMA

Chondroblastoma, a rare tumor, most commonly affects adolescents and young adults between the ages of 10 and 25 years, with a slight male predominance. Greater than 75% occur within the epiphysis of the major long bones, most commonly the femur, tibia, and humerus. Chondroblastomas can also involve the flat bones, such, talus, calcaneus, and patella.[17,24,25] When this lesion is found at unusual sites, such as skull or temporal bone, patients tend to be older (40–50 years old).[25] On plain films, chondroblastomas classically produce a small (3–6 cm), lytic, sharply demarcated, centrally or eccentrically placed lesion with a sclerotic rim of bone. The presence

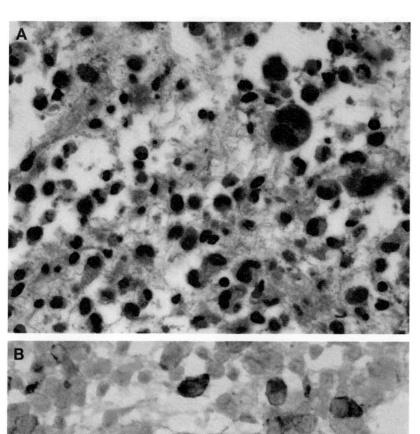

Fig. 2. (A) In this cellblock preparation from an aspirate of eosinophilic granuloma, all diagnostic features are identified, including many eosinophils, histiocytes, and multinucleate giant cells. (B) Immunohistochemical staining for CD1a is positive within the histiocytic cells of eosinophilic granuloma.

of matrix calcifications is a helpful, albeit not a constant, finding.[17]

FNA Cytology for Chondroblastoma

FNA of these lesions tend to produce cellular smears composed of a mixture of mononuclear cells and multinucleated giant cells. The cells can be loosely arranged or aggregate, creating a lobular appearance. The mononuclear chondroblasts are round to oval with moderate to scant, eosinophilic, and granular cytoplasm and well-defined cell borders (Fig. 3). The nuclei are often eccentrically located and demonstrate marked membrane irregularity, may show longitudinal grooves or clefts, and contain small but distinct nucleoli.[23,25,26] Two types of giant cells can be seen. The first are larger and contain many nuclei,

Fig. 3. Constituents of chondroblastoma include single chondroblasts with longitudinal grooves and multinucleate cells with similar nuclear grooving or infolding.

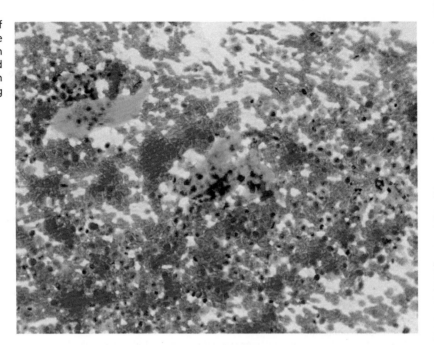

similar to osteoclast-like giant cells (OGCs) or those seen in giant cell tumor of bone (GCTB). The other type tends to be smaller and contain nuclei that are reminiscent of the surrounding mononuclear cell nuclei, with irregular contours and grooves.[24] Atypia, hyperchromasia, or mitotic activity should never be a prominent feature. Although not always present, the cells may appear to be floating in abundant myxoid/chondroid matrix, best depicted on Romanovsky staining.[10,24] An additional classic finding, yet uncommonly seen on aspirate smears, is focal calcification. According to Kilpatrick and Renner,[17] the identification of characteristic chondroblasts in an epiphyseal bone tumor with corroborative radiographic findings is sufficient for the diagnosis of chondroblastoma. The presence of chondroid matrix, giant cells, or calcifications is not needed for the diagnosis.

Differential Diagnosis for Chondroblastoma

The principal differential diagnoses include GCTB, chondromyxoid fibroma, Langerhans cell histiocytosis, and clear cell chondrosarcoma (CS). The mononuclear and multinucleated cells of a GCTB tend to be smaller with round, regular nuclei when compared with the cells of a chondroblastoma.[10] Table 1 discusses the main differential diagnoses and radiographic and cytologic differences of giant cell–rich tumors. Although the patient population is similar with chondromyxoid fibroma, these tumors tend to be metaphyseal in origin and produce smears with more abundant myxoid

fibrillar matrix and intermixed round to stellate-appearing, discohesive cells. In addition to usually affecting a younger population, the inflammatory milieu seen in Langerhans cell histiocytosis is typically absent in chondroblastomas. Distinction from a clear cell CS on imaging alone can be difficult, but those tumors typically present in the fourth to fifth decades of life, and cytologic preparations reveal round to oval cells with abundant clear cytoplasm; centrally placed, enlarged, round nuclei with prominent nucleoli; and a watery myxoid appearance in the background.[17,25]

CHONDROMYXOID FIBROMA

Chondromyxoid fibromas are tumors that comprise approximately only 1% to 2% of benign bone neoplasms. They have a marked predilection for the metaphyseal region of the long bones, in particular the proximal tibia, distal femur, and ilium. The most commonly effected population is male and between the ages of 10 and 30 years. Radiographically, these tumors form eccentric, sharply marginated, lucent lesions that cause thinning and expansion of the cortex.[17,27]

FNA Cytology for Chondromyxoid Fibroma

Cytologic smears tend to contain amorphous clumps of metachromatic chondroid matrix, best highlighted on Diff-Quik stain. Other components frequently identified in aspirates include giant cells and fragments of fibrous material (**Fig. 4**). Plump, round to stellate cells are often identified within

Table 1
Differential diagnosis for giant cell–rich lesions of bone

Diagnosis	Age	Common Location	Cytologic Appearance
ABC[a]	<20	Metaphysis; long bones and vertebrae	Scant cellularity, bloody background, fibroblasts, pigmented histiocytes, and individual OGCs
Giant Cell Tumor	20–40	Epiphysis (±metaphyseal extension); long bones and sacrum	Cellular smears, uniform spindled stromal cells and many intermixed OGCs; no atypia and no matrix production
Chondroblastoma	10–25	Epiphysis; long bones, acetabulum, and ilium	Cellular smears, uniform round chondroblasts with characteristic nuclear features (grooves and clefts), scattered OGC, ±myxoid matrix and/or calcifications
Fibrous Dysplasia[a]	10–30	Metaphysis/diaphysis; skull, long bones, and ribs	Scant cellularity, spindled cells with bland nuclei; rare OGCs; ±osteoid
OS (OGC rich)	<30	Metaphysis; long bones	Cellular smears, polygonal-shaped cells with eccentric nuclei, nuclear pleomorphism, abnormal mitotic activity, metachromatic matrix; many OGCs

[a] FNA is not recommended.
Abbreviations: ABC, aneurysmal bone cyst; OGC, osteoclast-like giant cell; OS, osteosarcoma.

or adjacent to the myxoid/chondroid matrix material. The nuclear features can be variable, with the majority displaying bland chromatin and small size and others exhibiting nuclear enlargement, smudgy chromatin, and atypia.[17,24,27] If present, the atypia should not cause confusion with malignant entities, such as CS, if special attention is given to the clinical presentation and radiographic findings. Mitotic figures are absent. Although the predominant cell population is mononuclear, a significant subpopulation of binucleated and multinucleated cells can be seen.[24]

Differential Diagnosis for Chondromyxoid Fibroma

In addition to CS, the cytologic differential diagnosis includes enchondroma and chondroblastoma. The presence of true hyaline cartilage, with lacunar spaces containing chondrocytes, essentially excludes the diagnosis of chondromyxoid fibroma.[27] This mature matrix production commonly is seen in examples of enchondroma and low-grade CS. Correlation with age of presentation, clinical symptoms, and radiographic appearance is crucial in further delineating that differential. In distinguishing chondromyxoid fibroma from chondroblastoma, knowledge of the tumor location (epiphysis vs metaphysis) is of utmost importance.

ENCHONDROMA

Enchondromas are benign cartilaginous neoplasms that tend to occur within the medullary cavity of small tubular bones, humerus, and femur. They can arise at any age, but most patients present between the ages of 10 and 30 years. These lesions are typically solitary, with multiple tumors associated with clinical syndromes, such as Ollier disease or Maffucci syndrome. Metaphyseal in location, these tumors demonstrate a sharply marginated, often lobular in contour, expansile, and lytic appearance on plain film. Evidence of matrix production is evident by the presence of variable punctuate calcifications.[17,24] In part due to the characteristic radiographic appearance, tissue biopsy, especially by conventional FNA sampling, is often avoided because the surrounding cortex is generally intact. If performed, usually by using intermediate-bore cutting needles, the main objective is often to confirm the presence of a cartilaginous neoplasm. What must be clearly understood is that on cytologic grounds alone, separation between an enchondroma and a low-grade CS is impossible. Correlation with radiographic appearance is required for the distinction.

FNA Cytology for Enchondroma

The smears demonstrate fragments or lobules of cartilage matrix, without a significant myxoid or watery appearance, that is most pronounced on Diff-Quik stain. Evaluation of the Papanicalaou stain enables the identification of scattered small, round, and uniformly bland chondrocytes within lacunar spaces (**Fig. 5**). The cells have modest amounts of cytoplasm and small nuclei with

Fig. 4. (A) An aspirated fragment of matrix from chondromyxoid fibroma with an inconspicuous population of small spindled cells. (B) The more fibrous component of chondromyxoid fibroma is illustrated here. Also note the isolated chondrocytes with mild cytologic atypia.

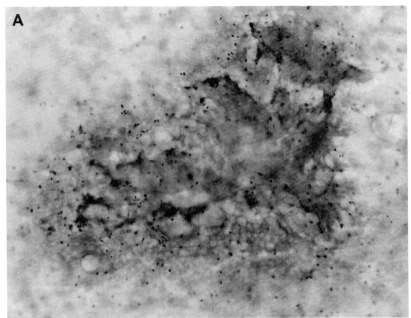

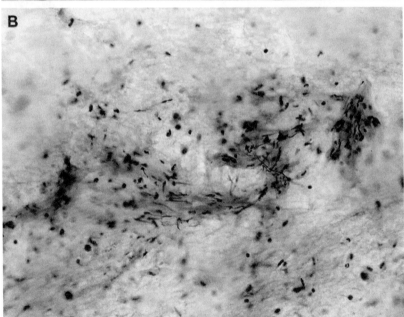

condensed chromatin. Binucleation is rarely encountered and mitotic activity is generally not seen.[17,24,28]

Differential Diagnosis for Enchondroma

The differential diagnosis is similar to that for chondromyxoid fibromas (discussed previously), which includes CS, chondromyxoid fibroma, and chondroblastoma.

GIANT CELL TUMOR OF BONE

GCTB is a locally aggressive low-grade neoplasm that generally arises in skeletally mature individuals, between the ages of 18 and 40 years.[10,17] Reports of metastatic disease exist, with reported rates of up to 5%; however, this has led to death in only a few patients. Even rarer are the reports of frank malignant transformation (1%–3%).[29,30] This tumor, which has also been called an

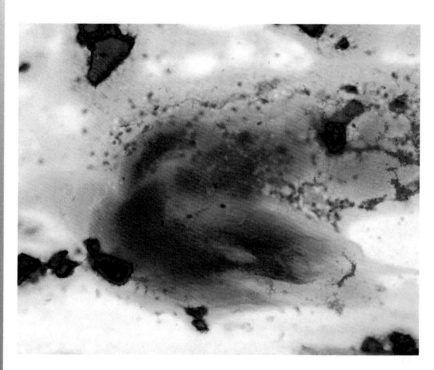

Fig. 5. Large intact fragment of paucicellular cartilage aspirated from an enchondroma.

osteoclastoma, demonstrates a slight female predominance. The majority of GCTB occur within the long bones, notably the distal femur, proximal tibia, distal radius, and proximal humerus. The sacrum, pelvic bones, and vertebral bodies, with the exception of the dorsal elements, can also be involved.[24] The radiographic and cytologic appearance of GCTB and brown tumor of hyperthyroidism are essentially indistinguishable and correlation with clinical and laboratory findings is necessary.[17] Classically, GCTB is centered within the epiphysis and can extend to involve the subarticular cortex and/or cross into the metaphyseal region. On radiograph, the tumor is frequently eccentric, geographic, and lytic with little to no surrounding sclerosis. Destruction of the cortex is a common finding with soft tissue extension.[10,17,24]

FNA Cytology for Giant Cell Tumor of Bone

Smears are typically markedly hypercellular with a bloody background. A dual cell population is evident with intermixed mononuclear cells and many multinucleated OGCs (**Fig. 6**). The stromal cells tend to have a uniform appearance, are ovoid to slightly spindled, and have a high nuclear to cytoplasmic ratio. The nuclei are round to elongated and regular with evenly distributed chromatin and inconspicuous nucleoli. Frequently, a syncytial appearance is seen when these cells aggregate or cluster. Significant atypia or marked/

atypical mitotic activity should not be present; if observed, the possibility of a giant cell–rich osteosarcoma (OS) should be considered. The nuclei of the giant cells are strikingly similar to the surrounding mononuclear cells. The number of nuclei can vary considerably, from few to more than 50. The cytoplasm is often vacuolated and may appear granular. Although dependent on the specimen, the OGCs should be a predominant component of the smears.[10,22,24]

Differential Diagnosis for Giant Cell Tumor of Bone

When considering the diagnosis of a GCTB, it must be distinguished it from nonossifying fibromas, chondroblastomas, chondromyxoid fibromas, giant cell–rich OSs, and some ABCs. In addition, the cytologic and histologic appearance of the brown tumor of hyperparathyroidism can be identical to that of GCTB.[17] As with all bone tumors, correlation with radiographic appearance is essential, because in addition to having fewer multinucleated giant cells, nonossifying fibromas are metaphyseal based and consistently demonstrate a sclerotic rim. Although most chondroblastomas arise in skeletally immature patients, there is potential overlap in clinical and radiographic findings. GCTB should not demonstrate chondroid matrix production, unless fracture callus is present. Additionally, the nuclear features of chondroblastomas

Fig. 6. Multinucleate giant cells are usually in abundance in aspirates of giant cell tumor. The nuclei of the giant cells are similar to the single cells in the background of the smears.

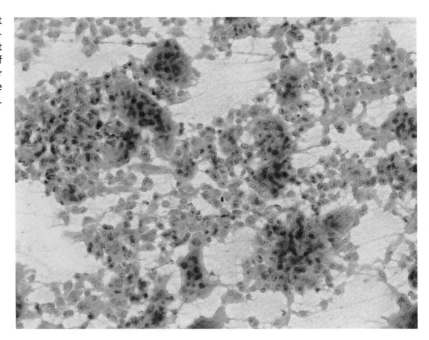

are distinct with irregular contours and frequent grooves. Similarly, abundant fibrillar matrix production and a less-prominent giant cell population are seen in cases of chondromyxoid fibroma. The separation of a GCTB and giant cell–rich OS is dependent on the evaluation of the mononuclear cells. Although some mitotic activity can be identified in both lesions, marked mitotic activity or atypical ones should not be observed in GCTB.[17,24] Additionally, GCTB lack the atypia and osteoid production that is seen in OSs. Correlation with radiographic appearance is also of great importance.[10] As with most giant cell–rich lesions, separation from an ABC may be impossible because secondary ABC-like changes are common. FNA of lesions that appear predominantly cystic should be avoided; however, if obtained, the presence of larger tissue fragments with a biphasic cell population and evenly distributed pattern of multinucleated giant cells exclude the diagnosis of a pure ABC.[24]

MALIGNANT LESIONS (PRIMARY)

OSTEOSARCOMA

OS represents one of the most common primary malignant tumors of bone. Children and adolescents are the most frequently affected individuals, but no age group is immune from this highly malignant neoplasm. In its classic form, OS appears as a metaphyseal-based destructive lesion of bone, often with early soft tissue extension.[17] Before the modern era, this was usually a lethal disease with early and frequent metastases to the lungs. With the introduction of successful chemotherapeutic agents against OS, many patients can often anticipate a much better chance of survival. Because state-of-the-art treatment now involves a neoadjuvant course of chemotherapy followed by definitive surgical treatment at a latter date, OS represents an ideal candidate for initial diagnosis by less invasive (ie, closed) biopsy techniques, such as FNA.[31]

FNA Cytology for Osteosarcoma

The cytologic appearance of OS is somewhat diverse, recapitulating the many varieties of OS encountered on histology. All diagnostic aspirates of OS, however, have two elements in common: extracellular matrix material and a cytologically malignant sarcomatous cell population. Matrix is best visualized in air-dried, Giemsa-based stains, such as Diff-Quik, where it stains a pink to magenta purple color (**Fig. 7A**). Alcohol-fixed preparations stained with either Papanicolaou or conventional hematoxylin-eosin have the advantage of revealing more nuclear detail, but the characteristics of the matrix material are minimized. In its most common form, matrix appears as an amorphous material intimately associated with small aggregates of tumor cells (see **Fig. 7B**). In

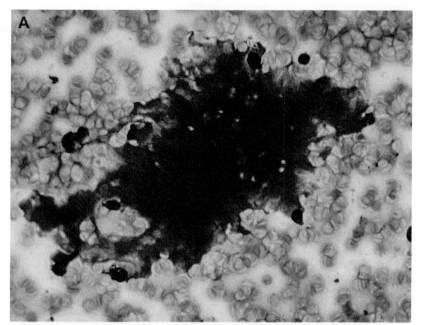

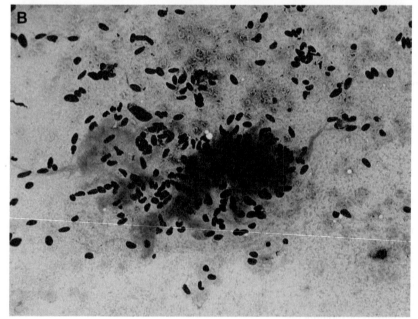

Fig. 7. Matrix material in aspirates of OS is usually less obvious than in those of the chondroid lesions. When matrix is identified, however, it often has the same color and consistency of chondroid matrix. (*A*) The unmineralized osteoid has a dense appearance with more of a ragged edge than the fibrillar appearance seen in chondroid lesions. (*B*) The matrix has more of a thin and wispy appearance.

color and texture, it can be next to impossible to distinguish from the chondroid type of extracellular matrix discussed previously and in the next section.[31,32] True osteoid, or ossified extracellular matrix, is a distinctly uncommon finding in aspirates, present in a minority of OS samples studied.[32–35] Most expert cytopathologists agree that the demonstration of osteoid in aspirates is not necessary for definitive diagnosis of OS by FNA.[32,33]

The cellular component of OS is likewise heterogeneous in appearance, again reflecting the many variant histologies. One of the more common appearances of the malignant osteoblast is of a large plasmacytoid cell (**Fig. 8A**). These are generally larger than normal plasma cells with

Fig. 8. Two different appearances of the sarcomatous cellular population of OS. (*A*) The cells are round to oval and highly pleomorphic. Multinucleate giant cells are a common finding. (*B*) The cells have much more cytoplasm and an epithelioid configuration but are still obviously malignant.

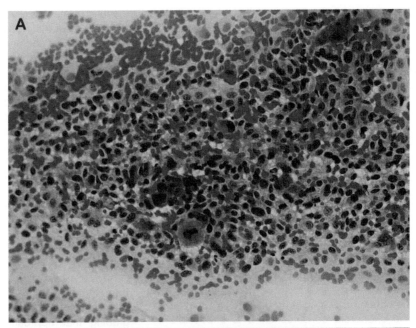

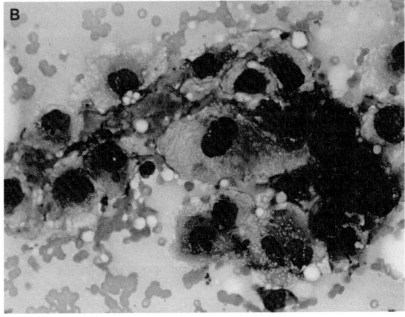

increases in the size of both the nucleus and cytoplasm. The cytoplasm often contains many small round vacuoles and osteoblast nuclei usually have one or more prominent nucleoli. The osteoblasts may also assume a spindled appearance or a frankly sarcomatous look that resembles that seen in high-grade undifferentiated sarcomas (see **Fig. 8**B). Ostoeclast-type giant cells are a frequent component of OS aspirates.[34,35]

Differential Diagnosis for Osteosarcoma

The main obstacle to successful diagnosis of OS by FNA is inadequacy of specimen. This is largely due to technical problems inherent in attempting to penetrate dense bone with a small-core needle.[36] If the aspirate of the suspected OS is technically adequate, the diagnosis is usually straightforward. Difficulties in interpretation arise when encountering some of the many variants. Aspirates of the chondroblastic variant of OS, for example, are often indistinguishable from those of CS.[28,37] Some of the well-differentiated variants of OS, parosteal OS in particular, can be difficult if not impossible to diagnose by FNA.[34,36]

CHONDROSARCOMA AND ITS VARIANTS

The cytologic diagnosis of chondroid neoplasms represents a challenging area even for the most experienced cytopathologists. The potential for misdiagnoses in this area include both underdiagnoses and overdiagnoses of malignancy on atypical-appearing chondroid aspirates. For example, an enchondroma is virtually indistinguishable from a low-grade CS on cytologic features alone. Also, many otherwise benign cartilaginous lesions, such as chondromyxoid fibroma, are notorious for displaying focal cytologic atypia of the chondroid constituents. It is impossible to overemphasize the importance of clinical and imaging correlation in this category. In many instances, these factors often trump the cytologic findings in importance in the formulation of a final diagnosis.

CS represents one of the more common primary malignant tumors of bone in the adult population. Unlike some of the other tumors described thus far, CS has a predilection for the axial skeleton (ribs, pelvis, and scapula) but occurs in the long bones as well.[17] The diagnosis of the conventional form of CS can frequently be made on imaging studies alone. And because the mainstay of treatment for CS is surgical excision, the biopsy step of the work-up of CS is often omitted. Also, as discussed previously, neither FNA or core biopsy can reliably distinguish a benign (enchondroma) lesion from a low-grade CS. Thus, small-biopsy techniques are largely used to confirm the cartilaginous nature of the neoplasm if the diagnosis is in question.

Aspirates of CS (and enchondromas as well) are characterized foremost by an abundance of extracellular chondroid matrix material. On air-dried and May-Grünwald-Giemsa–fixed stains, this appears as a spectacular magenta or fuscia colored film of various densities (Fig. 9A). Matrix material is less obvious on conventional alcohol-fixed preparations, usually identified as a pale gray or light blue material in the background (see Fig. 9B). Individual chondrocytes are identified both freely and in association with matrix. When present in association with matrix fragments, they are usually identified in small voids in the material, which correspond to the lacunaer spaces

identified histologically (Fig. 10A). Individual chondrocytes frequently possess slightly to modestly enlarged nuclei and are often binucleate or multinucleate. Although not a specific feature of malignancy, the presence of more-than-rare double or multinucleate chondrocytes should raise a suspicion that a low-grade CS is being sampled instead of a benign chondroma. Chondrocyte cytoplasm is usually abundant and often demonstrates small cookie cutter–like vacuoles (see Fig. 10B). Chondrocyte nuclei, best identified on fixed and conventionally stained (Papanicolaou or hematoxylin-eosin) preparations, frequently display convolutions and other nuclear irregularities that usually signify malignancy.

Cytologic Diagnosis of Chondrosarcoma

Grading of CS on cytologic material alone is a controversial practice.[38] Aside from issues arising from sampling, there has been no study to date that demonstrates the extent of reproducibility of grading that approaches that associated with complete histologic examination of a full resection specimen. Regardless, cytologic grading is probably a futile exercise because CSs are resected irrespective of grade.

Variants of CS include mesenchymal and clear cell subtypes. The cytologic features of the former have been described and illustrated in a small series of cases.[28,39] Given that mesenchymal CS is a biphasic neoplasm comprised of mature cartilage and a more primitive round cell component, it could be speculated that diagnosis by aspiration cytology or other small biopsy techniques would be difficult. Yet the combination of cartilaginous-type extracellular matrix with a small blue-cell component is a unique combination, which should suggest the correct diagnosis to an astute pathologist (Fig. 11). Cytologic descriptions of the clear cell variant of CS are restricted to single or small case reports.[28] Aspirates of dedifferentiated CS vary depending on the region sampled. Pleomorophic, spindled tumor cells characterize the dedifferentiated component whereas the conventional CS appears low grade. Difficulty in making this diagnosis on FNA is due to sampling one component and not the other.[40,41]

EWING SARCOMA

EWS represents the second most common primary neoplasm of bone after OS. The exact cell of origin for EWS is unknown but thought to be a mesenchymal stem cell capable of multilineage differentiation.[42] The majority of EWSs are characterized by a translocation involving the chromosomes 11 and 22. The EWS translocation

Fig. 9. The matrix material of CS often dominates the appearance of the aspirate. (*A*) The chondroid matrix appears thick and purple in color, a feature best seen in air-dried, Giemsa-stained preparations. (*B*) The same CS has very different appearance when the prepration is alcohol fixed and Papanicalaou stained, with a pale blue-green tint to the extracellular component.

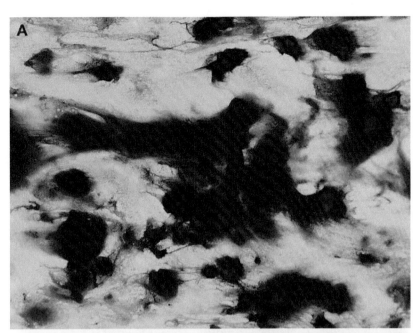

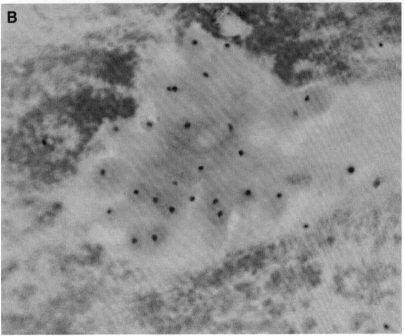

was the first ever identified in association with sarcoma and has since been demonstrated in several other neoplasms (peripheral neuroectodermal tumor, Askin tumor, desmoplastic small round-cell tumor). The presence of the translocation has led to their reclassification under an umbrella category known collectively as the EWS family of tumors.[42,43]

Histologically and cytologically, EWS tumors belong to the small, round, blue-cell group of neoplasms, which includes lymphoma/leukemia, neuroblastoma, and other neoplasms. Aspirates of EWS are usually very cellular with a dispersed population of uniform small round cells (**Fig. 12**). Individual tumor cells are usually 2 to 3 times larger than a mature lymphocyte and have a central

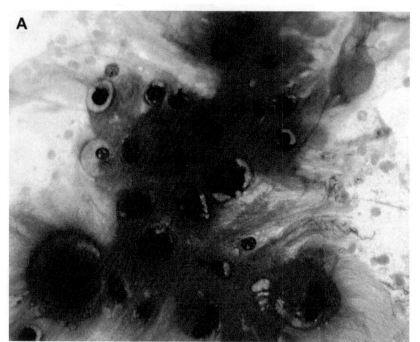

A

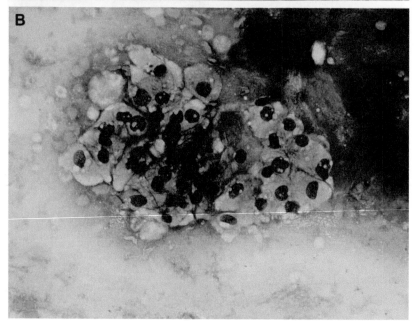

B

Fig. 10. (A) A small aggregate of fibrillar matrix material with malignant chondrocytes aspirated from a CS. In this instance there is obvious cytologic atypia of the chondrocyte nuclei. The lacunar spaces are also well preserved. (B) In this example, the chondrocyte cytoplasm is much more prominent. Note the small punched-out cookie cutter–type vacuoles.

nucleus with a small peripheral rim of cytoplasm. Nuclear chromatin is usually finely granular with small inconspicuous nucleoli. Rosettes are a feature often described in association with EWS or peripheral neuroectodermal tumor, but these are seldom demonstrable in FNA material.[24]

Cytologic Diagnosis of Ewing Sarcoma

Despite the characteristic appearance of EWS in histology or cytology, there are obstacles to a successful diagnosis.

First, EWS tumor cells are often fragile and large foci of tumor necrosis are often present. Small

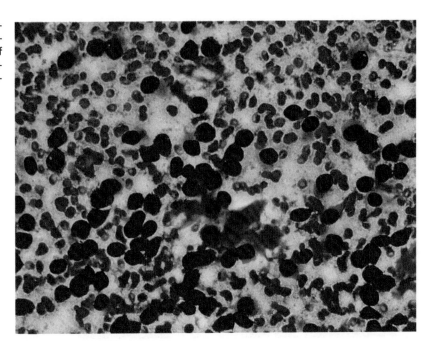

Fig. 11. Mesenchymal chondroma is characterized cytologically by the presence of extracellular chondromyxoid matrix as well as a population of small blue cells.

tissue biopsy techniques, including core biopsy and FNA, often sample only necrotic material. Nonviable cellular material is useless for the requisite ancillary studies needed to secure a diagnosis.

Second, many of the other so-called small, round, blue-cell tumors enter in the differential diagnosis of EWS and must be excluded. Although this is usually accomplished via judicious use of immunohistochemical, conventional histochemical, and flow cytometric analyses, there are still instances where the diagnosis may be problematic. Fortunately, the presence of the EWS-associated translocation can be exploited for diagnostic purposes. Cytologic preparations make excellent samples for molecular techniques (**Fig. 13**). The combination of FNA and in situ hybridization techniques are particularly well suited to each other because the combination allows for a direct visualization level of integrity to the diagnostic process.

CHORDOMA

Chordoma is a rare tumor thought to arise from the remnants of the embryonic notochord. This lesion is confined exclusively to the neuraxis with more than 50% in the midline sacral region. Although chordoma is a slow-growing lesion, it is nevertheless aggressive with a propensity for multiple recurrences and eventual metastases.[16]

Aspirates from chordoma are characterized by an abundance of extracellular matrix material.

The matrix has the same chondromyxoid appearance and staining quality as identified in smears from CS (**Fig. 14**A). In air-dried, Romanovsky-based preparations, the matrix is a striking magenta color. Extracellular matrix is less conspicuous on conventional, alcohol-fixed preparations, where it assumes a pale blue-gray to green color. Individual cells are scattered throughout the matrix material, either singly or in small loosely cohesive clusters.[24]

The histologic hallmark of chordoma is the physaliferous cell (from the Greek word for bubbles). In conventional histologic sections these bear some resemblance to lipoblasts with a clearing of the cytoplasm. This subcellular feature manifests itself differently in cytologic preparations. Here the cells are more likely to display many small vacuoles with a tendency to coalesce around the periphery of the cell cytoplasm. Individual cells tend to have large nuclei and are frequently binucleate (see **Fig. 14**B).[17]

Cytologic Diagnosis of Chordoma

Because of the characteristic anatomic location of this lesion, the cytologic diagnosis of chordoma tends to be straightforward. The main challenges to diagnosis occur when encountering variant of the usual histology. For instance, an aspirate from the chondroid variant of chordoma may be difficult to distinguish from a conventional CS. In this instance, immunohistochemical staining for

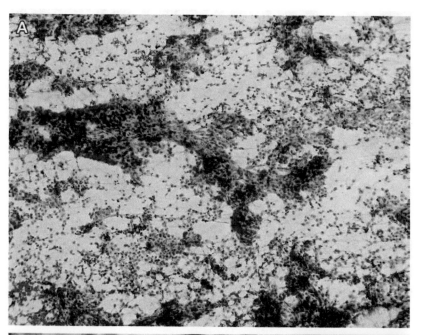

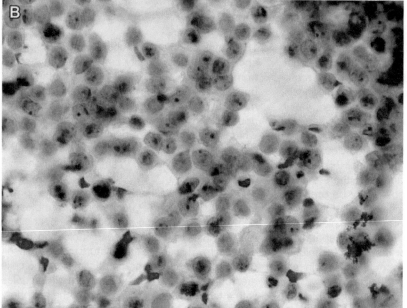

Fig. 12. (*A*) Low-power photomicrograph and (*B*) high-power photomicrograph of an aspirate of EWS. Aspirates are usually characterized by many dispersed and loosely aggregated small blue cells. Individual cells have a high nuclear to cytoplasmic ratio and often show signs of fragility, such as smearing of chromatin material. Isolated apoptotic cells are a common feature.

epithelial markers is immensely useful. Stains for keratin or epithelial membrane antigen are positive in the physaliferous cells of chordoma but negative in a CS. In addition, rare cases of chordoma dedifferentiate into a higher-grade lesion with a corresponding sarcomatous-like appearance.[44] The dedifferentiation phenomenon is unfortunately accompanied by a more aggressive clinical course as well.

HEMATOPOIETIC NEOPLASMS

PLASMACYTOMA/MYELOMA

Multiple myeloma represents a neoplastic proliferation of plasma cells that affects bone marrow and its ability to produce normal hematopoetic cells. Although almost all multiple myeloma patients have osseous lesions, a small fraction of patients

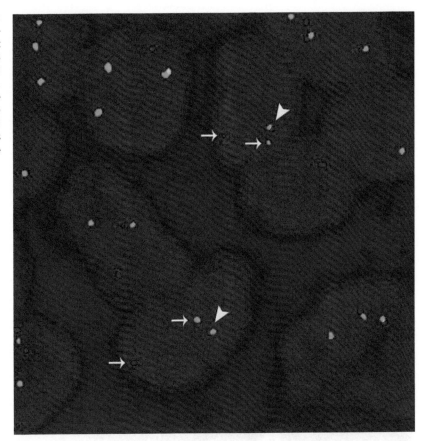

Fig. 13. Fluorescent in situ hybridization performed on a cytologic sample of EWS. The EWS translocation is identified with a break-apart probe. The presence of a single fusion signal (*arrowhead*) and two separate red and green signals (*arrows*) is indicative of the presence of a translocation.

present with a solitary bone plasmacytoma as the initial and perhaps only manifestation of disease.[45] These lesions are particularly common in the spine and patients may present with a spinal cord compression syndrome. In this scenario, FNA biopsy represents an attractive diagnostic modality becuase results are likely to be more rapid than with conventional methods of biopsy.

Cytologic Diagnosis of Plasmacytoma/Multiple Myeloma

The cytologic diagnosis of plasmacytoma/multiple myeloma is usually straightforward. Aspirates are often excessively bloody or hemorrhagic but usually yield a cellular population sufficient for diagnosis. The cells are monomorphic and dispersed. They have a typical plasma cell appearance with abundant bluish gray cytoplasm and an eccentrically placed nucleus (**Fig. 15**). Occasional mitoses and binucleate forms are often identified, a feature that can help confirm the malignant nature of the plasma cell infiltrate. In addition, cytologic specimens can be submitted

for light chain restriction analysis by either flow cytometric or immunohistochemical methods.[46,47]

LYMPHOMA

Primary lymphoma of bone is a rare lesion defined as a malignant lymphoid infiltrate of bone without concurrent involvement of lymph node or other sites. It is estimated that primary lymphoma of bone represents less than 5% of all extranodal lymphomas but probably a greater proportion of primary bone tumors (2%–7%). Symptoms are often vague with pain in the affected region with a destructive-appearing but otherwise nonspecific imaging study.[48]

The vast majority of PBLs are of the large B-cell type with rare isolated examples of follicular, anaplastic, and other subtypes.[46,48] This lesion occurs most frequently in older adults, and the clinical and radiographic differential frequently includes osseous metastases from an unknown primary. As such, these lesions are frequently subjected to FNA as an initial diagnostic modality.

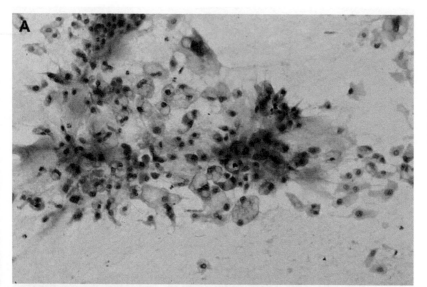

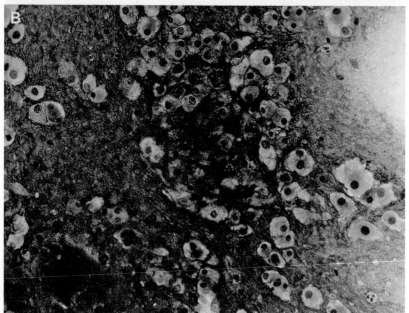

Fig. 14. The physalliferous cells of chordoma are best identified on alcohol-fixed stains. (A) The bubbly cytoplasm is apparent. A Diff-Quik, air-dried preparation (B) emphasizes the nature of the chondromyxoid matrix.

Cytologic Diagnosis of Lymphoma

Aspirates are usually modestly to markedly cellular with a dispersed population of small blue cells. In the typical PBL tumor, cells have a high nuclear-to-cytoplasmic ratio. Because the individual tumor cells are fragile, there may also be a significant smearing or crushing of cellular material resulting in wisps or strips of blue-stained nuclear material between intact tumor cells (Fig. 16). Irregular nuclear convolutions and irregular nucleoli are also frequent findings.[24] Tumor necrosis can be a major obstacle to obtaining a diagnosis via FNA. Viable cells are needed for ancillary studies, in particular immunophenotyping. Demonstration of a monoclonal lymphoid population can be done reliably with either immunohistochemical or flow cytometric analysis but the latter requires some foresight on part of the aspiration cytopathologist's part because this material needs to be submitted specifically to a flow cytometry laboratory for processing.

Fig. 15. A population of single round cells with eccentrically placed nuclei is characteristic of plasmacytoma.

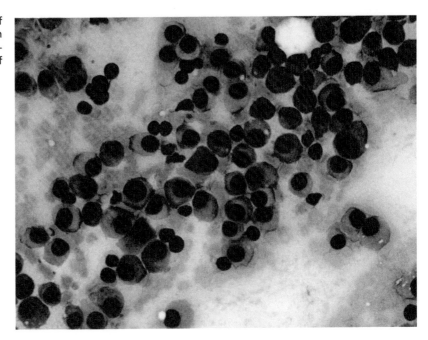

METASTATIC DISEASE

After the lung and liver, bone is the third most common site of metastatic disease. It is well known that involvement by metastatic disease is by far more common than any primary bone lesion.[49] FNA has been shown to be an excellent and highly accurate technique to assess for metastatic disease.[50–52] The most common sites of involvement include the axial skeleton, appendicular skeleton, and craniofacial region, in decreasing order of frequency. Patients typically present with pain, pathologic fracture, neuromuscular disturbances, and/or hematopoietic marrow dysfunction. In the

Fig. 16. Aspirate of lymphoma showing a dispersed population of monomorphic single cells.

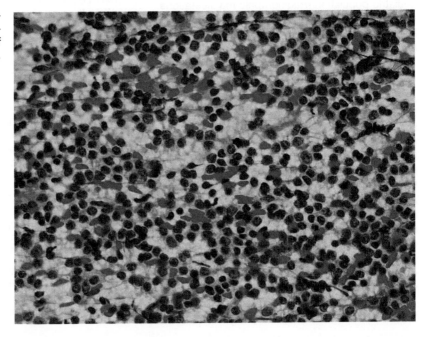

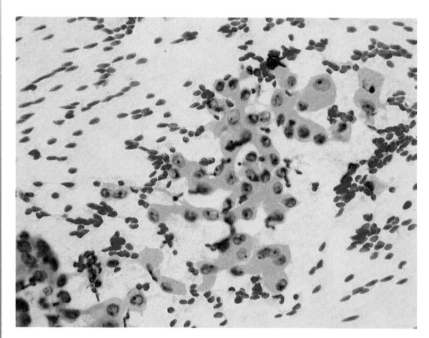

Fig. 17. In this FNA sample from a metastatic lung carcinoma, the tumor cells are loosely cohesive, suggesting a glandular configuration. They have obvious nuclear contour irregularities and small but prominent nucleoli.

adult population, the most frequently encountered metastatic malignancies include breast, lung, prostate, kidney, thyroid, and gastrointestinal tract carcinomas and melanomas.[50,51] Neuroblastoma, rhabdomyosarcoma, and retinoblastoma are most common secondary malignancies found within the pediatric population. Radiographic manifestations can be variable; however, most commonly these lesions have an aggressive, destructive, and lytic (or, less commonly, sclerotic) appearance.[17]

Cytologic Diagnosis of Metastatic Disease

Aspiration smears of metastatic carcinomas tend to be cellular and characterized by groups of cohesive tumor cells. Adenocarcinomas are by far the most common type of metastatic tumors to bone.[51] In smears, the epithelioid nature of the neoplasm is usually obvious. Individual cells often have abundant cytoplasm and nuclear features associated with malignancy. Classic cytologic indicators of malignancy include increased nuclear-to-cytoplasmic ratio, nuclear membrane irregularities, coarse chromatin, and/or prominent nucleoli (**Fig. 17**). The presence of keratinization (tadpole or strap cells), best depicted on Papanicolaou staining, is indicative of squamous cell carcinoma.

Other tumors also frequently metastasize to bone and are commonly subject to aspiration

Pitfalls
CYTOLOGIC DIAGNOSIS
OF BONE TUMORS

! The sampling and subsequent distinction between osteoid and chondroid matrix is difficult on cytologic preperations.

! Some benign chondroid lesions, in particular chondromyxoid fibroma and chondroblastoma, may have subtle cytologic atypia of the chondrocytes. This should not be overinterpreted as a sign of malignancy.

! The brown tumor of hyperparathyroidism appears cytologically identical to GCTB. When a giant cell tumor appears in an unusual location or has an atypical appearance on imaging, the possibility of hyperparathyroidism-associated brown tumor should be considered.

! The chondroblastic variant of OS appears similar to CS on FNA. Patient age, lesion location, and imaging appearance should always be considered when rendering a diagnosis of a chondroid lesion in a young patient.

! Osteoblasts frequently appear plasmacytoid in cytologic preparations. It is easy to misidentify a plasmacytoid cell, particularly when they are few in number.

cytology for confirmation of diagnosis. Some tumors, namely colorectal, prostate, and kidney, have distinctive cytologic features and usually do not represent much of a diagnostic challenge. Neuroendocrine neoplasms tend to be composed of a bland, uniform cell population and can often be difficult to separate from lymphoid lesions. The presence of nuclear molding and many apoptotic bodies should arouse suspicion of a small cell type of carcinoma, such as that classically associated with lung origin. Cytologic samples from metastatic melanoma tend to be composed of large, epithelioid to polygonal cells with abundant cytoplasm and prominent nucleoli. Although rare, the presence of intracytoplasmic pigment and/or nuclear pseudoinclusions is supportive. If available, the use of immunohistochemical stains on paraffin-embedded cellblocks is a powerful tool that may provide additional information regarding cell lineage and site of tumor origin.[17,24]

REFERENCES

1. Layfield LJ, Dodd LG, Hirschowitz S, et al. Fine-needle aspiration of primary osseous lesions: a cost effectiveness study. Diagn Cytopathol 2010;38:239–43.

2. Ward WG, Savage P, Boles CA, et al. Fine-needle aspiration biopsy of sarcomas and related tumors. Cancer Control 2001;8:232–8.

3. Ruhs SA, el-Khoury GY, Chrischilles EA. A cost minimization approach to the diagnosis of skeletal neoplasms. Skeletal Radiol 1996;25:449–54.

4. Kreicbergs A, Bauer HC, Brosjo O, et al. Cytological diagnosis of bone tumours. J Bone Joint Surg Br 1996;78:258–63.

5. Ward WG Sr, Kilpatrick S. Fine needle aspiration biopsy of primary bone tumors. Clin Orthop Relat Res 2000;373:80–7.

6. Coley BL, Sharp GS, Ellis EB. Diagnosis of bone tumors by aspiration. Am J Surg 1931;13:215–24.

7. Lalli AF. Roentgen-guided aspiration biopsies of skeletal lesions. J Can Assoc Radiol 1970;21:71–3.

8. Khalbuss WE, Teot LA, Monaco SE. Diagnostic accuracy and limitations of fine-needle aspiration cytology of bone and soft tissue lesions: a review of 1114 cases with cytological-histological correlation. Cancer Cytopathol 2010;118:24–32.

9. Yamamoto T, Nagira K, Marui T, et al. Fine-needle aspiration biopsy in the initial diagnosis of bone lesions. Anticancer Res 2003;23:793–7.

10. Layfield LJ. Cytologic diagnosis of osseous lesions: a review with emphasis on the diagnosis of primary neoplasms of bone. Diagn Cytopathol 2009;37:299–310.

11. El-Khoury GY, Terepka RH, Mickelson MR, et al. Fine-needle aspiration biopsy of bone. J Bone Joint Surg Am 1983;65:522–5.

12. Layfield LJ, Armstrong K, Zaleski S, et al. Diagnostic accuracy and clinical utility of fine-needle aspiration cytology in the diagnosis of clinically primary bone lesions. Diagn Cytopathol 1993;9:168–73.

13. Dollahite HA, Tatum L, Moinuddin SM, et al. Aspiration biopsy of primary neoplasms of bone. J Bone Joint Surg Am 1989;71:1166–9.

14. Wedin R, Bauer HC, Skoog L, et al. Cytological diagnosis of skeletal lesions. Fine-needle aspiration biopsy in 110 tumours. J Bone Joint Surg Br 2000;82:673–8.

15. Huening MA, Reddy S, Dodd LG. Fine-needle aspiration of fibrous dysplasia of bone: a worthwhile endeavor or not? Diagn Cytopathol 2008;36:325–30.

16. Bullough PG. Orthopaedic pathology. Philadelphia: Mosby/Elsevier; 2009.

17. Kilpatrick SE, Renner JB. Diagnostic musculoskeletal surgical pathology: clinicoradiologic and cytologic correlations. Philadelphia: Elsevier, Inc; 2004. p. 393.

18. White LM, Schweitzer ME, Deely DM, et al. Study of osteomyelitis: utility of combined histologic and microbiologic evaluation of percutaneous biopsy samples. Radiology 1995;197:840–2.

19. Lupovitch A, Elie JC, Wysocki R. Diagnosis of acute bacterial osteomyelitis of the pubis by means of fine needle aspiration. Acta Cytol 1989;33:649–51.

20. Kilpatrick SE. Fine needle aspiration biopsy of Langerhans cell histiocytosis of bone: are ancillary studies necessary for a "definitive diagnosis"? Acta Cytol 1998;42:820–3.

21. Pohar-Marinsek Z, Us-Krasovec M. Cytomorphology of Langerhans cell histiocytosis. Acta Cytol 1996;40: 1257–64.

22. Akerman M, Domanski HA, Jonsson K. Fine needle aspiration of bone tumours: the clinical, radiological, cytological approach. In: Orell SR, editor. Basel (Switzerland): Karger; 2010. p. 91.

23. Kilpatrick SE, Pike EJ, Geisinger KR, et al. Chondroblastoma of bone: use of fine-needle aspiration biopsy and potential diagnostic pitfalls. Diagn Cytopathol 1997;16:65–71.

24. Layfield LJ. Cytopathology of bone and soft tissue tumors. New York: Oxford University Press, Inc; 2002. p. 266.

25. Fanning CV, Sneige NS, Carrasco CH, et al. Fine needle aspiration cytology of chondroblastoma of bone. Cancer 1990;65:1847–63.

26. Jain M, Kaur M, Kapoor S, et al. Cytological features of chondroblastoma: a case report with review of the literature. Diagn Cytopathol 2000;23:348–50.

27. Bergman S, Madden CR, Geisinger KR. Fine-needle aspiration biopsy of chondromyxoid fibroma: an investigation of four cases. Am J Clin Pathol 2009; 132:740–5.

28. Walaas L, Kindblom LG, Gunterberg B, et al. Light and electron microscopic examination of fine-needle aspirates in the preoperative diagnosis of

cartilaginous tumors. Diagn Cytopathol 1990;6: 396–408.

29. Anract P, De Pinieux G, Cottias P, et al. Malignant giant-cell tumours of bone. Clinico-pathological types and prognosis: a review of 29 cases. Int Orthop 1998;22:19–26.

30. Campanacci M, Baldini N, Boriani S, et al. Giant-cell tumor of bone. J Bone Joint Surg Am 1987;69:106–14.

31. Kilpatrick SE, Ward WG, Bos GD, et al. The role of fine needle aspiration biopsy in the diagnosis and management of osteosarcoma. Pediatr Pathol Mol Med 2001;20:175–87.

32. Nicol KK, Ward WG, Savage PD, et al. Fine-needle aspiration biopsy of skeletal versus extraskeletal osteosarcoma. Cancer 1998;84:176–85.

33. White VA, Fanning CV, Ayala AG, et al. Osteosarcoma and the role of fine-needle aspiration. A study of 51 cases. Cancer 1988;62:1238–46.

34. Dodd LG, Scully SP, Cothran RL, et al. Utility of fine-needle aspiration in the diagnosis of primary osteosarcoma. Diagn Cytopathol 2002;27:350–3.

35. Klijanienko J, Caillaud JM, Orbach D, et al. Cyto-histological correlations in primary, recurrent, and metastatic bone and soft tissue osteosarcoma. Institut Curie's experience. Diagn Cytopathol 2007;35: 270–5.

36. Domanski HA, Akerman M. Fine-needle aspiration of primary osteosarcoma: a cytological-histological study. Diagn Cytopathol 2005;32:269–75.

37. Dodd LG. Fine-needle aspiration of chondrosarcoma. Diagn Cytopathol 2006;34:413–8.

38. Lerma E, Tani E, Brosjo O, et al. Diagnosis and grading of chondrosarcomas on FNA biopsy material. Diagn Cytopathol 2003;28:13–7.

39. Trembath DG, Dash R, Major NM, et al. Cytopathology of mesenchymal chondrosarcomas: a report and comparison of four patients. Cancer 2003;99:211–6.

40. Estrada-Villasenor E, Rico-Martinez G, Linares-Gonzalez LM. Diagnosis of a dedifferentiated chondrosarcoma of the pelvis by fine needle aspiration. A case report. Acta Cytol 2010;54:217–20.

41. Rinas AC, Ward WG, Kilpatrick SE. Potential sampling error in fine needle aspiration biopsy of dedifferentiated chondrosarcoma: a report of 4 cases. Acta Cytol 2005;49:554–9.

42. Ludwig JA. Ewing sarcoma: historical perspectives, current state-of-the-art, and opportunities for targeted therapy in the future. Curr Opin Oncol 2008; 20:412–8.

43. Sanati S, Lu DW, Schmidt E, et al. Cytologic diagnosis of Ewing sarcoma/peripheral neuroectodermal tumor with paired prospective molecular genetic analysis. Cancer 2007;111:192–9.

44. Layfield LJ, Liu K, Dodd LG, et al. "Dedifferentiated" chordoma: a case report of the cytomorphologic findings on fine-needle aspiration. Diagn Cytopathol 1998;19:378–81.

45. Dimopoulos MA, Moulopoulos LA, Maniatis A, et al. Solitary plasmacytoma of bone and asymptomatic multiple myeloma. Blood 2000;96:2037–44.

46. Silverman JF, McLeod DL, Park HK. Fine-needle aspiration cytology of hematopoietic lesions from multiple sites. Diagn Cytopathol 1990;6:252–7.

47. Soderlund V, Tani E, Skoog L, et al. Diagnosis of skeletal lymphoma and myeloma by radiology and fine needle aspiration cytology. Cytopathology 2001;12:157–67.

48. Bhagavathi S, Micale MA, Les K, et al. Primary bone diffuse large B-cell lymphoma: clinicopathologic study of 21 cases and review of literature. Am J Surg Pathol 2009;33:1463–9.

49. Mundy GR. Mechanisms of bone metastasis. Cancer 1997;80:1546–56.

50. Treaba D, Assad L, Govil H, et al. Diagnostic role of fine-needle aspiration of bone lesions in patients with a previous history of malignancy. Diagn Cytopathol 2002;26:380–3.

51. Bommer KK, Ramzy I, Mody D. Fine-needle aspiration biopsy in the diagnosis and management of bone lesions: a study of 450 cases. Cancer 1997; 81:148–56.

52. Mehrotra R, Singh M, Singh PA, et al. Should fine needle aspiration biopsy be the first pathological investigation in the diagnosis of a bone lesion? An algorithmic approach with review of literature. Cytojournal 2007;4:9.

BENIGN BONE-FORMING TUMORS: APPROACH TO DIAGNOSIS AND CURRENT UNDERSTANDING OF PATHOGENESIS

Shefali Bhusnurmath, MD, Benjamin Hoch, MD*

KEYWORDS

• Osteoma • Osteoid osteoma • Osteoblastoma • Osteosarcoma

ABSTRACT

The diagnosis of benign bone-forming tumors continues to be based on the traditional approach to bone tumor diagnosis using knowledge of the spectrum of histopathologic features seen in these tumors in combination with clinical and radiological correlation. This review emphasizes the pathologic features and the clinical and radiological features that the surgical pathologist must have a working understanding of to make an accurate diagnosis and avoid confusion with other lesions, particularly osteosarcomas. New and persistent challenges facing the practicing pathologist and our current understanding of the cytogenetic and molecular abnormalities involved in the pathogenesis of these tumors are discussed.

OVERVIEW

It has been imperative that the practicing surgical pathologist has knowledge no only of the histopathologic features of a bone tumor, but also of the clinical presentation and imaging features in order to arrive at a correct diagnosis. The diagnosis of osteoma, osteoid osteoma, and osteoblastoma continues to be based on this approach. As such, this review focuses on the clinical, radiological, and pathologic features that surgical pathologists must have working knowledge of to accurately classify these tumors as part of

Key Points
BONE-FORMING TUMORS

• The diagnosis of benign bone-forming tumors continues to be based on the knowledge of the spectrum of histopathologic features in combination with clinical and radiological correlation.

• Distinguishing osteoblastomas from osteosarcomas, recognizing pseudosarcomatous change in an osteoblastoma, and working with limited tissue in trying to diagnose osteoid osteomas are still the greatest challenges for the pathologist.

• There is limited understanding of the cytogenetic and molecular abnormalities that result in the pathogenesis of benign bone tumors and that could be used for ancillary diagnostic studies.

Department of Pathology, University of Washington, 1959 NE Pacific Street, Box 356100, Room NE110, Seattle, WA 98195, USA
* Corresponding author.
E-mail address: bhoch@u.washington.edu

Surgical Pathology 5 (2012) 101–116
doi:10.1016/j.path.2011.07.010
1875-9181/12/$ – see front matter © 2012 Elsevier Inc. All rights reserved.

a multidisciplinary approach. In addition, the authors comment on challenges and practical issues pertaining to making a diagnosis and highlight new developments in the management of these neoplasms that impact the practicing pathologist. The authors also discuss the current understanding of the molecular and cytogenetic abnormalities that pertain to the pathogenesis of these neoplasms and that may one day serve as ancillary diagnostic tools.

OSTEOMAS

Skeletal osteomas are benign tumors composed of dense cortical bone that arise on the surface of bones. They generally can be placed into 2 major categories: (1) sinonasal/skull osteoma and (2) long bone osteoma (parosteal osteoma). The exact incidence of osteomas is uncertain because most cases are incidentally discovered.[1] The incidence of sinonasal osteomas has been reported to be 3% in patients undergoing computerized tomography (CT) imaging for sinonasal symptoms.[2] Long bone osteomas are exceedingly rare.[3]

LOCATION OF OSTEOMAS

Sinonasal/skull osteomas usually arise on the surfaces of the cranial vault, jaw, and orbit, or within the paranasal sinuses where they most frequently involve the frontal sinus.[1,4] Up to 86% of long bone osteomas arise in the lower extremity but may also

affect the humerus and vertebral column.[3,5] Osteomas are typically isolated lesions, but multiple osteomas can be a manifestation of Gardner syndrome.[2,4,6]

CLINICAL FEATURES OF OSTEOMAS

Osteomas affect all age groups, but are most commonly diagnosed in adults around the fourth and fifth decade of life.[4] The male-to-female ratio has been reported to range from 1.7 to 2.6: 1.0 for sinonasal osteomas.[2] There is not a definite sex predilection of long bone osteomas.[3,5] They are often asymptomatic; but if they are larger and situated in a vital location, osteomas can cause sinusitis, visual disturbances, spinal cord compression, otitis media, and headaches.[4,7,8] Osteomas of the pelvic bones and long bones often present with pain.[3,9]

RADIOLOGICAL FEATURES OF OSTEOMAS

On plain films or CT imaging, an osteoma appears as a round to lobular, homogeneous radiodensity with a smooth contour on the cortical surface usually measuring less than 3 cm with no involvement of the underlying bone (Fig. 1).[1,3] In the sinonasal region, osteomas tend to form polypoid intracavitary growths. Some sinonasal osteomas may have central areas of radiolucency that correlate with microscopic features indistinguishable from osteoblastomas.[10] In long bone, it can be

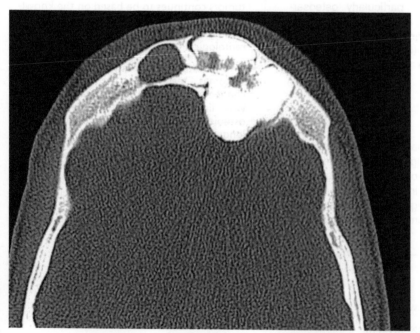

Fig. 1. CT of an osteoma of the frontal sinus demonstrates characteristic homogeneous density of cortical bone, smooth contour, intracavitary growth, and no involvement of the underlying bone. The central areas of lucency correspond to cancellous bone or osteoblastoma-like areas within the tumor.

difficult to distinguish osteomas from parosteal osteosarcomas by imaging studies.

GROSS PATHOLOGY OF OSTEOMAS

Grossly, osteomas are round or oval, tan-white, bosselated masses that are attached to the underlying bone by a broad base or a small stalk. They are most often composed of compact, white-tan cortical bone. Sinonasal osteomas can have variable amounts of compact and cancellous bone, and cases with osteoblastoma-like features have dense cortical bone surrounding areas of red-brown soft bone.

MICROSCOPIC PATHOLOGY OF OSTEOMAS

Histologically, osteomas are composed of sheets of cortical bone that blend with the underlying cortex (Fig. 2). The cortical bone is usually made up of lamellar bone, but many woven bone can be seen in more actively growing lesions. The osseous surfaces show minimal osteoblastic or osteoclastic activity, and the osteocytes are small and inconspicuous. Osteoblastoma-like areas seen in sinonasal osteomas consist of interanastomosing trabeculae of woven bone rimmed by osteoblasts and occasional osteoclasts associated with a loose fibrovascular stroma (Fig. 3).

DIFFERENTIAL DIAGNOSIS OF OSTEOMAS

Based on histopathology alone, the differential diagnosis of an osteoma may include normal cortical bone, osteoblastoma, low-grade parosteal osteosarcoma, and other surface lesions with a component of cortical bone formation, such as an osteochondroma or reactive hyperostosis secondary to an adjacent tumor. The cortical bone of an osteoma is thicker than normal cortex and usually has increased numbers of Haversian canals with greater size variation. Distinguishing an osteoblastoma in the craniofacial region from a sinonasal osteoma with osteoblastoma-like areas can be difficult. The latter areas are very similar to an osteoblastoma, but an osteoma usually has a large component of cortical bone not seen in an osteoblastoma. An osteochondroma may lose its cartilage cap in adulthood and look like fragments of cortical and cancellous bone on microscopic examination, leading one to consider an osteoma in the differential diagnosis. The spongiosa of an osteochondroma frequently contains remnants of calcified cartilage deposited during the growth phase of the lesion, a finding not present in an osteoma. Radiological correlation should also allow for proper classification by identifying continuity between the osteochondroma and the underlying host bone.[11] Hyperostosis of bone as seen adjacent to neoplasms, such as meningioma, can be distinguished from an osteoma by more active remodeling of the

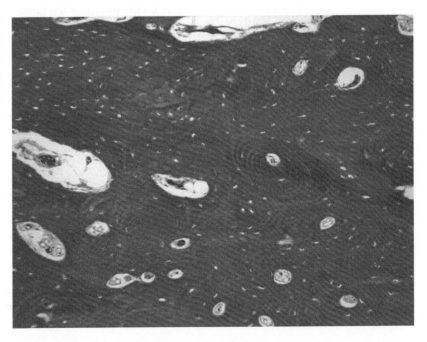

Fig. 2. Histologically, osteomas are generally consist mostly of lamellar cortical bone. The Haversian canals may be more numerous compared with normal cortex and can vary more in size.

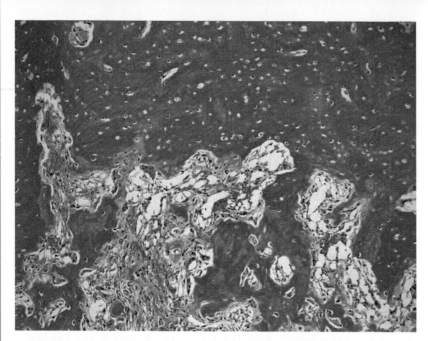

Fig. 3. Active osteomas can have abundant woven cortical bone (*top*). Osteoblastoma-like areas are occasionally seen in sinonasal osteomas (*bottom*).

Differential Diagnosis
BONE-FORMING TUMORS

Tumor	Compared with	Helpful Distinguishing Features
Osteoma	Osteoblastoma	• Osteoma contains large component of cortical bone not seen in osteoblastoma • Osteoblastoma is very rare in the paranasal sinuses, nasal cavity, and orbit where osteoma commonly arises
	Osteochondroma	Osteochondroma contains remnants of calcified cartilage not present in osteoma
	Low-grade parosteal osteosarcoma	Osteosarcoma contains a proliferating fibroblastic spindle cell component between bone trabeculae, within Haversian canals, or on the surface of the tumor not present in osteoma
Osteoid Osteoma	Osteoblastoma	*Osteoblastoma has:* • generally increased cellularity • larger size • lack of marked reactive sclerosis
	Osteosarcoma	*Osteosarcoma:* • is larger than osteoid osteoma • demonstrates cytologic atypia combined with mitotic activity • has infiltrative growth pattern with entrapment of host cancellous bone
Osteoblastoma	Osteoid osteoma	*Osteoid osteoma has* • Smaller size • More commonly affects long bones, particularly in the lower extremity • Has zone of reactive sclerosis around a nidus
	Osteoma	• Has predilection for the sinonasal bones • Mostly composed of cortical bone
	Osteosarcoma	• Has infiltrative growth pattern with entrapment of host cancellous bone • Demonstrated cytological atypia combined with mitotic activity (may be lacking in osteoblastoma-like osteosarcoma)

hyperostotic bone, lack of the very dense cortical bone of an osteoma, and clinicoradiological correlation. Finally, the most clinically relevant lesion in the differential diagnosis is a low-grade parosteal osteosarcoma. A parosteal osteoma is much less common than a parosteal osteosarcoma, but the two tumors may be impossible to differentiate from each other radiographically and on gross examination. Furthermore, a small minority of parosteal osteosarcomas are histologically composed of a predominance of cortical bone virtually identical to an osteoma. Parosteal osteosarcoma is diagnosed by recognizing a proliferating fibroblastic spindle cell component between the bone trabeculae, within Haversian canals, or on the surface of the tumor.

DISCUSSION OF OSTEOMAS

Practically speaking, the diagnosis of an osteoma of the sinonasal region is generally not problematic when the histopathologic findings can be correlated with imaging studies. However, in routine practice, this is often not the case. In such circumstances, a descriptive diagnosis of "dense cortical bone consistent with sinonasal osteoma in the appropriate clinical and radiological setting" is probably sufficient. In contrast, one must be very careful in entertaining a diagnosis of a parosteal osteoma given the difficulty in distinguishing it from a parosteal osteosarcoma. These lesions need to be extensively sampled (resection specimen) to rule out the possibility of a parosteal osteosarcoma.

The pathogenesis of an osteoma is still uncertain and speculative. Historically, developmental, traumatic, and an infectious causes have been put forth for osteomas of the sinonasal region.[2,12] Given the benign nature of osteomas, there has not been an intensive effort to elucidate its molecular pathogenesis. The association of osteomas as a part of Gardner syndrome suggests a link to abnormalities of the APC gene and related molecular pathways.[13] Rare examples of familial osteomas unrelated to Gardner syndrome have been reported, suggesting the existence of a dominantly inherited predisposition to osteoma formation.[14] In addition, RFB retrovirus has been associated with the induction of osteomas.[12] However, there is no specific molecular abnormality known to cause most sporadic osteomas.

OSTEOID OSTEOMAS

Osteoid osteoma is a benign osteogenic tumor of small size (usually <1 cm) that accounts for approximately 13.5% of benign bone tumors and 2% to 3% of all primary bone tumors.[6,15,16] It usually occurs in the cortex of long bones and causes characteristic nocturnal pain that is relieved by non–steroidal antiinflammatory drugs (NSAIDs). Lesions consist of a central neoplastic proliferation of bone-forming osteoblastic cells, termed the nidus, which is surrounded by a wide zone of reactive sclerotic host bone. When an osteoid osteoma develops within cancellous bone, there may only be a thin rim of reactive sclerosis. Infrequent cases with more than one nidus have been reported; however, multiple osteoid osteomas in separated bones are exceedingly rare.[6,17–19]

LOCATION OF OSTEOID OSTEOMAS

More than half of the cases occur in the long bones of the lower extremity, with the proximal femur being the most common location.[20] In long bone, the lesion is usually diaphyseal or metadiaphyseal and arises in the cortex. A minority are intramedullary. A total of 10% to 25% of the cases occur in the spine, with a predilection for the posterior vertebral elements.[21,22] Epiphyseal and intraarticular tumors are rare.[16,23,24] Despite the predilection for the lower extremity, any bone may be affected.[6,24–29]

CLINICAL FEATURES OF OSTEOID OSTEOMAS

Patients with osteoid osteomas are young, with most patients aged 10 to 30 years. Males are more frequently affected than females. Up to 80% of cases present with the pathognomonic symptom of nocturnally aggravated pain that responds to NSAIDs.[28,30,31] In fact, the tumor has been shown to express high levels of prostaglandins that are presumed to be the cause of pain. Cyclooxygenase 2 (a target of NSAIDs) has been implicated as one of the mediators of the increased production of prostaglandins.[32] Less than 2% of patients present with no pain.[33] Spinal lesions may cause painful scoliosis.[21] Synovitis may occur if located within a joint.[27]

RADIOGRAPHIC FEATURES OF OSTEOID OSTEOMAS

On plain radiographs, the nidus is a small (1 cm or less) oval or round radiolucent area surrounded by dense cortical bone or periosteal reaction (Fig. 4). The amount of reactive bone may vary from minimal, particularly with intramedullary and intraarticular lesions, to extensive sclerosis. The nidus is demonstrated in up to 85% of the cases.[34] CT is the ideal imaging modality for delineating a small nidus or when intense reactive sclerosis may

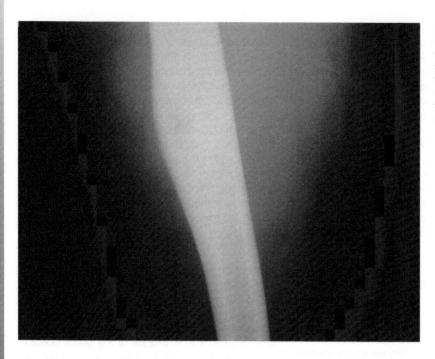

Fig. 4. Typical radiographic appearance of an osteoid osteoma of the femur consisting of a region of cortical thickening (sclerosis) in the diaphysis with a small central area of lucency (the nidus).

obscure the lesion.[16,35] Magnetic resonance imaging with gadolinium enhancement may also be used to help localize the nidus.[36]

GROSS PATHOLOGY OF OSTEOID OSTEOMAS

An osteoid osteoma looks like a round or oval focus of red to pink (when fresh) to brown (when fixed) granular bone sharply demarcated from the surrounding thickened cortical bone. The color of the nidus is related to its vascularity. A specimen radiograph should be performed if the nidus cannot be grossly identified. Today, with radiofrequency ablation being the mainstay of treatment, such intact gross specimens are rare.

MICROSCOPIC PATHOLOGY OF OSTEOID OSTEOMAS

Histologically, the nidus is a well-circumscribed focus of haphazardly intersecting trabeculae of variably mineralized woven bone that are rimmed by benign osteoblasts and scattered osteoclasts (**Fig. 5**). The trabeculae are generally short and thin, but can be broad and sclerotic. Osteoblasts lining trabeculae are of uniform size and shape with eccentric amphophilic cytoplasm and the nuclei have open chromatin and small nucleoli. Scattered enlarged osteoblasts may be seen, but nuclear pleomorphism and high mitotic activity are not present. The intertrabecular space is filled by loose fibrous tissue that contains slightly dilated

capillaries. The surrounding reactive bone is consists of dense cortical or trabecular bone exhibiting variable amounts of woven and lamellar bone and evidence of osteoblastic-osteoclastic remodeling (**Fig. 6**). The synovitis associated with intraarticular tumors can have lymphoplasmacytic inflammation with lymphoid aggregates reminiscent of rheumatoid arthritis.

DIFFERENTIAL DIAGNOSIS OF OSTEOID OSTEOMAS

Other lesions to be considered in the differential diagnosis based on the radiographic features and/or histopathology, or both include stress fracture, Brodie abscess, osteoblastoma, and osteosarcoma. Stress fracture seem similar to an osteoid osteoma on imaging studies.[11,37] Histologically, stress fracture show extensively remodeled cortical bone with associated woven bone formation, or if a frank fracture has occurred, there will be overt fracture callus. Reactive bone in stress fracture lacks the small irregular trabeculae of osteoid osteomas. A Brodie abscess (osteomyelitis) is also commonly considered in the clinical and radiographic differential diagnosis of an osteoid osteoma. Microscopically, the two lesions lack any similarity, but the peripheral sclerotic rim surrounding a Brodie abscess may be indistinguishable from the reactive zone of an osteoid osteoma.

Fig. 5. The nidus of osteoid osteoma is generally composed of short, thin, haphazardly intersecting bone trabeculae with variable mineralization. Some areas may have thicker trabeculae (*left*). Osteoblastic cells are uniform in size and shape and accompanied by scattered osteoclasts (*center*).

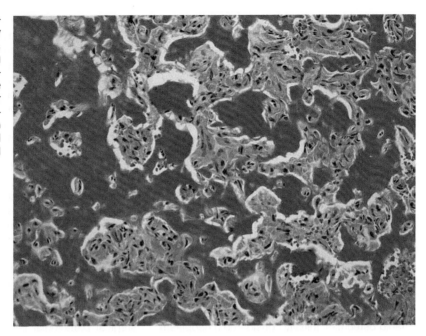

Osteoblastoma is most often considered in the differential diagnosis because the microscopic appearance of an osteoid osteoma and an osteoblastoma can be indistinguishable. An osteoblastoma differs by virtue of its generally increased cellularity, larger size, and lack of marked reactive sclerosis. More subtle distinguishing histologic features include broader, less tightly woven, and longer bone trabeculae and greater vascularity. Mitoses may be more frequent. Immunohistochemical stains for neurofilament and S-100 protein can readily identify nerve fibers within osteoid osteomas, whereas osteoblastomas lack these structures.[4] Clinically, osteoblastomas preferentially involve the axial skeleton and usually do not exhibit the characteristic pattern of nocturnal

Fig. 6. Reactive bone surrounding the nidus of osteoid osteoma is consists of thickened cortical bone (*top*) or trabecular bone (*bottom*) with a reactive fibrous stroma and evidence of remodeling, including osteoblastic and osteoclastic activity, increased amounts of woven bone, and irregular cement lines.

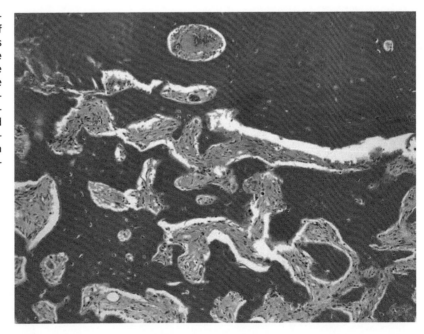

pain. Lesions should be classified as an osteoid osteoma or osteoblastoma depending on the overall clinical, radiological, and histopathologic features. In borderline cases, an arbitrary size cutoff of 1.5 cm has historically been used.

An osteosarcoma must always be considered in the differential diagnosis of a bone-forming tumor. In general, an osteosarcoma is larger, demonstrates cytologic atypia combined with mitotic activity, and has an infiltrative growth pattern with the entrapment of host cancellous bone.

DISCUSSION OF OSTEOID OSTEOMAS

Osteoid osteoma was first described as a distinct entity by Jaffe[38] in a report of 5 cases published in 1935. In 2 subsequent reports by Jaffe published in 1940 and 1945, respectively, 57 more cases were recorded, establishing this tumor in the lexicon of surgical pathology.[39,40] Historically, there has been debate over the precise nature of osteoid osteomas. Initially considered a neoplasm by Jaffe, other investigators have proposed a reactive or reparative process citing its limited growth potential and the ability to spontaneously regress in some cases.[38,39,41–43] Today, most pathologists accept the initial assertion that this tumor is a neoplasm. Cytogenetic studies have been performed on only a few cases and have found clonal cytogenetic abnormalities, including alterations involving chromosome 22q, a region containing genes involved in cell proliferation that is commonly affected in a variety of other neoplasms.[44,45]

Given the histopathologic similarities between osteoid osteoma and osteoblastoma, there has been a long-standing debate over the relationship between these two entities. Such debate has been fueled by rare cases of an osteoid osteoma transforming into an osteoblastoma.[46] In simplest terms, an osteoid osteoma is a small tumor with limited growth potential and a characteristic clinical presentation that usually affects long bones of the lower extremity. In contrast, an osteoblastoma has unlimited growth potential, subtle histopathologic differences, a nonspecific clinical presentation, and a predilection for the axial skeleton. To date, there has been no evidence of a molecular link between these two neoplasms.[45]

The treatment of osteoid osteomas aims at the removal or destruction of the nidus. Traditionally, an en bloc resection would be performed. Current treatment consists of less-invasive techniques, such as radiofrequency ablation.[47–49] The significance of minimally invasive procedures to the surgical pathologist lies in the scant amount of tissue available for microscopic examination. Inconclusive pathologic findings may occur in up to 67.5% of cases whereby the clinical and radiological findings are thought to be typical of an osteoid osteoma.[47] This rate is mostly explained by the lack of sampling of the nidus. Higher rates of a positive diagnosis are obtained with larger needles.[49] If the nidus is sampled, even when the biopsy material is rather limited, one can make the diagnosis or at least suggest it in the appropriate radiological context (Fig. 7). The most

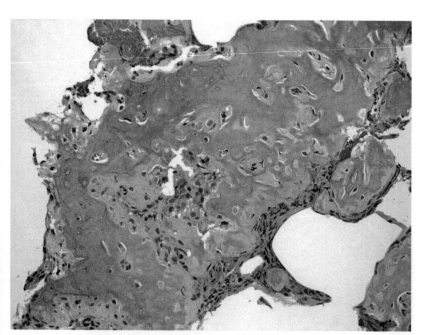

Fig. 7. Limited needle biopsy sampling of osteoid osteoma with radiofrequency ablation can be a diagnostic challenge. Here fragments of irregular bone trabeculae associated with clusters of benign osteoblasts supports the diagnosis.

common lesion presumed to be an osteoid osteoma and treated as such is a Brodie abscess followed by a chondroblastoma, eosinophilic granuloma, and fibrous dysplasia.[47] Although the need for preablation needle biopsy is a subject of debate, it is generally advised to establish a pathologic diagnosis. As such, the practicing pathologist will continue to struggle with limited material in the diagnosis of an osteoid osteoma.

OSTEOBLASTOMAS

An osteoblastoma is a benign neoplasm that accounts for 1% of primary bone tumors and 3% of all benign bone tumors and histologically resembles the nidus of an osteoid osteoma, but usually lacks reactive sclerosis. It is further characterized by having greater growth potential (>2 cm) and risk for local recurrence (10%–20%).[1,28,50] Clinically, an osteoblastoma has a different skeletal distribution and commonly lacks the nocturnal pain of an osteoid osteoma. An osteoblastoma may be indolent or locally aggressive, even resulting in the demise of patients on rare occasions. Such biologic behavior has resulted in the introduction of terms, such as *aggressive osteoblastoma* and *malignant osteoblastoma*. The spectrum of what constitutes an osteoblastoma is further broadened by the documentation of other subtypes, including *multifocal osteoblastoma*, *pseudomalignant osteoblastoma*, and *osteoblastomatosis*.

LOCATION OF OSTEOBLASTOMAS

The three most common sites of involvement are the spinal column (21%–33%), long tubular bones (26%–38%), and jaw (10%).[40,51–54] In the appendicular skeleton, the metaphysis is most commonly involved followed by the diaphysis.[52,54] Approximately half of the cases are cortically based and the other half arises in cancellous bone.[52–54] Vertebral tumors most commonly arise in the posterior elements. Vertebral body involvement alone is infrequent.[52–54]

CLINICAL FEATURES OF OSTEOBLASTOMAS

Osteoblastomas are most commonly seen in adolescents and young adults, with up to 75% of patients younger than 25 years.[52] Similar to an osteoid osteoma, an osteoblastoma has a predilection for males, with a male-to-female ratio of at least 2:1.[52,54] Patients often present with pain at the affected site that usually does not have a nocturnally accentuated pattern. Spinal osteoblastomas may present with neurologic findings and progressive scoliosis.[51,55] Intraarticular osteoblastomas presenting with osteoarthritis and synovitis have also been reported.[56] Severe systemic manifestations, including weight loss, fever, and anemia, can be seen in exceptionally rare cases.[57]

RADIOGRAPHIC FEATURES OF OSTEOBLASTOMAS

On plain films, an osteoblastoma appears as a circumscribed lytic lesion with a mineralized bone matrix evident in at least half of the cases (Fig. 8).[52–54] Most osteoblastomas are sharply marginated and have a peripheral rim of thin sclerotic bone and remain confined to the bone. However, up to 25% can have features that mimic a malignant bone tumor, such as cortical destruction, periosteal reaction, and large size.[54] Aneurysmal bone cyst changes can occur, particularly in spinal lesions, producing a blow-out appearance. Rare cases occur on the surface of bone and may be confused with an osteosarcoma (Fig. 9).

GROSS PATHOLOGY OF OSTEOBLASTOMAS

Because most osteoblastomas are treated by curettage, the tissue is received piecemeal and is composed of bloody, red-tan, gritty, and friable fragments. In intact cases, the tumor is sharply demarcated from the adjacent bone. Reactive sclerosis is usually minimal, appearing as a thin rim of dense, white-tan bone surrounding a red-brown tumor. The average size is 3.0 to 3.5 cm, but some cases can be greater than 10 cm.[52,55]

MICROSCOPIC PATHOLOGY AND SUBTYPES OF OSTEOBLASTOMAS

Conventional Osteoblastomas

Microscopically, an Osteoblastoma is similar to an osteoid osteoma, but there can be a broader spectrum of bone formation, including cords and clusters of activated osteoblasts with minimal osteoid, lace-like osteoid, broad anastomosing trabeculae of woven bone, and sheets of woven bone (Fig. 10). Neoplastic bone is lined by plump osteoblasts that can vary from large immature-appearing cells with eccentric basophilic granular cytoplasm, a perinuclear Hof (Golgi apparatus), and a large vesicular nucleus with distinct nucleoli to mature osteoblasts that are smaller with less cytoplasm and smaller nuclei. Mitotic activity is usually low, and atypical mitoses are not seen. The interface with host bone is well defined, often with the tumor showing peripheral bone maturation.[52] Osteoblastomas can show expansion into the soft tissue, but will still be surrounded by

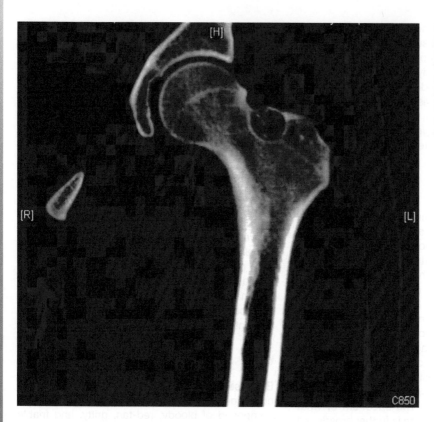

Fig. 8. Circumscribed lytic lesion in the metaphyseal region of the proximal femur with thin rim of reactive sclerotic bone and evidence of bone-like matrix mineralization supports a radiological diagnosis of osteoblastoma.

a thin shell of reactive bone. Very rare cases contain a cartilaginous matrix.[58]

Aggressive (Epithelioid) Osteoblastomas

Dorfman[59] first suggested the term aggressive osteoblastoma in 1972. Then in 1984, Dorfman and Weiss,[51] in a study of 43 conventional osteoblastomas and 15 aggressive osteoblastomas, noticed consistent differences between the two entities; the latter was locally aggressive but with a nonmetastasizing behavior. The distinctive histologic feature of an aggressive osteoblastoma is large epithelioid osteoblasts with abundant eosinophilic cytoplasm either rimming bone trabeculae or in cellular sheets and clusters (**Fig. 11**).[51,55] The trabeculae may seem wider and more irregular than those of a conventional osteoblastoma. Close to half of the cases can have lace-like or sheet-like bone. Mitotic activity can range from 1 to 4 per 20 high power fields (HPF). Importantly, there is a lack of marked stromal pleomorphism, atypical mitoses, necrosis, and bone invasion. Today, the term *aggressive osteoblastoma* is most appropriately used for cases with both the histopathologic features and locally aggressive growth (recurrence). In the absence of clinically aggressive behavior, *epithelioid osteoblastoma* may be a more appropriate diagnosis for cases with large numbers of epithelioid osteoblasts. It is important to remember that occasional larger epithelioid-appearing osteoblasts can be seen in conventional osteoblastoma. Some investigators attribute the aggressiveness of osteoblastomas to location (eg, flat bone lesions) and not particular histologic features.[60]

Malignant Osteoblastomas

Malignant osteoblastoma was the term given to 8 cases described by Schwajowicz[61] in 1976 that had a more histologically aggressive appearance. However, the use of the term malignant was not substantiated either pathologically or clinically. Today, these lesions can be considered part of the spectrum of changes seen in aggressive osteoblastomas and the term *malignant osteoblastoma* should not be used.

Pseudomalignant Osteoblastomas

Pseudomalignant osteoblastoma is defined as an osteoblastoma with characteristic clinical, radiological, and histopathologic features that contain cells with large, sometimes multilobulated nuclei with smudgy, dark chromatin and vacuolated cytoplasm in the absence of mitotic figures (**Fig. 12**).

Fig. 9. Surface osteoblastoma of the posterior distal femur may be radiologically interpreted as a surface osteosarcoma making clinicopathologic correlation difficult.

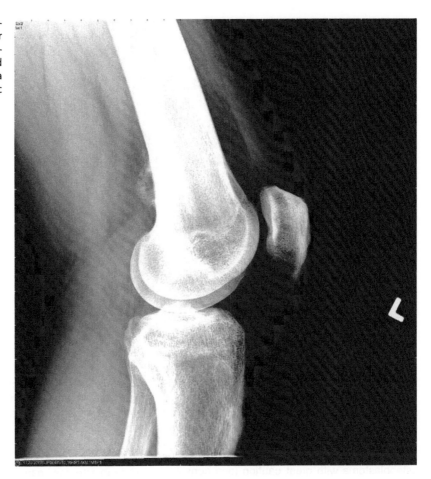

Fig. 10. Generally, areas of osteoblastoma are indistinguishable from osteoid osteoma, but there can be a broader spectrum of bone formation, including lace-like bone (*bottom center*) to broad trabeculae and sheets of neoplastic bone (*left* and *upper right*).

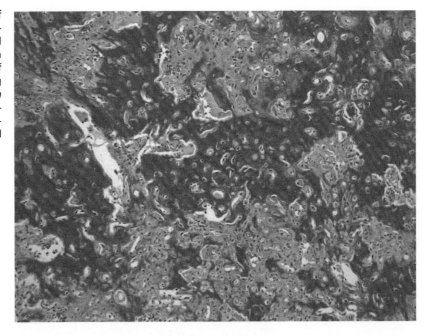

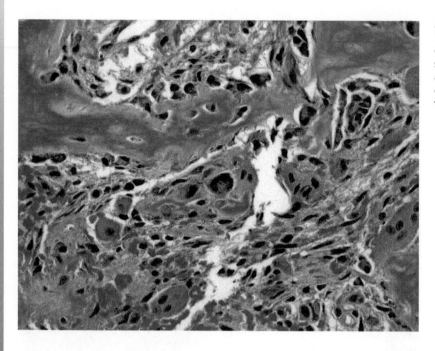

Fig. 11. Enlarged epithelioid osteoblasts with abundant cytoplasm (*center*) are seen in large numbers in aggressive osteoblastoma or very focally in conventional osteoblastoma.

Mirra and colleagues[62] first recognized this in 1976. Subsequently, Cheung and colleagues[63] reported a similar case, and they stressed that absolutely no mitoses were seen and the patient had long-term disease-free follow-up. One should only entertain a diagnosis of pseudosarcomatous osteoblastoma with great caution (and consultation), and the diagnosis should be reserved for cases with typical clinicopathological features of an osteoblastoma that histologically contain cells with degenerative atypia and lack mitotic activity and atypical mitoses.

Multifocal Osteoblastomas

Osteoblastomas can be multifocal, occurring either as multiple foci within a single region of

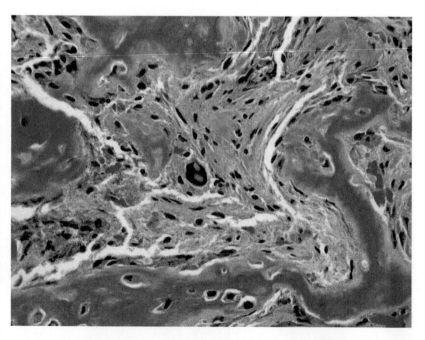

Fig. 12. Pseudomalignant cells in osteoblastoma have large nuclei with very dark and smudgy-appearing chromatin (*center*). In this case, the degenerative cell also has intranuclear cytoplasmic inclusions.

bone or multiple foci in separate bones. In 1970, Schwajowicz and Lemos[64] described 4 cases that were composed of several discrete foci of osteoblastoma within a sclerotic region of a single bone, which they designated as *multifocal sclerosing osteoblastoma*. Although these were large tumors, given the small size of the separate foci of the osteoblastoma and the association with surrounding sclerotic bone, arguably such cases may be better described as *multifocal osteoid osteoma*. Rare cases of multifocal lesions within separate bones have been reported.[65] In 2007, Filippi and colleagues[66] described 26 cases of what they termed *epithelioid multinodular osteoblastoma* that most commonly involved the jaw bones and were made up of multiple nodules of epithelioid osteoblasts associated with a lacy, blue bone matrix and frequent formation of sheets of cells with no matrix.

Osteoblastomatosis

Kyriakos and colleagues[67] have recently put forth the term *osteoblastomatosis* to describe exceedingly rare cases consisting of numerous multiple lytic lesions within individual or separate bones that histologically resemble an osteoblastoma.[67,68] They postulate that osteoblastomatosis represents a distinct clinicopathologic entity based primarily on the fact that the radiographic features mimic a multifocal vascular lesion, but the lesions are essentially indistinguishable from osteoblastoma on microscopic examination.

Malignant Transformation of Osteoblastomas

Malignant transformation has been reported with at most 16 adequately documented cases reported in the literature.[61,69,70] Defining what constitutes malignant transformation is complicated by the fact that osteoblastomas can be locally aggressive and cases of osteosarcoma can be difficult to distinguish from osteoblastomas (osteoblastoma-like osteosarcoma). True transformation to malignancy should be considered when a high-grade osteosarcoma with metastatic potential arises at the site of a previous osteoblastoma that originally had characteristic histopathologic and radiological features.

DIFFERENTIAL DIAGNOSIS OF OSTEOBLASTOMAS

As previously discussed, the distinction between an osteoid osteoma and an osteoblastoma can be problematic. These tumors exist on a spectrum from small lesions with reactive bone sclerosis to very large tumors with no host reaction. Using clinical, radiological, and pathologic features, lesions toward each end of the spectrum can readily be classified (eg, 0.5 cm lytic lesion in the femur with marked host bone sclerosis [osteoid osteoma] or a large destructive lesion in the spine with no host reaction and more florid bone production [osteoblastoma]). Lesions in the middle of the spectrum that have equivocal clinicopathologic features continue to be arbitrarily classified based on size, with tumors larger than 1.5 cm called osteoblastomas.

Extensive areas of reactive bone formation resembling an osteoblastoma can be seen in a primary aneurysmal bone cyst and more rarely in other benign bone tumors, such as giant cell tumor and chondromyxoid fibroma. The underlying tumor is usually readily recognized as a distinct mass separate from the secondary reactive bone formation. As previously discussed, sinonasal osteomas with osteoblastoma-like areas can be distinguished from osteoblastomas by the identification of dense cortical bone. An osteoblastoma is also very rare in the paranasal sinuses, nasal cavity, and orbit where an osteoma commonly arises. An osteoblastoma-like osteosarcoma histologically is virtually identical to an osteoblastoma.[60,71] The histologic feature that separates the two is the presence of an infiltrative growth pattern between the host bone trabeculae or the invasion of Haversian canals. Conventional osteosarcomas may have focal areas that are virtually indistinguishable from osteoblastomas, but will have regions with marked cytologic atypia, high mitotic activity, and patterns of bone formation typically seen in conventional osteosarcoma.

DISCUSSION OF OSTEOBLASTOMAS

Osteoblastic tumors were first described in the literature almost 80 years ago.[72] By the middle of the last century, osteoblastomas had been established as a distinct entity and a possible relationship with osteoid osteomas had been recognized.[73–75] However, difficulties in distinguishing it from osteoid osteomas and osteosarcomas and challenges in understanding its biologic potential and pathogenesis remain. From a clinical standpoint, the most important task is to exclude osteosarcomas. However, with limited sampling it may not be possible to distinguish osteoblastoma from osteosarcoma, particularly osteoblastoma-like osteosarcomas. In this circumstance, a diagnosis of "atypical bone forming neoplasm" can be made along with a comment that additional sampling is required to rule out an osteosarcoma. One also needs to be mindful that a minority of conventional osteoblastomas and surface (subperiosteal) osteoblastomas may be radiologically interpreted as osteosarcomas causing problematic clinicopathological correlation. Expert consultation should be sought if there is any doubt.

Only a few cases of osteoblastomas have been studied by cytogenetic analysis.[50,75–79] To date, these studies have shown that a variety of chromosomal abnormalities can be found, but no specific characteristic translocation has been identified. However, involvement of chromosomes 1 and 14 may be recurrent in osteoblastomas.[77,78] Molecular abnormalities of p53 and retinoblastoma genes and highly complex karyotypes typical of osteosarcomas are not seen in osteoblastomas suggesting no relationship between these two. In contrast, abnormalities of 17 p have been documented in osteosarcomas and osteoblastomas suggesting that in some cases there may be progression from an osteoblastoma to an osteosarcoma (malignant transformation).[76] Truly understanding the pathogenesis of osteoblastoma and its relationship to osteoid osteoma and osteosarcoma requires cytogenetic and molecular analysis of many cases with detailed clinical correlation and follow-up, which has not been performed to date. As such, it seems that we will continue to struggle with osteoblastoma and its relationship to osteoid osteomas and osteosarcoma for some years to come.

SUMMARY

The diagnosis of benign bone-forming tumors continues to be based on histologic examination combined with clinical and radiological correlation. This approach should allow for the appropriate classification of most cases. However, some areas remain challenging, including distinguishing osteoblastomas from osteosarcomas, recognizing pseudosarcomatous change in osteoblastomas, or grappling with limited tissue in trying to diagnose osteoid osteomas. There is very limited understanding of the cytogenetic and molecular abnormalities that result in the pathogenesis of these tumors and that could serve as ancillary diagnostic studies. As such, we will continue the current diagnostic approach, at least into the near future.

REFERENCES

1. White LM, Kandel R. Osteoid-producing tumors of bone. Semin Musculoskelet Radiol 2000;4(1):25–43.
2. Erdogan N, Demir U, Songu M, et al. A prospective study of paranasal sinus osteomas in 1,889 cases: changing patterns of localization. Laryngoscope 2009;119(12):2355–9.
3. Bertoni F, Unni KK, Beabout JW, et al. Parosteal osteoma of bones other than of the skull and face. Cancer 1995;75(10):2466–73.
4. Nielsen GP, Rosenberg AE. Update on bone forming tumors of the head and neck. Head Neck Pathol 2007;1(1):87–93.
5. Peyser AB, Makley JT, Callewart CC, et al. Osteoma of the long bones and the spine. A study of eleven patients and a review of the literature. J Bone Joint Surg Am 1996;78(8):1172–80.
6. Unni KK, Inwards CY. Mayo Foundation for medical E, research. Dahlin's bone tumors: general aspects and data on 10,165 cases. Philadelphia: Wollters Kluwer Health/Lippincott Williams & Wilkins; 2010.
7. Wang W, Kong L, Dong R, et al. Osteoma in the upper cervical spine with spinal cord compression. Eur Spine J 2006;15(Suppl 5):616–20.
8. Pau A, Chiaramonte G, Ghio G, et al. Solitary intracranial subdural osteoma: case report and review of the literature. Tumori 2003;89(1):96–8.
9. Soler Rich R, Martinez S, de Marcos JA, et al. Parosteal osteoma of the iliac bone. Skeletal Radiol 1998; 27(3):161–3.
10. McHugh JB, Mukherji SK, Lucas DR. Sino-orbital osteoma: a clinicopathologic study of 45 surgically treated cases with emphasis on tumors with osteoblastoma-like features. Arch Pathol Lab Med 2009;133(10):1587–93.
11. Greenspan A. Benign bone-forming lesions: osteoma, osteoid osteoma, and osteoblastoma. Clinical, imaging, pathologic, and differential considerations. Skeletal Radiol 1993;22(7):485–500.
12. Gimbel W, Schmidt J, Brack-Werner R, et al. Molecular and pathogenic characterization of the RFB osteoma virus: lack of oncogene and induction of osteoma, osteopetrosis, and lymphoma. Virology 1996;224(2):533–8.
13. Bisgaard ML, Bulow S. Familial adenomatous polyposis (FAP): genotype correlation to FAP phenotype with osteomas and sebaceous cysts. Am J Med Genet A 2006;140(3):200–4.
14. Ruggieri M, Pavone V, Polizzi A, et al. Familial osteoma of the cranial vault. Br J Radiol 1998; 71(842):225–8.
15. Kitsoulis P, Mantellos G, Vlychou M. Osteoid osteoma. Acta Orthop Belg 2006;72(2):119–25.
16. Papathanassiou ZG, Megas P, Petsas T, et al. Osteoid osteoma: diagnosis and treatment. Orthopedics 2008;31(11):1118.
17. Glynn JJ, Lichtenstein L. Osteoid-osteoma with multicentric nidus. A report of two cases. J Bone Joint Surg Am 1973;55(4):855–8.
18. De Santis E, Rosa MA, Pannone A. Review of 115 cases of osteoid osteoma. Arch Putti Chir Organi Mov 1989;37(1):209–18.
19. Solarino G, Scialpi L, De Vita D, et al. Multiple osteoid osteoma. A clinical case. Chir Organi Mov 2004;89(2):161–6.

20. Kransdorf MJ, Stull MA, Gilkey FW, et al. Osteoid osteoma. Radiographics 1991;11(4):671–96.

21. Zileli M, Cagli S, Basdemir G, et al. Osteoid osteomas and osteoblastomas of the spine. Neurosurg Focus 2003;15(5):E5.

22. Saccomanni B. Osteoid osteoma and osteoblastoma of the spine: a review of the literature. Curr Rev Musculoskelet Med 2009;2(1):65–7.

23. Simon WH, Beller ML. Intracapsular epiphyseal osteoid osteoma of ankle joint. A case report. Clin Orthop Relat Res 1975;108:200–3.

24. Destian S, Hernanz-Schulman M, Raskin K, et al. Case report 468. Epiphyseal osteoid osteoma distal end of femur. Skeletal Radiol 1988;17(2):141–3.

25. Al Shaikhi A, Hebert-Davies J, Moser T, et al. Osteoid osteoma of the capitate: a case report and literature review. Eplasty 2009;9:e38.

26. Shukla S, Clarke AW, Saifuddin A. Imaging features of foot osteoid osteoma. Skeletal Radiol 2010;39(7): 683–9.

27. Cassard X, Accadbled F, De Gauzy JS, et al. Osteoid osteoma of the elbow in children: a report of three cases and a review of the literature. J Pediatr Orthop B 2002;11(3):240–4.

28. Jones AC, Prihoda TJ, Kacher JE, et al. Osteoblastoma of the maxilla and mandible: a report of 24 cases, review of the literature, and discussion of its relationship to osteoid osteoma of the jaws. Oral Surg Oral Med Oral Pathol Oral Radiol Endod 2006;102(5):639–50.

29. Rahsepar B, Nikgoo A, Fatemitabar SA. Osteoid osteoma of subcondylar region: case report and review of the literature. J Oral Maxillofac Surg 2009;67(4):888–93.

30. Goto T, Shinoda Y, Okuma T, et al. Administration of nonsteroidal anti-inflammatory drugs accelerates spontaneous healing of osteoid osteoma. Arch Orthop Trauma Surg 2011;131(5):619–25.

31. Khan A, Muthusamy C, Turnbull I, et al. Osteoid osteoma imaging. emedicine; 2009.

32. Mungo DV, Zhang X, O'Keefe RJ, et al. COX-1 and COX-2 expression in osteoid osteomas. J Orthop Res 2002;20(1):159–62.

33. Jackson RP, Reckling FW, Mants FA. Osteoid osteoma and osteoblastoma. Similar histologic lesions with different natural histories. Clin Orthop Relat Res 1977;128:303–13.

34. Lee EH, Shafi M, Hui JH. Osteoid osteoma: a current review. J Pediatr Orthop 2006;26(5):695–700.

35. Ghanem I. The management of osteoid osteoma: updates and controversies. Curr Opin Pediatr 2006;18(1):36–41.

36. Zampa V, Bargellini I, Ortori S, et al. Osteoid osteoma in atypical locations: the added value of dynamic gadolinium-enhanced MR imaging. Eur J Radiol 2009;71(3):527–35.

37. Unni KK, American Registry of P, Armed Forces Institute of P. Tumors of the bones and joints. Washington, DC: American Registry of Pathology in collaboration with the Armed Forces Institute of Pathology; 2005.

38. Jaffe HL. "Osteoid-osteoma" a benign osteoblastic tumor composed of osteoid and atypical bone. Arch Surg 1935;31(5):709–28.

39. Jaffe HL, Lichtenstein L. Osteoid-osteoma: further experience with this benign tumor of bone: with special reference to cases showing the lesion in relation to shaft cortices and commonly misclassified as instances of sclerosing non-suppurative osteomyelitis or cortical-bone abscess. J Bone Joint Surg Am 1940;22(3):645–82.

40. Jaffe HL. Osteoid-osteoma of bone. Radiology 1945; 45(4):319–34.

41. Moberg E. The natural course of osteoid osteoma. J Bone Joint Surg Am 1951;33(A:1):166–70.

42. Golding JS. The natural history of osteoid osteoma; with a report of twenty cases. J Bone Joint Surg Br 1954;36(2):218–29.

43. Cabot RC, Mallory TB, Castleman B, et al. Case 31432. N Engl J Med 1945;233(17):508–10.

44. Baruffi MR, Volpon JB, Neto JB, et al. Osteoid osteomas with chromosome alterations involving 22q. Cancer Genet Cytogenet 2001;124(2):127–31.

45. Dal Cin P, Sciot R, Samson I, et al. Osteoid osteoma and osteoblastoma with clonal chromosome changes. Br J Cancer 1998;78(3):344–8.

46. Pieterse AS, Vernon-Roberts B, Paterson DC, et al. Osteoid osteoma transforming to aggressive (low grade malignant) osteoblastoma: a case report and literature review. Histopathology 1983;7(5):789–800.

47. Becce F, Theumann N, Rochette A, et al. Osteoid osteoma and osteoid osteoma-mimicking lesions: biopsy findings, distinctive MDCT features and treatment by radiofrequency ablation. Eur Radiol 2010; 20(10):2439–46.

48. Rosenthal DI, Alexander A, Rosenberg AE, et al. Ablation of osteoid osteomas with a percutaneously placed electrode: a new procedure. Radiology 1992;183(1):29–33.

49. Laredo JD, Hamze B, Jeribi R. Percutaneous biopsy of osteoid osteomas prior to percutaneous treatment using two different biopsy needles. Cardiovasc Intervent Radiol 2009;32(5):998–1003.

50. Roessner A, Metze K, Heymer B. Aggressive osteoblastoma. Pathol Res Pract 1985;179(3):433–8.

51. Dorfman HD, Weiss SW. Borderline osteoblastic tumors: problems in the differential diagnosis of aggressive osteoblastoma and low-grade osteosarcoma. Semin Diagn Pathol 1984;1(3):215–34.

52. Lucas DR, Unni KK, McLeod RA, et al. Osteoblastoma: clinicopathologic study of 306 cases. Hum Pathol 1994;25(2):117–34.

53. Kroon HM, Schurmans J. Osteoblastoma: clinical and radiologic findings in 98 new cases. Radiology 1990;175(3):783–90.

54. McLeod RA, Dahlin DC, Beabout JW. The spectrum of osteoblastoma. AJR Am J Roentgenol 1976; 126(2):321–5.

55. Lucas DR. Osteoblastoma. Arch Pathol Lab Med 2010;134(10):1460–6.

56. Abolghasemian M, Rezaie M, Behgoo A, et al. Exostosis-like intra-articular periosteal osteoblastoma: a rare case. Am J Orthop (Belle Mead NJ) 2010; 39(6):E50–3.

57. Mirra JM, Cove K, Theros E, et al. A case of osteoblastoma associated with severe systemic toxicity. Am J Surg Pathol 1979;3(5):463–71.

58. Bertoni F, Unni KK, Lucas DR, et al. Osteoblastoma with cartilaginous matrix. An unusual morphologic presentation in 18 cases. Am J Surg Pathol 1993; 17(1):69–74.

59. Dorfman HD. Proceedings: malignant transformation of benign bone lesions. Proc Natl Cancer Conf 1972; 7:901–13.

60. Della Rocca C, Huvos AG. Osteoblastoma: varied histological presentations with a benign clinical course. An analysis of 55 cases. Am J Surg Pathol 1996;20(7):841–50.

61. Schajowicz F, Lemos C. Malignant osteoblastoma. J Bone Joint Surg Br 1976;58(2):202–11.

62. Mirra JM, Kendrick RA, Kendrick RE. Pseudomalignant osteoblastoma versus arrested osteosarcoma: a case report. Cancer 1976;37(4):2005–14.

63. Cheung FM, Wu WC, Lam CK, et al. Diagnostic criteria for pseudomalignant osteoblastoma. Histopathology 1997;31(2):196–200.

64. Schajowicz F, Lemos C. Osteoid osteoma and osteoblastoma. Closely related entities of osteoblastic derivation. Acta Orthop Scand 1970;41(3):272–91.

65. Adler CP. Multifocal osteoblastoma of the hand. Skeletal Radiol 2000;29(10):601–4.

66. Zon Filippi R, Swee RG, Krishnan Unni K. Epithelioid multinodular osteoblastoma: a clinicopathologic analysis of 26 cases. Am J Surg Pathol 2007;31(8):1265–8.

67. Kyriakos M, El-Khoury GY, McDonald DJ, et al. Osteoblastomatosis of bone. A benign, multifocal osteoblastic lesion, distinct from osteoid osteoma and osteoblastoma, radiologically simulating a vascular tumor. Skeletal Radiol 2007;36(3):237–47.

68. O'Connell JX, Rosenthal DI, Mankin HJ, et al. A unique multifocal osteoblastoma-like tumor of the bones of a single lower extremity. Report of a case. J Bone Joint Surg Am 1993;75(4):597–602.

69. Kunze E, Enderle A, Radig K, et al. Aggressive osteoblastoma with focal malignant transformation and development of pulmonary metastases. A case report with a review of literature. Gen Diagn Pathol 1996;141(5–6):377–92.

70. Wozniak AW, Nowaczyk MT, Osmola K, et al. Malignant transformation of an osteoblastoma of the mandible: case report and review of the literature. Eur Arch Otorhinolaryngol 2010;267(6):845–9.

71. Bertoni F, Unni KK, McLeod RA, et al. Osteosarcoma resembling osteoblastoma. Cancer 1985;55(2):416–26.

72. Jaffe HL, Mayer L. An osteoblastic osteoid tissue-forming tumor of a metacarpal bone. Arch Surg 1932;24(4):550–64.

73. Dahlin DC, Johnson EW Jr. Giant osteoid osteoma. J Bone Joint Surg Am 1954;36(3):559–72.

74. Lichtenstein L. Benign osteoblastoma; a category of osteoid-and bone-forming tumors other than classical osteoid osteoma, which may be mistaken for giant-cell tumor or osteogenic sarcoma. Cancer 1956;9(5):1044–52.

75. Jaffe HL. Benign osteoblastoma. Bull Hosp Joint Dis 1956;17(2):141–51.

76. Mascarello JT, Krous HF, Carpenter PM. Unbalanced translocation resulting in the loss of the chromosome 17 short arm in an osteoblastoma. Cancer Genet Cytogenet 1993;69(1):65–7.

77. Angervall L, Persson S, Stenman G, et al. Large cell, epithelioid, telangiectatic osteoblastoma: a unique pseudosarcomatous variant of osteoblastoma. Hum Pathol 1999;30(10):1254–9.

78. Giannico G, Holt GE, Homlar KC, et al. Osteoblastoma characterized by a three-way translocation: report of a case and review of the literature. Cancer Genet Cytogenet 2009;195(2):168–71.

79. Baker AC, Rezeanu L, Klein MJ, et al. Aggressive osteoblastoma: a case report involving a unique chromosomal aberration. Int J Surg Pathol 2010; 18(3):219–24.

OSTEOSARCOMA: DIFFERENTIAL DIAGNOSTIC CONSIDERATIONS

Adriana L. Gonzalez, MD*, Justin M.M. Cates, MD, PhD

KEYWORDS

• Bone-forming tumors • Osteosarcoma • Osteoblastoma

ABSTRACT

Accurate diagnosis of bone-forming tumors, including correct subclassification of osteogenic sarcoma is critical for determination of appropriate clinical management and prediction of patient outcome. The morphologic spectrum of osteogenic sarcoma is extensive, however, and its histologic mimics are numerous. This review focuses on the major differential diagnoses of the specific subtypes of osteosarcoma, presents summaries of various diagnoses, and provides tips to overcoming pitfalls in diagnosis.

OVERVIEW

In the past decade, several excellent articles have been published focusing on different aspects of osteogenic sarcoma (OGS), including its epidemiology,[1–7] morphologic variants,[8,9] etiology, cytogenetics and molecular biology,[10–23] clinical management,[24–31] prognostic markers,[32–36] and even prosection of bone specimens and recommendations for tumor reporting.[37,38]

Common throughout these various fields is the principle that OGS is a diverse disease entity—clinically, anatomically, and pathologically. For example, older patients with secondary OGS are at high risk for poor outcomes.[4,39–41] In contrast, low-grade variants (parosteal and low-grade intraosseous OGS) tend to result in favorable outcomes after complete surgical resection alone.[9,42–44] Accordingly, diagnosis and subclas-

sification determine the histologic grade, an important parameter in both the American Joint Committee on Cancer TNM staging system and the Musculoskeletal Tumor Society/Enneking staging system for bone tumors.[38,45–47] Although the diagnosis of bone-forming tumors can be straightforward in many cases, it becomes problematic when there are issues with biopsy sampling, unusual variations in tumor histology, or discrepancies with radiographic findings. In this article, we discuss the most common histologic mimics for each subtype of OGS, with an emphasis on the differentiating features.

CONVENTIONAL OSTEOGENIC SARCOMA

The sine qua non for the diagnosis of OGS is production of osteoid matrix by malignant tumor cells (Fig. 1A), regardless of the amount produced, which can range from dense matrix deposition seen in the sclerotic variant of osteoblastic OGS and well-formed lamellar trabeculae that can mimic a benign process, to inconspicuous amounts of matrix elaborated by tumor cells in fibroblastic or small cell OGS.[48–50] Although this definition of OGS is straightforward, in practice the histologic findings of OGS are protean and its clinicomorphologic spectrum can be confusing (Table 1).[8,48]

As might be surmised, identification of osteoid deposition is critical for the pathologic evaluation of bone tumors. Unfortunately, osteoid is, at times, difficult to identify with certainty and can present in

Disclosure statement: The authors have no conflicts of interest to disclose.
Department of Pathology, Microbiology and Immunology, Vanderbilt University School of Medicine, 3rd Floor, Medical Center North, C-3321, Nashville, TN 37232-2561, USA
* Corresponding author.
E-mail address: adriana.gonzalez@vanderbilt.edu

Surgical Pathology 5 (2012) 117–146
doi:10.1016/j.path.2011.07.011
1875-9181/12/$ – see front matter © 2012 Published by Elsevier Inc.

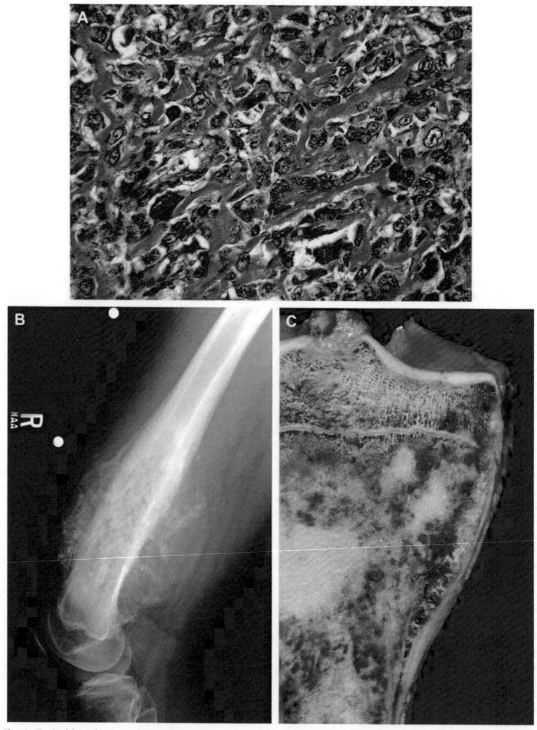

Fig. 1. Typical histologic, radiographic, and gross characteristics of osteosarcoma. (*A*) The deposition of osteoid matrix by cytologically malignant mesenchymal cells is definitional for osteosarcoma (original magnification ×400). (*B*) Lateral radiograph of an ill-defined, mixed lytic and sclerotic lesion of the distal femur transgressing the cortex and inciting an aggressive periosteal response, diagnostic of a malignant process. (*Courtesy of* John J. Block, MD, Nashville, TN.) (*C*) Intramedullary osteosarcoma of the proximal tibial metaphysis with destruction of adjacent cortex, lifting of periosteum, and generation of reactive periosteal bone formation (Codman triangle) best seen at the distal aspect of the tumor.

Table 1
World Health Organization classification of osteogenic tumors[a]

Osteoid osteoma	
Osteoblastoma	
Osteosarcoma (OGS)	
Conventional	(80%)
Osteoblastic	(>50%)
Chondroblastic	($\approx$25%)
Fibroblastic	($\approx$20%)
Telangiectatic	(3%–4%)
Small cell	(1%–2%)
Low-grade central (intraosseous)	(1%–2%)
Secondary	(3%–5%)
Juxtacortical or surface variants	(7%–8%)
Parosteal	(5%–6%)
Periosteal	(1%–2%)
High-grade surface	(<1%)

[a] Numbers in parentheses indicates approximate percentage among all osteogenic sarcoma (OGS).

a variety of patterns within malignant bone tumors. Morphologically, osteoid is densely eosinophilic, homogeneous, or glassy and is typically not arranged in long, linear bundles as is nonosseous, fibrillar collagen. The pattern of osteoid deposition by malignant cells is variable; most often it is delicate and anastomosing (the so-called "filigree" or "lacelike" pattern) and closely associated with tumor cells. Other patterns include dense confluent sheets of matrix (sclerotic pattern) and, rarely, thick trabeculae that can mimic normal bone. The distinction between osteoid and sclerotic collagen (which can undergo dystrophic mineralization) is subjective, however. In these cases, the relationship between the matrix and the neoplastic cells should be evaluated. Whereas osteoblastic cells appear intimately admixed with and surrounded by osteoid matrix, stromal cells adjacent to nonosseous collagen instead appear compressed by the adjacent matrix.[9,51] Fibrin can also mimic osteoid, but is usually more fibrillar, does not polarize, and is associated with hemorrhage or necrosis.[52]

That radiographic correlation is critical in the diagnosis of bone-forming lesions cannot be overemphasized. Variability in histology and limited architectural patterns observable on biopsy and curettage samples create significant challenges in diagnosis, and the radiographic findings are the surgical pathologist's substitute for a gross pathologic evaluation. Not only can the anatomic location of the tumor and its predominant matrix (or the absence thereof) be ascertained, but an impression of its biologic behavior can be surmised from its effect on the host bone and the response of the host bone to the tumor (see **Fig. 1**B).[53] First and foremost, the infiltrative growth pattern of most OGS results in poorly demarcated lesional margins, in contrast to most benign lesions of bone. Quite often, cortical destruction and tumor extension into soft tissue is associated with a periosteal response (ie, Codman triangles, "sunburst" or "onion-skin" patterns of new bone formation) (see **Fig. 1**C). In many cases, the differential diagnosis of a bone tumor can be limited to a few possibilities based solely on its radiographic characteristics. Needless to say, accurate diagnosis of biopsy specimens from bone-producing lesions requires careful consideration of radiographic findings.[9]

Conventional cases of OGS are intramedullary tumors and by definition high grade. They are subclassified based on the predominant matrical component as either osteoblastic, chondroblastic, or fibroblastic; however, many tumors show a combination of patterns and may not fit neatly into one of these histologic subtypes. Although subclassification of conventional OGS does not appear to be of prognostic significance, it is useful in framing the differential diagnosis (**Table 2**).[9,48]

CONVENTIONAL OGS, OSTEOBLASTIC TYPE VERSUS OSTEOBLASTOMA

Osteoblastic OGS is the most common histologic subtype and shows a predominance of lacelike bony matrix without significant chondroid or fibrous matrix. The tumor cells are usually epithelioid, often growing in clusters or sheets, and intermixed with osteoid. Although typically arising in the medullary cavity of the metaphysis of appendicular long bones, aggressive growth often results in extension beyond the metaphysis and destruction of cortical bone with involvement of subperiosteal tissues and a periosteal reaction by the time of clinical presentation.

In contrast, osteoblastoma is a rare, benign, bone-forming tumor that may arise in the cortex, medulla, or periosteal tissues of almost any bone, particularly those of the axial skeleton.[54–56] Osteoblastomas may reach impressive sizes (>10 cm), and mimic osteoblastic or sclerosing OGS both radiographically and histologically. In most cases, radiographic features argue against a malignant diagnosis, especially when the lesion

Table 2
Differential diagnosis: conventional osteosarcoma

Osteosarcoma Subtype	Differential Diagnosis
Osteoblastic osteosarcoma • Usually meta(dia)physis of appendicular skeleton • Sheets of atypical cells producing osteoid matrix • Permeative growth pattern with entrapment of preexisting bone • Soft tissue extension • High mitotic rate, ± atypical mitotic figures	Osteoblastoma • Well-circumscribed, often with peripheral rim of reactive bone • Loose fibrovascular stroma without intertrabecular sheets of cells • Osteoblastic rimming of bony trabeculae • No atypical mitoses Fracture callus • History of trauma or likelihood of pathologic fracture • Uniform, reactive cellular morphology • Organized, purposeful matrix deposition • Granulation tissue-like stroma • Transition from immature osteoid to bony spicules lined by osteoblasts • Hyaline cartilage or fibrocartilage merging with reactive woven bone
Chondroblastic osteosarcoma • Usually younger patient (<25 years) • High-grade cartilaginous lobules • Periphery of chondroid nodules are hypercellular • Chondroid nodules merge with spindled, sarcomatous stroma • Neoplastic osteoid/bone within or between chondroid nodules	Conventional skeletal chondrosarcoma • Older patient (usually >40 years) • Malignant cartilage, often myxoid, permeating adjacent bone marrow or soft tissue • No bone or osteoid matrix produced by tumor cells • Enchondral ossification of chondroid nodules may be present Dedifferentiated chondrosarcoma • Older patient (>50 years) • Abrupt transition between chondrosarcoma and high-grade, nonchondroid sarcoma with or without bone production
Fibroblastic osteosarcoma • Cytologically malignant spindle cells in fascicular or storiform arrays • At least focal osteoid or chondroid matrix deposition by tumor cells	Fibrosarcoma/Undifferentiated pleomorphic sarcoma • Skeletal sarcoma without osteoid or chondroid matrix production by tumor cells Desmoplastic fibroma • Cytologically bland fibrous tumor resembling soft tissue fibromatosis • No osteoid or chondroid matrix production by tumor cells

is seen to be well circumscribed, confined to the involved bone, or surrounded by a rim of peripheral sclerosis. Aggressive radiographic features, however, such as lack of circumscription, cortical destruction, and periosteal new bone formation, may be seen in osteoblastoma.[57,58]

Histologic features that favor the diagnosis of osteoblastoma include a well-circumscribed lesional border that often merges with a peripheral rim of reactive woven bone (**Fig. 2**A), an intertrabecular stroma composed of loose fibrovascular tissue (not densely populated by randomly oriented, monotonous osteoblastic cells as in OGS), osteoblastic rimming of bony trabeculae by a single layer of uniform osteoblasts (even if epithelioid; see later in this article), and the absence of intertrabecular osteoid deposition.[52,55,56,59,60] Mitotic activity is inconspicuous and atypical mitotic figures are not observed. Lesional necrosis is an ominous finding, unless seen in association with fracture. Cytologic atypia is not present, except in rare cases with degenerative cellular changes (pseudoanaplasia) (see **Fig. 2**B).[52,55,61] In these unusual cases, the lack

Fig. 2. Osteoblastoma versus osteoblastoma-like osteosarcoma. (*A*) Osteoblastoma demonstrating well-circumscribed border with lesional trabeculae merging with rim of reactive woven bone at periphery of tumor (original magnification ×20). (*B*) Pseudoanaplastic osteoblastoma with enlarged, hyperchromatic nuclei and smudgy chromatin. Note lack of intertrabecular osteoblastic proliferation and mitotic activity, supporting the interpretation of degenerative-type atypia (original magnification ×200).

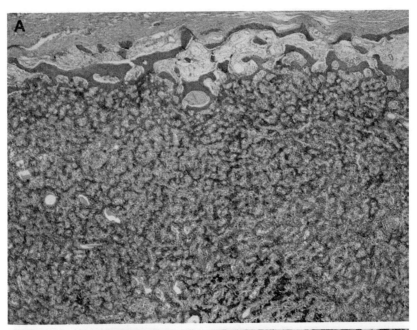

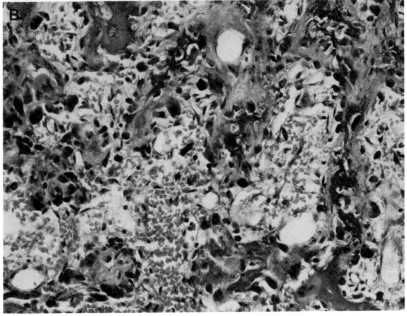

of mitotic activity and hypercellular stroma argue for a benign diagnosis.[52] Although osteoblastomas can rarely produce a chondroid matrix (even in the absence of fracture), this finding is more often indicative of OGS.[52,62] Dorfman and Czerniak[60] point out that, although these and other atypical histologic features (such as intricate, lace-like, or broad sheets of osteoid deposition; hypercellular stroma consisting of sheets of spindle cells; or increased stromal mitoses [more than 4 per 20 high-power fields, but no atypical mitotic figures]) may occasionally be seen in isolation within an individual tumor, their presence should at least raise the possibility of malignancy and prompt reevaluation of the radiologic findings and a thorough search for evidence of an infiltrative growth pattern.

The controversial entity of "aggressive osteoblastoma" is discussed in detail in many sources.[52,59,60,63,64] These rare tumors are

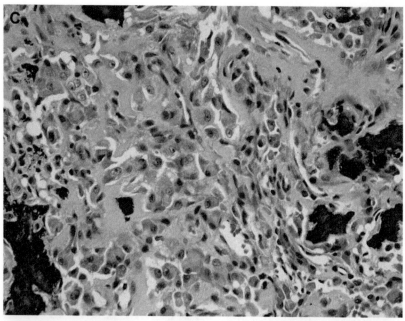

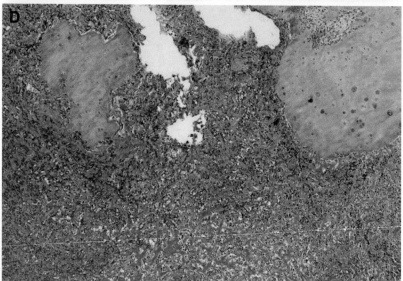

Fig. 2. (*C*) Aggressive osteoblastoma with intratrabecular sheets of uniform epithelioid osteoblasts and "blue spiculated bone" (original magnification ×200). (*D*) Osteoblastoma-like osteosarcoma demonstrating invasion and destruction of adjacent cartilage. Elsewhere in this case, conspicuous mitotic activity, tumoral necrosis, and sheetlike deposition of osteoid were present, supporting the diagnosis of malignancy (original magnification ×40).

characterized by increased cellularity and sheets of epithelioid osteoblasts (defined as osteoblasts twice the size of normal osteoblasts, polygonal in shape, and containing a large vesicular nucleus with prominent nucleoli), sometimes with sheet-like osteoid deposition, stromal mitoses, or immature-appearing "blue spiculated bone" (see **Fig. 2**C). They are distinguished from OGS by the lack of atypical mitotic figures, cellular anaplasia, abundant lace-like osteoid deposition, and host bone permeation.[52,60]

When one is faced with a borderline osteoblastic lesion, it is also important to recall the rare "osteoblastoma-like OGS" variant described by Bertoni and colleagues.[65,66] In these cases, the malignant cells can line immature bony trabeculae in a single layer and appear deceptively bland; however, careful study may demonstrate a permeative or infiltrative growth pattern, increased cellularity, and decreased vascularity of the intertrabecular stroma and scattered mitotic figures, all of which are suggestive of malignancy (see **Fig. 2**D).[65]

Chromosomal analysis has not been successful in identifying karyotypic markers of osteoblastoma[54,55]; however, a recent study showed that immunohistochemical staining for cyclooxygenase-2 (COX2) may be a useful marker for osteoblastoma. Whereas staining for COX2 was limited to the chondroblastic component of 6 of 26 OGS, all osteoblastomas were strongly and diffusely positive.[67]

In summary, an infiltrative or permeative growth pattern with lesional matrix deposition between and surrounding preexisting host bone trabeculae and the absence of a zone of reactive woven bone merging with host bone at the host-tumor interface are perhaps the most helpful diagnostic criteria for OGS (see **Fig. 2**).[52] One caveat to remember is that the multinodular growth pattern of some osteoblastomas may simulate a permeative pattern of growth, once again exemplifying the importance of radiographic correlation in the evaluation of bone specimens.[56,57,65,66]

CONVENTIONAL OGS, OSTEOBLASTIC TYPE VERSUS OSTEOID OSTEOMA

Generally, the distinction between osteoid osteoma and OGS is relatively straightforward clinically and radiographically. Osteoid osteoma is by definition a small (smaller than 2 cm), circumscribed lesion with a central nidus and a variable degree of peripheral sclerosis.[52] It would be unusual for an OGS to come to clinical attention when smaller than 2 cm in size, and particularly unusual to be as sharply delimited as osteoid osteoma. Studies of chromosomal abnormalities in osteoid osteoma are limited, but these tumors appear to be characterized by partial deletions of chromosomes 22q and 17q,[68] and lack the degree of karyotypic abnormalities seen in conventional OGS.[20,21]

CONVENTIONAL OGS, OSTEOBLASTIC TYPE VERSUS FRACTURE CALLUS

The early phases of reactive matrix-producing lesions, such as stress fractures or hypertrophic fracture callus, are pseudosarcomatous in light of their hypercellularity, reactive cellular atypia, exuberant mitotic activity, and permeative histologic growth pattern.[52] The reactive woven bone being produced, however, is usually oriented in a purposeful manner and in some semblance of order, whereas neoplastic bone is completely haphazard and unorganized.[51,60] The bony spicules are usually rimmed by a prominent single layer of uniform, albeit reactive-appearing osteoblasts notably different in morphology from nonosteoblastic mesenchymal cells. In contrast, the neoplastic

bone of OGS lacks such obvious osteoblastic rimming and osteogenic cells are not as readily distinguished from adjacent nonosteogenic stromal cells (**Fig. 3**A, B).[51,52,60] Although the intertrabecular stroma may be edematous and composed of reactive-appearing, mitotically active fibroblasts/myofibroblasts admixed with numerous small immature vessels reminiscent of granulation tissue, the stroma in OGS is more fibrous, lacks prominent vessels, and instead is populated by randomly oriented, atypical spindle cells that show variable degrees of hyperchromasia and anisonucleosis.[52] The cartilage in fracture callus may be hyaline type or fibrocartilaginous and often merges with adjacent reactive woven bone (see **Fig. 3**C).[60] Instead, the malignant cartilage in OGS is almost always hyaline (with or without myxoid degeneration), contains atypical chondrocytes, and merges with hypercellular and atypical stroma or undergoes enchondral ossification. Paradoxically, extensive permeation of skeletal muscle is more indicative of a benign reactive process than a malignant one.[52] The presence of significant nuclear atypia and atypical mitotic figures excludes the diagnosis of reactive bone, however. As usual in orthopedic pathology, correlation of the histologic features with the clinical history and radiologic findings can prevent a serious misdiagnosis.[9]

CONVENTIONAL OGS, CHONDROBLASTIC TYPE, VERSUS CONVENTIONAL SKELETAL CHONDROSARCOMA

Plain radiographs of both chondroblastic OGS and chondrosarcoma may show characteristic rings, arcs, or "popcorn" calcifications, indicative of chondroid matrix undergoing enchondral mineralization (**Fig. 4**A). The clinical setting is often helpful in this differential diagnosis, however. Whereas OGS occurs predominantly in adolescents, chondrosarcoma is much more common in middle-aged to elderly adults[1,5]; however, it should be recalled that the age-specific incidence rate of OGS is bimodal and this diagnosis should not be disregarded in older adults.[1,4,7,39,69,70]

Chondroblastic OGS is characterized by high-grade cytologic atypia within chondroid nodules, the periphery of which become more cellular and merge with a sarcomatous stromal component that usually harbors a variable amount of neoplastic osteoid deposition (see **Fig. 4**B).[48,50,52,55,60] In contrast, the malignant cartilage of skeletal chondrosarcoma is not associated with neoplastic bone production, but instead may undergo enchondral ossification or dystrophic mineralization of the chondroid lobules (see **Fig. 4**C).[51,60]

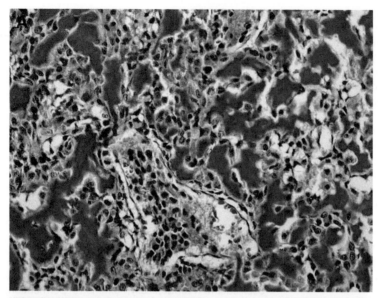

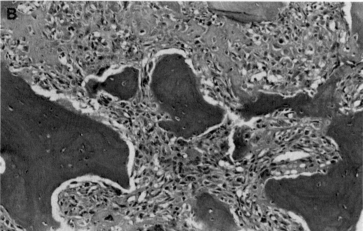

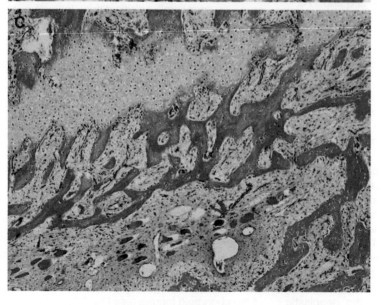

Fig. 3. Conventional osteosarcoma versus fracture callus. (*A*) Irregular and haphazard osteoid matrix being produced by a monotonous and mitotically active cell population that densely populates the intertrabecular stroma (original magnification ×200). (*B*) Osteoblastic osteosarcoma infiltrating between and destroying preexisting host bone trabeculae (original magnification ×100). (*C*) Fracture callus with immature reactive hyaline cartilage and woven bone deposition. Note organized, purposeful pattern of matrix deposition, background granulation tissue-like stroma, and overrun skeletal muscle fibers (original magnification ×40).

Fig. 4. Chondroblastic osteosarcoma versus skeletal chondrosarcoma. (*A*) Lateral radiograph of chondroblastic osteosarcoma demonstrating intramedullary lobulated, "popcorn"-type calcifications typical of the mineralization pattern of a chondroid matrix. Note the associated cortical irregularity and periosteal reaction, suggestive of an aggressive process. (*Courtesy of* John J. Block, MD, Nashville, TN.)

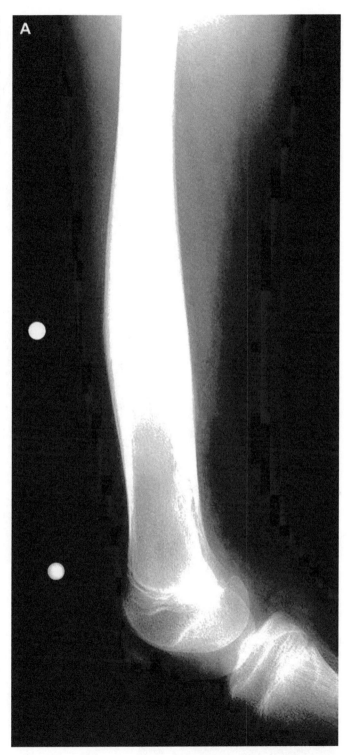

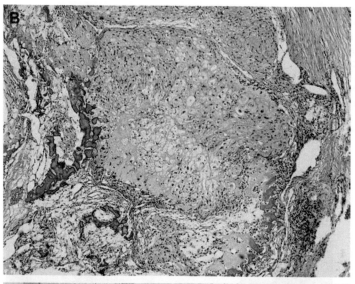

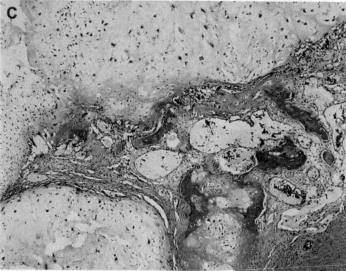

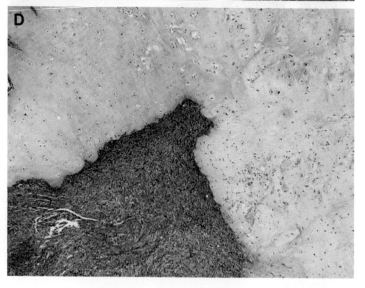

Fig. 4. (*B*) In chondroblastic osteosarcoma, the periphery of the chondroid nodules is hypercellular and often merges into adjacent sarcomatous stroma. The presence of focal neoplastic osteoid deposition confirms the diagnosis of osteosarcoma (original magnification ×100). (*C*) In contrast, the chondroid nodules of conventional skeletal chondrosarcoma lack peripheral spindling and instead may undergo enchondral ossification. There is no deposition of osteoid by neoplastic cells (original magnification ×40). (*D*) Dedifferentiated chondrosarcoma shows an abrupt transition from malignant hyaline cartilage to high grade, non-chondroid sarcoma (original magnification ×40).

In occasional cases, the distinction between OGS and chondrosarcoma may be difficult despite consideration of the clinical, radiographic, and histologic features. Recent reports of potential diagnostic markers, such as ezrin (EZR) and galectin-1 (GAL1), are therefore of interest. Although the cartilaginous components of chondroblastic OGS were positive for EZR in 10 of 16 cases, none of more than 100 conventional-type chondrosarcomas expressed EZR.[71] The investigators suggest that despite its limited sensitivity, in this clinical setting, EZR staining is diagnostic for OGS. In contrast, although GAL1 appears to be more sensitive for chondroblastic OGS (positive in 92% of cases), focal and weak expression may be seen in 18% of chondrosarcomas.[72]

CONVENTIONAL OGS, CHONDROBLASTIC TYPE, VERSUS DEDIFFERENTIATED CHONDROSARCOMA

Areas of OGS can be present in dedifferentiated chondrosarcoma, complicating the distinction from chondroblastic OGS. However, dedifferentiated chondrosarcoma typically affects older adults and, in many cases, a precursor chondroid neoplasm can be documented either radiographically or pathologically.[52] Although the cartilage of dedifferentiated chondrosarcoma is most often of low histologic grade, in some cases it can be more cytologically atypical and mimic that of chondroblastic OGS. The critical distinguishing histologic feature between these tumors is the nature of the interface between the chondroid matrix and the nonchondroid sarcomatous component. Dedifferentiated chondrosarcomas appear truly biphasic, with a sharp and abrupt transition from neoplastic cartilage to a nonchondroid sarcoma (see Fig. 4D). In contrast, chondroblastic OGS will show an admixture of or gradual transition between the 2 components, with condensation of spindle cells at the periphery of the chondroid nodules merging with and apparently arising from adjacent spindle cell sarcoma.[52,60] Diagnostic markers useful in the distinction of chondroblastic OGS and conventional chondrosarcoma are of no utility, because, in many cases, the high-grade sarcomatous components of dedifferentiated chondrosarcoma are positive for GAL1 and EZR.[71,72]

CONVENTIONAL OGS, CHONDROBLASTIC TYPE, VERSUS CLEAR CELL CHONDROSARCOMA

Clear cell chondrosarcoma is a rare tumor and one of the few tumors with characteristic involvement of the epiphysis (with more than half of cases involving the proximal femur). This tumor usually occurs in slightly older patients than chondroblastic OGS, although there is overlap in the age distributions. The tumor is composed of sheets of rather distinctive clear cells with osteoclast-like giant cells and associated intralesional bone production reminiscent of osteoblastoma. The lack of conspicuous mitotic activity and osteoid deposition by the malignant cellular component excludes the diagnosis of OGS.[52,60] The neoplastic cartilage in 10 clear cell chondrosarcomas was reported to be negative for EZR by immunohistochemistry, suggesting that this marker may have utility in distinguishing this tumor from chondroblastic OGS.[71]

CONVENTIONAL OGS, FIBROBLASTIC TYPE, VERSUS FIBROSARCOMA OF BONE, UNDIFFERENTIATED PLEOMORPHIC SARCOMA OF BONE, AND PRIMARY LEIOMYOSARCOMA OF BONE

Fibroblastic OGS is composed predominantly of atypical spindle cells arranged in various patterns (most often interlacing fascicles or herringbone or storiform patterns) associated with focal neoplastic osteoid matrix, regardless of how limited in extent (Fig. 5A).[50] It is acknowledged that the distinction between fibroblastic OGS and fibrosarcoma of bone can be subjective and is highly dependent on adequate sampling.[55] The same may be said of primary undifferentiated pleomorphic sarcoma (UPS) of bone and UPS-like fibroblastic OGS (see Fig. 5B).[9,51,55,73] These types of skeletal sarcomas seem to arise more frequently in association with preexisting conditions (secondary skeletal sarcomas), such as Paget disease, bone infarction, or prior radiation therapy. Fortunately, the distinction between UPS of bone and UPS-like osteosarcoma may not be critical for patient management or prognosis, because studies have shown similar metastasis-free survival rates and histologic responses to chemotherapy.[74,75] Primary leiomyosarcoma of bone usually shows morphologic or immunohistochemical features of smooth muscle differentiation (see Fig. 5C).[76] Fibroblastic OGS is more cytologically atypical and mitotically active than desmoplastic fibroma and low-grade intraosseous (central) OGS.[60]

MORPHOLOGIC OSTEOSARCOMA SUBTYPES

The current World Health Organization classification recognizes 3 morphologic variants of intramedullary OGS: telangiectatic, small cell, and

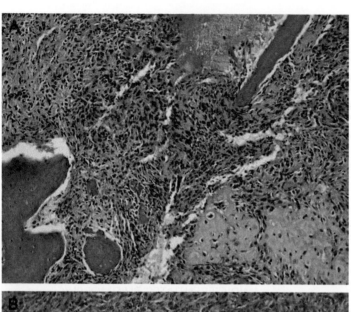

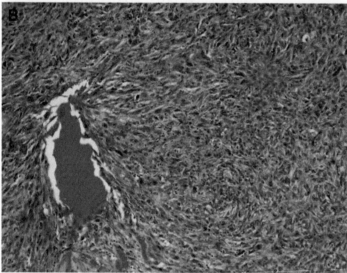

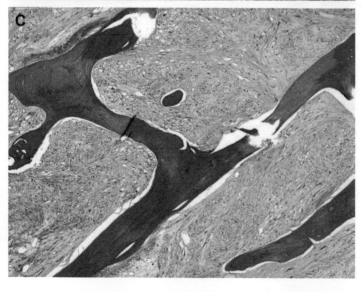

Fig. 5. Fibroblastic osteosarcoma versus nonosteogenic skeletal sarcomas. (A) Fibroblastic osteosarcoma with focal osseous and chondroid matrix deposition at bottom of field (original magnification ×200). (B) Undifferentiated pleomorphic sarcoma of bone infiltrating host bone trabeculae without deposition of osteoid or chondroid matrix by neoplastic cells (original magnification ×100). (C) Leiomyosarcoma of bone with infiltrative growth pattern and morphologic evidence of smooth muscle differentiation (original magnification ×40).

low-grade central (intraosseous) OGS. In addition, there are a number of rarer subtypes not specifically categorized in this classification scheme.[8] Each subtype has specific histologic mimics that comprise the differential diagnosis (Table 3).

TELANGIECTATIC OGS VERSUS ANEURYSMAL BONE CYST

Grossly, both telangiectatic OGS and aneurysmal bone cyst (ABC) are cystic and hemorrhagic lesions that can expand and extend beyond the confines of the bone of origin (Fig. 6A). The low-power microscopic appearances of telangiectatic OGS and ABC can also be identical, with septa of variable thickness containing reactive woven bone and osteoclast-like giant cells. In telangiectatic OGS, however, the septa contain atypical tumor cells with striking pleomorphism, mitotic activity, atypical mitotic figures, tumoral necrosis and focal neoplastic osteoid deposition (often quite limited in extent) (see Fig. 6B).[9,55,60,77] In contrast, the septa in ABC are composed of reactive, mitotically

---

Table 3
Differential diagnosis: morphologic variants of osteosarcoma

Osteosarcoma Subtype	Differential Diagnosis
Telangiectatic osteosarcoma • Similar tumor location to conventional OGS • Radiographically lytic and destructive (appears cystic) • Significant anaplasia of cells within cyst walls • Conspicuous mitoses, ± atypical mitotic figures • Subtle, focal osteoid deposition • Tumoral necrosis	Aneurysmal bone cyst • Benign, but can be large and expansile • May be secondary to other lesions (eg, chondroblastoma, fibrous dysplasia, giant cell tumor) • No cytologic atypia, lesional necrosis or atypical mitotic figures • Admixed inflammatory cells • Osteoid often present parallel to cyst wall and not associated with atypical cells
Small cell osteosarcoma • Radiographs show permeative pattern similar to other infiltrative small cell malignancies • Round to spindled cells, usually more pleomorphic and larger than those of tumors in differential diagnosis • Minimal osteoid deposition ± chondroid matrix • Cytoplasmic CD99 staining in some cases • Negative for t(11;22) or *EWSR1* gene rearrangement	Ewing sarcoma/primitive neuroectodermal tumor • Usually smaller, more uniform cells than small cell OGS • No truly spindled tumor cells or cellular anaplasia • No osteoid or chondroid matrix production by tumor cells • Membranous CD99 staining • Presence of t(11;22) or *EWSR1* gene rearrangement
Low-grade intraosseous osteosarcoma • Well-developed bony trabeculae and fibrous stroma • Bland to mildly atypical cells with tapered nuclei • Permeative growth pattern entrapping adjacent host bone trabeculae • Focal cortical destruction/soft tissue extension • Amplification of chromosome 12q13-15	Fibrous dysplasia • Fibrous stroma with plump, oval to elongated fibroblasts with smooth nuclear outlines and no significant cytologic atypia • Usually thinner, shorter or more delicate trabeculae of woven bone • No permeation of surrounding tissues Desmoplastic Fibroma • Similar to soft tissue desmoid fibromatosis • No bone or osteoid production by tumor cells
Giant cell-rich osteosarcoma • Skeletally immature patient (usually) • Metaphyseal/metadiaphyseal location • Cytologically malignant cells associated with osteoid deposition • Abundant admixed benign osteoclast-like giant cells may obscure malignant features	Giant cell tumor of bone • Epiphyseal location; skeletally mature patient • Reactive/metaplastic bone formation, numerous mitotic figures, lesional necrosis and lymphovascular invasion may be seen • Evenly placed osteoclast-like giant cells amid uniform mononuclear cells • No osteoid or chondroid matrix production by tumor cells, no anaplasia

Abbreviation: OGS, osteogenic sarcoma.

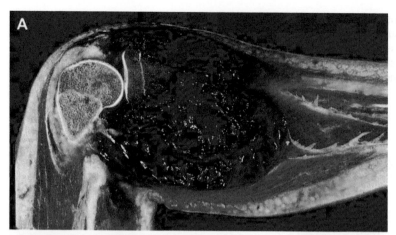

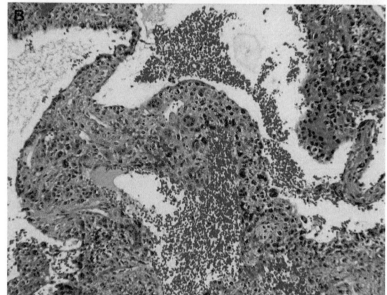

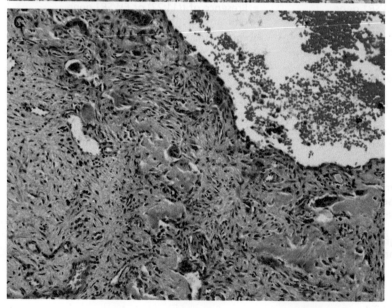

Fig. 6. Telangiectatic osteosarcoma versus aneurysmal bone cyst. (*A*) The diagnosis of telangiectatic osteosarcoma is partially based on the presence of multiple blood-filled spaces and intervening spongy tissue observed on gross pathologic evaluation. (*B*) Anaplastic tumor cells within the fibrous septa of a telangiectatic osteosarcoma (original magnification ×100). (*C*) Aneurysmal bone cyst with reactive granulation-like tissue, metaplastic ossification with osteoblastic rimming, and osteoclast-like giant cells within cyst walls (original magnification ×100).

active spindle cells with admixed inflammatory cells, reactive osteoid deposition, and granulation-like tissue, lacking overt cytologic atypia and extensive lesional necrosis (see **Fig. 6C**).[52] Because areas of ABC-like change may predominate in curettage specimens of telangiectatic OGS, the lesion should be thoroughly sampled before malignancy is excluded.

Demographics are not generally helpful in distinguishing ABC from telangiectatic OGS; however, whereas the posterior elements of the vertebrae, the small bones of the hands and feet, and craniofacial bones are common sites for ABC or its solid variant (sometimes referred to as giant cell reparative granuloma), these would be unusual locations for telangiectatic OGS.[60,78] Recently, a characteristic chromosomal anomaly involving 17p13 (site of the USP6 gene locus) has been reported in more than 60% of ABCs, which may eventually serve as a useful diagnostic marker.[79,80]

SMALL CELL OGS VERSUS OTHER SMALL ROUND CELL TUMORS OF BONE

The cytologic features of this rare variant of OGS may closely mimic Ewing sarcoma/primitive neuroectodermal tumor (ES/PNET), lymphoma, mesenchymal chondrosarcoma, or metastatic small round cell tumors.[81,82] The tumor cells in small cell OGS may be round or short spindle cells with minimal cytoplasm and hyperchromatic nuclei and can range from small to intermediate size.[8,82] With adequate sampling, close inspection of the tumor stroma discloses the presence of scant osteoid deposition between tumor cells (**Fig. 7A**).[9,82–84] The possibility that "tumor osteoid" is instead actually intercellular fibrin deposition often seen in ES/PNET should always be considered.[55,81,84] Demonstration of osteonectin or osteocalcin immunoreactivity within the intercellular matrix may be helpful in this regard.[83] The tendency for the tumor cells in small cell OGS to show variation in size and assume a spindled morphology is also helpful, as these features are not typical of either ES/PNET or lymphoma (see **Fig. 7B**). When tumor cartilage is present in small cell OGS, it is usually of intermediate to high histologic grade, and not the mature, low-grade type of hyaline cartilage seen in mesenchymal chondrosarcoma.[85] Conversely, when bone formation is seen in mesenchymal chondrosarcoma, it is either the result of enchondral ossification of hyaline cartilage or is metaplastic in origin.[52] Immunohistochemistry can be useful in excluding ES/PNET (FLI1-positive), mesenchymal chondrosarcoma (SOX9-positive), and lymphoma (CD45-positive).

In the appropriate clinical setting, lymphoblastic lymphoma should be excluded by immunohistochemical (IHC) staining for terminal deoxynucleotidyltransferase (TdT), as this tumor may coexpress CD99 and FLI1 in the absence of CD45 and CD20.[82] Also, it should be recalled that CD56 and CD99 can be expressed in both small cell OGS and ES/PNET[82]; however, CD99 staining in OGS is not usually membranous, as in ES/PNET. Preliminary evidence suggests that podoplanin (D2–40) may also be a useful diagnostic marker in this setting, staining small cell OGS (2 of 2 cases), but not ES/PNET (5 cases).[86] Molecular studies documenting the presence of one of the known genetic alterations of ES/PNET (ie, rearrangement of EWSR1 on chromosome 22q12) are extremely helpful in difficult cases, such as those with increased pleomorphism or artifactual spindling of tumor cells (see **Fig. 7C**).[55,81] The differential diagnosis with other small cell tumors of bone has recently been reviewed.[82,84]

LOW-GRADE INTRAOSSEOUS (CENTRAL) OGS VERSUS FIBROUS DYSPLASIA, OSTEOFIBROUS DYSPLASIA, AND DESMOPLASTIC FIBROMA

The low-grade intraosseous OGS is a rare and deceptively benign-appearing fibrous tumor associated with well-formed bony trabeculae and is often misdiagnosed as fibrous dysplasia or, less often, as desmoplastic fibroma.[52,87–89] It is histologically similar to parosteal osteosarcoma except for its anatomic location (see later in this article). Each of these tumors is characterized by abundant, relatively hypocellular collagenous or moderately cellular fibrous stroma (**Fig. 8**). The degree of osteoid production in low-grade intraosseous OGS is variable. Chondroid differentiation may also occur in this tumor, but is usually focal.[87–89] Although close scrutiny may disclose coarse trabeculae composed of admixed woven and lamellar bone, subtle cytologic atypia, and rare mitotic figures in low-grade intraosseous OGS (features not typically seen in fibrous dysplasia), these findings are easily overlooked.[8,52,55,60] Therefore, unless the periphery of the lesion is sampled where infiltration and permeation of preexisting host bone trabeculae may be observed, the tumor is likely to be histologically misinterpreted as fibrous dysplasia. Radiographic correlation is critical in these cases, as fibrous dysplasia will not show poorly marginated borders or aggressive growth patterns, such as cortical destruction and soft tissue extension.[8,55,60,78,87,88] Nevertheless, some cases of low-grade intraosseous

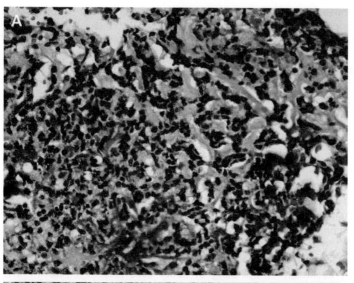

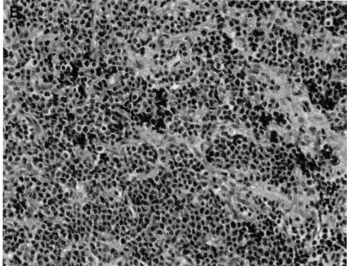

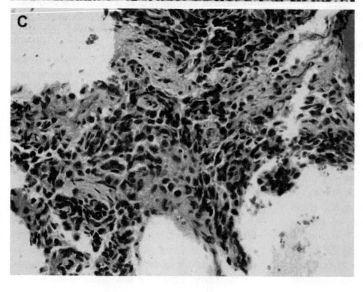

Fig. 7. Small cell osteosarcoma versus ES/PNET. (*A*) Small cell osteosarcoma with focal osteoid production by tumor cells that are slightly more pleomorphic than those typically seen in ES/PNET (original magnification ×200). (*B*) Typical ES/PNET with monotonous cell population showing little variation in size and no evidence of matrix production despite thorough sampling (original magnification ×100). (*C*) ES/PNET with focal spindling of tumor cells secondary to crush artifact during biopsy. Rearrangement of the *EWSR1* locus was confirmed by fluorescence in situ hybridization in this case (original magnification ×200).

Fig. 8. Low-grade intraosseous osteosarcoma versus fibrous dysplasia. (*A*) Low-grade intraosseous osteosarcoma with mature-appearing trabeculae of woven bone and moderately cellular fibrous stroma. In the absence of an infiltrative growth pattern, this tumor may be indistinguishable from fibrous dysplasia (original magnification ×40). Careful inspection may identify occasional cells with subtle nuclear enlargement and hyperchromasia (inset, original magnification ×200). (*B*) Fibrous dysplasia of bone with thin, delicate bony trabeculae and cellular fibrous stroma. Distinction from a malignant fibro-osseous proliferation may not be possible without radiographic and clinical correlation (original magnification ×200). (*C*) Desmoplastic fibroma of bone resembles desmoid fibromatosis of soft tissue and in contrast to low-grade intraosseous osteosarcoma, shows no osteoid deposition (original magnification ×200).

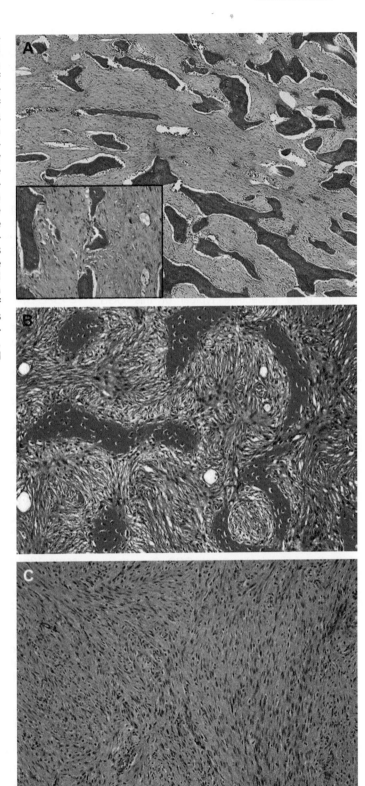

OGS will lack obvious radiographic signs of malignancy.[9,42]

It should also be recalled that low-grade intraosseous OGS is one of the few malignant bone-forming tumors that will occasionally display prominent osteoblast rimming.[52,87] This finding may raise the possibility of osteofibrous dysplasia (ossifying fibroma), but this lesion almost always involves the cortex of the tibia or fibula in young children.[52,78] Desmoplastic fibroma resembles desmoid fibromatosis of soft tissue, and is distinguished from low-grade intraosseous OGS by the complete absence of tumoral osteoid deposition, although non-neoplastic, reactive woven bone may be seen at the invasive front (see Fig. 8C).[60,87] Bone formation in fibroblastic OGS is typically much less extensive than that seen in low-grade intraosseous OGS, without the thick, mature bone trabeculae typical of this OGS subtype.[60]

A proportion (15%–65%) of low-grade intraosseous OGS cases are positive for amplification of chromosome 12q13-14, a molecular aberration that appears to be of diagnostic utility.[21,42,90] Indeed, subsequent studies have suggested that IHC for CDK4 and MDM2 are also useful markers in the differential diagnosis of this OGS variant.[91]

GIANT CELL-RICH OGS VERSUS GIANT CELL TUMOR OF BONE

Some cases of giant cell tumor of bone (GCT) show histologic features of malignancy, such as a high mitotic rate, tumor necrosis, and even lymphovascular invasion, which can complicate the distinction from giant cell–rich OGS. Sometimes the age of the patient and anatomic location of the tumor can assist in the differential diagnosis; an epiphyseal tumor in a skeletally mature patient is much more likely to be a GCT than a giant cell–rich OGS.[52,55,60,92] The production of metaplastic or reactive-type woven bone is well known to occur in GCT, particularly at its peripheral aspects (Fig. 9)[52]; however, osteoid deposited in irregular clumps or sheets without associated reactive osteoblasts should alert the observer to the possibility of a giant cell–rich OGS.[52,93] The presence of a cartilage matrix in the absence of fracture callus should also raise this suspicion.[52] Marked nuclear atypia and/or atypical mitotic figures help to confirm this impression (see Fig. 9).[55,60,92] Rare cases with a high-grade spindle cell sarcoma arising in association with an otherwise typical GCT are perhaps best considered primary malignant GCT, but if identified, the presence of an associated osteosarcomatous component should be reported for treatment purposes. Of potential diagnostic significance is a recent study demonstrating podoplanin (D2–40) expression in 22 of 26 OGS and only 1 of 7 GCT.[86]

JUXTACORTICAL AND SURFACE VARIANTS

Accurate classification of surface or juxtacortical OGS is important for clinical management, as these OGS variants are characterized by different biologic behavior (Table 4).[94] The current World Health Organization classification can be used to define low-grade (parosteal OGS), intermediate-grade (periosteal OGS), and high-grade tumors (dedifferentiated parosteal OGS and high-grade surface OGS) (see Table 1).[38,43,95,96]

PAROSTEAL OGS VERSUS FIBROUS DYSPLASIA

This surface OGS is histologically low grade, similar to low-grade intraosseous OGS except for its anatomic location and typically dense pattern of mineralization. Besides its marked predilection for the posterior aspect of the distal femoral or proximal tibial metaphysis, this tumor is also characterized by its mushroom-type growth pattern resulting in circumferential growth with minimal periosteal reaction or intramedullary extension (Fig. 10A, B).[43,55] Its histologic hallmark is production of thick, often parallel, arrays of bony trabeculae associated with a moderately cellular fibrous stroma (see Fig. 10C).[43,55] In some cases, the woven bone may focally mature into lamellar bone.[52,94] Like low-grade intraosseous OGS, parosteal OGS also shows amplification of chromosome 12q13-15 in most cases.[21,43,55,97] As for low-grade intraosseous OGS, IHC for CDK4 and MDM2 may be useful in difficult cases.[91,98] Although this tumor is considered low grade and typically has an excellent prognosis, careful gross and microscopic evaluation of the specimen should be performed to exclude the possibility of dedifferentiation, particularly in recurrent tumors, which usually manifests as a histologically high-grade OGS, fibrosarcoma, or UPS.[50,94]

PAROSTEAL OGS VERSUS OSTEOCHONDROMA

Nodules of tumor cartilage are sometimes present within parosteal OGS, either intermixed with the neoplastic bone or arrayed along the peripheral aspect of the tumor, where it may mimic the cartilaginous cap of an osteochondroma (see Fig. 10D); however, the chondrocytes within malignant cartilage caps are atypical and fail to

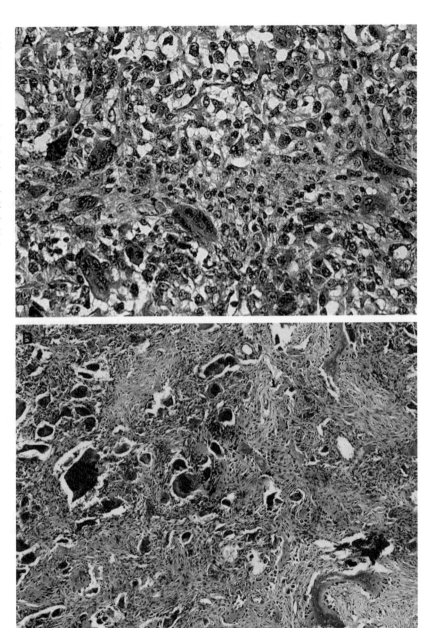

Fig. 9. Giant cell–rich osteosarcoma versus giant cell tumor of bone. (*A*) Giant cell–rich osteosarcoma with focal osteoid deposition (top of field) by cytologically atypical stromal cells with admixed benign osteoclast-like giant cells (original magnification ×200). (*B*) Giant cell tumor of bone with focal metaplastic ossification and no significant degree of cytologic atypia or abnormal mitotic figures (original magnification ×40).

demonstrate the orderly maturation into lamellar bone seen in osteochondroma.[43,55,60] In addition, in the absence of traumatic injury, the intertrabecular spaces of osteochondroma are not composed of fibrous stroma, but rather fatty or hematopoietic marrow.[8,60] Cross-sectional radiographic studies usually demonstrate continuity between the medullary cavity of the involved bone and the stalk of osteochondroma, whereas the cortical bone underlying parosteal OGS is intact.[60]

PAROSTEAL OGS VERSUS HETEROTOPIC OSSIFICATION

Heterotopic ossification can be easily distinguished because it is not attached to the underlying bone, and regardless of the maturation stage of the lesion, the stroma is not dense and fibrous, as in parosteal OGS.[55] Radiographically, heterotopic ossification tends to be more radiodense at its

Table 4
Differential diagnosis: surface/juxtacortical osteosarcoma

Osteosarcoma Subtype	Differential Diagnosis
Parosteal osteosarcoma (low grade) • Similar to low-grade intraosseous OGS, but arises from outer layer of periosteum • Strong predilection for posterior aspect of distal femur • No periosteal reaction • Hypocellular fibrous stroma with mild cytologic atypia • Long parallel streamers of well-formed bone • May have disorganized cartilage at periphery • Amplification of chromosome 12q13-15 • May undergo dedifferentiation to high-grade osteosarcoma	Osteochondroma • Benign outgrowth of bone and cartilage recapitulating growth plate • Cartilaginous cap undergoes orderly maturation to bone • Continuity between stalk and with medullary cavity of involved bone can be demonstrated grossly or radiographically • Fatty or hematopoietic bone marrow; no fibrous intertrabecular stroma • Normal mature cortical and trabecular bone Heterotopic ossification • Not attached to bone • Zonated architecture with cellular spindled stroma in center and maturing bone at periphery Surface osteoma • Mature trabecular and cortical bone with fatty or hematopoietic bone marrow • No fibrous intertrabecular stroma
Periosteal osteosarcoma (intermediate grade) • Histologically similar to chondroblastic osteosarcoma • Arises from inner layer of periosteum, without medullary involvement	Chondroblastic osteosarcoma • Intramedullary tumor that may extend outside the bone and show periosteal elevation, but not arising from periosteum Periosteal chondrosarcoma • Rare tumor in older patient; no periosteal reaction • May show enchondral ossification but no tumor osteoid
High-grade surface osteosarcoma • Histologically resembles conventional high-grade OGS, usually osteoblastic or fibroblastic type	Reactive surface lesions • Can be hypercellular and mitotically active • Lack unequivocal cellular anaplasia • Show organization or zonation pattern • Often arise on bones of acral skeleton

periphery, as opposed to the increased central density seen in parosteal OGS.[60]

PAROSTEAL OGS VERSUS SURFACE OSTEOMA

Surface osteomas are composed of mature cortical and cancellous lamellar bone with intertrabecular hematopoietic bone marrow or fat and lack the dense fibrous stroma and cartilaginous foci seen in parosteal OGS.[52,55,60,99] Radiographic features may be distinctive as well, as osteoma has a circumscribed, uniformly and densely sclerotic lesional border whereas parosteal OGS often shows variable radiographic density at its periphery.[100]

PAROSTEAL OGS VERSUS HIGH-GRADE SURFACE OSTEOSARCOMA

High-grade surface OGS is a very rare subtype of surface OGS, almost always involving long bones.[94,101] Typical cases resemble conventional intramedullary OGS of osteoblastic or fibroblastic type, and lack the low-grade, densely mineralized component of parosteal OGS. In addition, high-grade surface OGS has a broad attachment to the underlying cortex, such that a radiolucent zone between the tumor and cortical bone is not seen, as in parosteal OGS; however, it should also be recalled that approximately 25% of parosteal OGS undergoes dedifferentiation to high-grade OGS

Fig. 10. Parosteal osteosarcoma versus osteochondroma. (*A*) Lateral radiograph of parosteal osteosarcoma showing classic anatomic location (posterior distal femur) of this well-defined and densely mineralized lesion. Note the mushroom-type growth pattern and absence of periosteal response. (*Courtesy of* John J. Block, MD, Nashville, TN.) (*B*) Parosteal osteosarcoma arises from the periosteal surface and grows circumferentially around the cortex with minimal, if any involvement of medullary cavity.

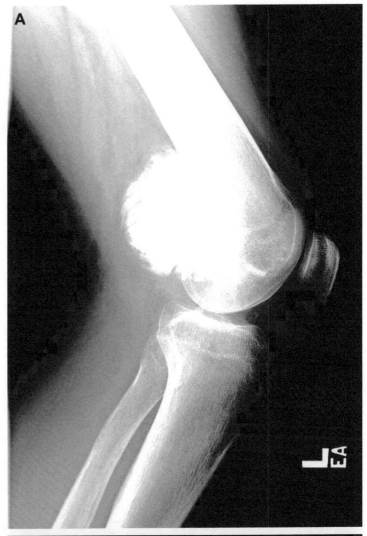

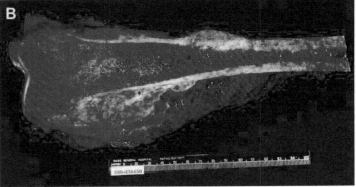

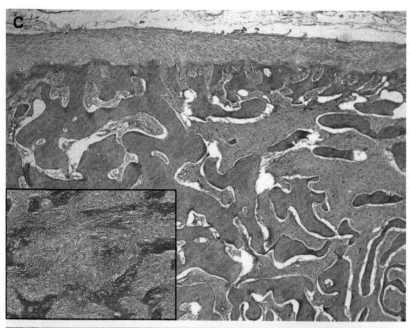

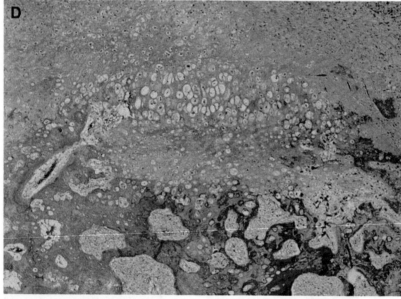

Fig. 10. (*C*) Parosteal osteosarcoma histologically resembles low-grade intraosseous osteosarcoma and lacks the mature cortical and cancellous lamellar bone and fatty marrow characteristic of surface osteoma (original magnification ×40). It is also one of the few malignant bone-forming lesions that can demonstrate pronounced osteoblastic rimming (inset, original magnification ×100). (*D*) A subset of parosteal osteosarcoma has a peripheral cartilaginous cap. Distinction from osteochondroma is based on the presence of cytologic atypia in the cartilaginous or fibrous cap, a fibrous intertrabecular stroma and an intact underlying cortex (original magnification ×100).

(particularly in recurrent lesions).[102–104] Therefore, the presence of a high-grade component should always be searched for when evaluating juxtacortical bone-forming lesions.

PERIOSTEAL OGS VERSUS CHONDROBLASTIC OGS

Periosteal OGS is an intermediate-grade chondroblastic OGS that most often originates from the cortex of the diaphysis or metaphysis of the tibia or femur in adolescents and young adults.[50,95] The prototypical case presents radiographically as a relatively small (often around 3 cm) concave lucency of the cortex with mineralized bone spicules oriented perpendicular to the cortical surface (so-called "sunburst" pattern) and an aggressive periosteal reaction.[49,50,60] The cut surface is typically chondroid with irregular areas of mineralization. Gross evaluation confirms origin from the periosteum with complete or near complete lack of intramedullary involvement, thereby excluding the diagnosis of intramedullary chondroblastic OGS (**Fig. 11A**).[60] Histologically, it resembles conventional chondroblastic OGS, with lobules of malignant cartilage harboring easily recognized cytologic atypia and mitotic activity (see **Fig. 11B**). Neoplastic bone spicules may be seen either within or at the periphery of the chondroid lobules, often arrayed perpendicular to the cortical surface, accounting for its distinctive radiologic appearance (see **Fig. 11C**).[49,50,94,95]

PERIOSTEAL OGS VERSUS HIGH-GRADE SURFACE OSTEOSARCOMA

When the tumor matrix of high-grade surface OGS is predominantly osteoblastic or fibroblastic,

distinction from periosteal OGS is straightforward[60,94,101]; however, rare cases with abundant chondroblastic differentiation may be very difficult to distinguish from periosteal OGS. For practical purposes, if the degree of cytologic atypia is severe, the tumor should be considered high grade, and by definition, not diagnostic of periosteal OGS, which is an intermediate-grade sarcoma.[95,96]

PERIOSTEAL OGS VERSUS JUXTACORTICAL/ PERIOSTEAL CHONDROSARCOMA AND OSTEOCHONDROMA

Periosteal OGS and juxtacortical/periosteal chondrosarcoma arise from the periosteum and produce abundant neoplastic cartilage, sometimes

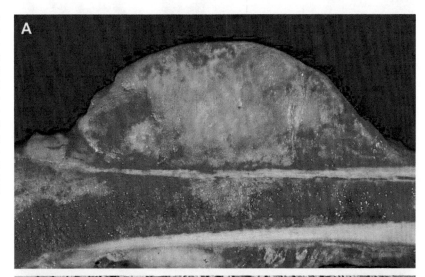

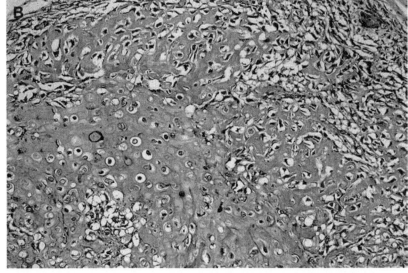

Fig. 11. Periosteal osteosarcoma versus periosteal chondrosarcoma. (*A*) Periosteal osteosarcoma arises from the periosteum, has a glistening, chondroid cut surface, and can generate a reactive periosteal response (seen at the right aspect of the tumor). (*B*) Histologically, periosteal osteosarcoma resembles chondroblastic osteosarcoma (original magnification ×200).

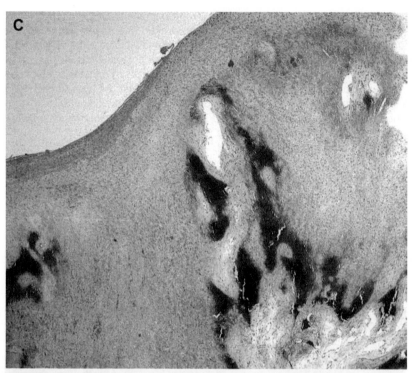

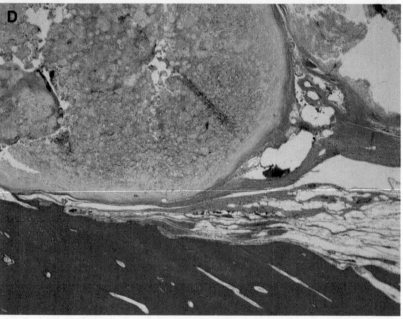

Fig. 11. (*C*) Ossification of matrix within and adjacent to the chondroid nodules generates perpendicular spicules of intralesional bone, which are helpful in the radiographic differential diagnosis (original magnification ×20). (*D*) In contrast, periosteal chondrosarcoma is characteristically a low-grade lesion, lacks associated neoplastic osteoid, and generates a minimal periosteal response (original magnification ×20).

Fig. 12. Surface osteosarcoma versus reactive surface lesions. (*A*) Parosteal myositis ossificans usually demonstrates some degree of zonation and never shows unequivocal cytologic atypia. In this case, an immature-appearing, hypercellular, and mitotically active fibrous proliferation (*top left*) merges with areas of dense woven bone deposition (*bottom right*) (original magnification ×100). (*B*) Bizarre parosteal osteochondromatous proliferation is characterized by a proliferative and hypercellular cartilage cap undergoing enchondral ossification to "blue bone" and bony trabeculae within a loose fibrovascular stroma (original magnification ×40). (*C*) Subungual exostosis is histologically similar to other reactive surface lesions but often appears more mature with well-formed bony trabeculae (original magnification ×100).

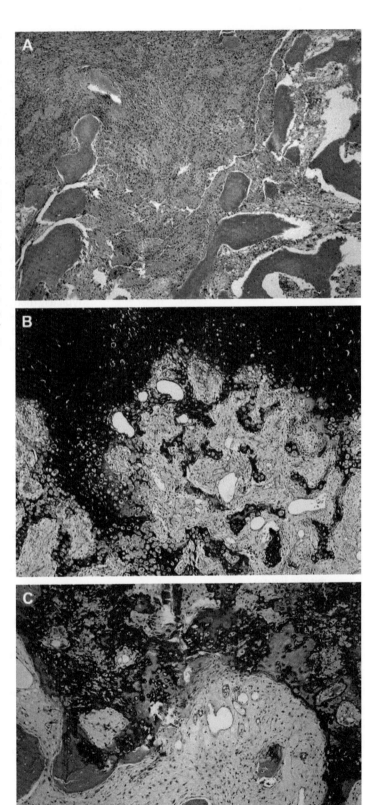

generating a difficult differential diagnosis. Periosteal chondrosarcoma affects older patients, however, and shows subtle radiographic differences (coarser and more extensive peripheral mineralization and minimal periosteal reaction).[60] Histologically, the cartilage of periosteal chondrosarcoma is relatively mature, predominantly low grade, and associated with enchondral or reactive ossification (see Fig. 11D), whereas the chondroid matrix of periosteal osteosarcoma is of higher histologic grade, shows peripheral hypercellularity, and merges with adjacent spindle cell stroma, similar to conventional chondroblastic OGS.[51,52,55,60,105]

In contrast with osteochondroma, the neoplastic cartilage of periosteal OGS shows cytologic atypia and lacks orderly enchondral ossification of subjacent bony trabeculae seen in osteochondroma. In addition, communication of the fatty marrow of the stalk and the underlying medullary cavity characteristic of osteochondroma does not occur in periosteal OGS.

JUXTACORTICAL OGS VERSUS REACTIVE SURFACE LESIONS

Reactive surface lesions, such as parosteal myositis ossificans, florid periostitis, bizarre parosteal osteochondromatous proliferation (BPOP, Nora lesion), acquired osteochondroma (turret exostosis), and subungual exostosis can mimic a variety of OGS subtypes (Fig. 12); however, they all lack bona fide nuclear anaplasia, demonstrate some degree of zonation or organization (histologically or radiographically), and tend to involve acral bones, which help to exclude the diagnosis of malignancy in most cases.[60] For instance, although the proliferative cartilage seen in BPOP is hypercellular and can be cytologically atypical, examination of the lesion at low power demonstrates zones of enchondral ossification typically merging with immature trabeculae (sometimes composed of curious "blue bone") and intervening bland, paucicellular fibrovascular tissue (see Fig. 12B).[55,60]

Box 1
Common pitfalls in the diagnosis of osteosarcoma

- Missing an osteosarcoma:
  - Examine the tumor under high-power magnification to exclude the presence of malignant cells associated with osteoid production, particularly in cystic and giant cell–rich lesions
  - Always correlate histologic findings with radiographic features
- Mistaking osteoblastoma for OGS:
  - Correlate with the clinical history and radiographic features
  - Examine the peripheral aspects (if sampled) for histologic evidence of permeative, infiltrative growth
  - Look for atypical osteoblasts focally in sheets filling intertrabecular spaces and displaying atypical mitotic figures
- Distinguishing chondroblastic OGS from chondrosarcoma:
  - Hypercellular spindle cells merging with sarcomatous stroma at the periphery of the chondroid nodules favors OGS
  - Look for diagnostic neoplastic bone deposition in between chondroid lobules
- Mistaking fibroblastic OGS for another type of skeletal sarcoma:
  - Look for subtle or focal chondro-osseous matrix deposition within the fibrous stroma
  - Rule out other sarcomas with IHC, if indicated
- Mistaking telangiectatic OGS for aneurysmal bone cyst
  - Examine the cyst walls carefully for the presence of atypical cells or atypical mitotic figures
- Mistaking low-grade OGS for benign lesions:
  - Be aware of the clinicopathologic features of low-grade OGS
  - Look for histologic evidence of a permeative, infiltrative growth pattern with entrapment of pre-existing bone trabeculae
  - Look for subtle nuclear enlargement or hyperchromasia and scattered mitotic figures

SUMMARY

The myriad of radiographic and histologic manifestations of OGS sometimes generates difficult diagnostic problems. There exist many pseudo-sarcomatous lesions that closely mimic the various subtypes of OGS, as well as relatively rare, deceptively benign, low-grade variants of OGS. Errors can be easily made when strict diagnostic criteria are not applied or when a diagnosis is rendered without correlation with pertinent radiographic findings (Box 1).

REFERENCES

1. Damron TA, Ward WG, Stewart A. Osteosarcoma, chondrosarcoma, and Ewing's sarcoma: National Cancer Data Base Report. Clin Orthop Relat Res 2007;459:40–7.
2. Eyre R, Feltbower RG, Mubwandarikwa E, et al. Epidemiology of bone tumours in children and young adults. Pediatr Blood Cancer 2009;53(6): 941–52.
3. Mascarenhas L, Siegel S, Spector L, et al. Malignant bone tumors. In: Bleyer A, O'Leary M, Barr R, et al, editors. Cancer epidemiology in older adolescents and young adults 15 to 29 years of age, including SEER incidence and survival: 1975-2000. Bethesda (MD): National Cancer Institute; 2006. NIH Pub. No. 06–5767. p. 97–109.
4. Mirabello L, Troisi RJ, Savage SA. Osteosarcoma incidence and survival rates from 1973 to 2004: data from the Surveillance, Epidemiology, and End Results Program. Cancer 2009;115(7):1531–43.
5. Ries LA, Young JL, Keel GE, et al. Cancers of the bone and joint. Bethesda (MD): National Cancer Institute; 2007. SEER Program, NIH Pub. No. 07–6215.
6. Stiller CA, Bielack SS, Jundt G, et al. Bone tumours in European children and adolescents, 1978-1997. Report from the automated childhood cancer information system project. Eur J Cancer 2006;42(13): 2124–35.
7. Ottaviani G, Jaffe N. The epidemiology of osteosarcoma. Cancer Treat Res 2010;152:3–13.
8. Klein MJ, Siegal GP. Osteosarcoma: anatomic and histologic variants. Am J Clin Pathol 2006;125(4): 555–81.
9. Raymond AK, Jaffe N. Osteosarcoma multidisciplinary approach to the management from the pathologist's perspective. Cancer Treat Res 2010; 152:63–84.
10. Bridge JA, Sandberg AA. Cytogenetic and molecular genetic techniques as adjunctive approaches in the diagnosis of bone and soft tissue tumors. Skeletal Radiol 2000;29(5):249–58.
11. Fuchs B, Pritchard DJ. Etiology of osteosarcoma. Clin Orthop Relat Res 2002;397:40–52.
12. Gorlick R. Current concepts on the molecular biology of osteosarcoma. Cancer Treat Res 2010; 152:467–78.
13. Gorlick R, Khanna C. Osteosarcoma. J Bone Miner Res 2010;25(4):683–91.
14. Geryk-Hall M, Hughes DP. Critical signaling pathways in bone sarcoma: candidates for therapeutic interventions. Curr Oncol Rep 2009;11(6): 446–53.
15. Hayden JB, Hoang BH. Osteosarcoma: basic science and clinical implications. Orthop Clin North Am 2006;37(1):1–7.
16. Kansara M, Thomas DM. Molecular pathogenesis of osteosarcoma. DNA Cell Biol 2007;26(1):1–18.
17. Khanna C. Novel targets with potential therapeutic applications in osteosarcoma. Curr Oncol Rep 2008;10(4):350–8.
18. Ottaviani G, Jaffe N. The etiology of osteosarcoma. Cancer Treat Res 2010;152:15–32.
19. Papachristou D, Papavassiliou A. Osteosarcoma and chondrosarcoma: new signaling pathways as targets for novel therapeutic interventions. Int J Biochem Cell Biol 2007;39(5):857–62.
20. Ragland BD, Bell WC, Lopez RR, et al. Cytogenetics and molecular biology of osteosarcoma. Lab Invest 2002;82(4):365–73.
21. Sandberg AA, Bridge JA. Updates on the cytogenetics and molecular genetics of bone and soft tissue tumors: osteosarcoma and related tumors. Cancer Genet Cytogenet 2003;145(1):1–30.
22. Wachtel M, Schafer BW. Targets for cancer therapy in childhood sarcomas. Cancer Treat Rev 2010; 36(4):318–27.
23. Wang LL. Biology of osteogenic sarcoma. Cancer J 2005;11(4):294–305.
24. Bielack S, Carrle D, Casali PG. Osteosarcoma: ESMO clinical recommendations for diagnosis, treatment and follow-up. Ann Oncol 2009;20(Suppl 4):137–9.
25. Bielack SS, Carrle D. State-of-the-art approach in selective curable tumors: bone sarcoma. Ann Oncol 2008;19(Suppl 7):vii155–60.
26. Ferrari S, Palmerini E, Staals EL, et al. The treatment of nonmetastatic high grade osteosarcoma of the extremity: review of the Italian Rizzoli experience. Impact on the future. Cancer Treat Res 2010; 152:275–87.
27. Heare T, Hensley MA, Dell'Orfano S. Bone tumors: osteosarcoma and Ewing's sarcoma. Curr Opin Pediatr 2009;21(3):365–72.
28. Jaffe N. Osteosarcoma: review of the past, impact on the future. The American experience. Cancer Treat Res 2010;152:239–62.
29. Biermann JS, Adkins DR, Benjamin RS, et al. National Comprehensive Cancer Network Bone Cancer Panel. Bone cancer. J Natl Compr Canc Netw 2010;8(6):688–712.

30. Saeter G. Osteosarcoma: ESMO clinical recommendations for diagnosis, treatment and follow-up. Ann Oncol 2007;18(Suppl 2):ii77–8.

31. Ta H, Dass C, Choong P, et al. Osteosarcoma treatment: state of the art. Cancer Metastasis Rev 2009; 28(1–2):247–63.

32. Bakhshi S, Radhakrishnan V. Prognostic markers in osteosarcoma. Expert Rev Anticancer Ther 2010; 10(2):271–87.

33. Bielack SS, Kempf-Bielack B, Delling G, et al. Prognostic factors in high-grade osteosarcoma of the extremities or trunk: an analysis of 1,702 patients treated on neoadjuvant cooperative osteosarcoma study group protocols. J Clin Oncol 2002;20(3): 776–90.

34. Bramer JA, van Linge JH, Grimer RJ, et al. Prognostic factors in localized extremity osteosarcoma: a systematic review. Eur J Surg Oncol 2009;35(10): 1030–6.

35. Clark JC, Dass CR, Choong PF. A review of clinical and molecular prognostic factors in osteosarcoma. J Cancer Res Clin Oncol 2008;134(3):281–97.

36. Kim SY, Helman LJ. Strategies to explore new approaches in the investigation and treatment of osteosarcoma. Cancer Treat Res 2010;152:517–28.

37. Abdul-Karim FW, Bauer TW, Kilpatrick SE, et al. Recommendations for the reporting of bone tumors. Hum Pathol 2004;35(10):1173–8.

38. Rubin BP, Antonescu CR, Gannon FH, et al. "Protocol for the examination of specimens from patients with tumors of bone" College of American Pathologists (CAP) Cancer Protocols and Checklists. Available at: http://www.cap.org. Accessed October 15, 2010.

39. Benjamin RS, Patel SR. Pediatric and adult osteosarcoma: comparisons and contrasts in presentation and therapy. Cancer Treat Res 2010;152: 355–63.

40. Longhi A, Errani C, Gonzales-Arabio D, et al. Osteosarcoma in patients older than 65 years. J Clin Oncol 2008;26(33):5368–73.

41. Deyrup AT, Montag AG, Inwards CY, et al. Sarcomas arising in Paget disease of bone: a clinicopathologic analysis of 70 cases. Arch Pathol Lab Med 2007;131(6):942–6.

42. Inwards CY, Knuutila S. Low grade central osteosarcoma. In: Fletcher CD, Unni KK, Mertens F, editors. World Health Organization classification of tumours: pathology and genetics of tumours of soft tissue and bone. Lyon (France): IARC Press; 2002. p. 275–6.

43. Unni KK, Knuutila S. Parosteal osteosarcoma. In: Fletcher CD, Unni KK, Mertens F, editors. World Health Organization classification of tumours: pathology and genetics of tumours of soft tissue and bone. Lyon (France): IARC Press; 2002. p. 279–81.

44. Han I, Oh JH, Na YG, et al. Clinical outcome of parosteal osteosarcoma. J Surg Oncol 2008;97(2): 146–9.

45. Edge SB, Byrd DR, Compton CC, et al. AJCC cancer staging manual. 7th edition. New York: Springer; 2010.

46. Enneking WF, Spanier SS, Goodman MA. A system for the surgical staging of musculoskeletal sarcoma. Clin Orthop Relat Res 1980;153: 106–20.

47. Reith JD. Protocols for the examination and reporting of bone and soft tissue tumors–letter. Arch Pathol Lab Med 2007;131:680–1.

48. Raymond AK, Ayala AG, Knuutila S. Conventional osteosarcoma. In: Fletcher CD, Unni KK, Mertens F, editors. World Health Organization classification of tumours: pathology and genetics of tumours of soft tissue and bone. Lyon (France): IARC Press; 2002. p. 264–70.

49. Dahlin DC, Unni KK. Osteosarcoma of bone and its important recognizable varieties. Am J Surg Pathol 1977;1(1):61–72.

50. Unni KK, Dahlin DC. Osteosarcoma—pathology and classification. Semin Roentgenol 1989;24(3):143–52.

51. Carter JR, Abdul-Karim FW. Pathology of childhood osteosarcoma. In: Rosenberg HS, Bernstein J, Newton WA, editors, Perspectives in pediatric pathology, vol. 9. New York: S. Karger Ag; 1987. p. 133–70.

52. Mirra JM, Picci P, Gold RH. Bone tumors: clinical, radiologic, and pathologic correlations. Philadelphia: Lea & Febiger; 1989.

53. Klein MJ. Radiographic correlation in orthopedic pathology. Adv Anat Pathol 2005;12(4):155–79.

54. Malcolm AJ, Schiller AL, Schneider-Stock R. Osteoblastoma. In: Fletcher CD, Unni KK, Mertens F, editors. World Health Organization classification of tumours: pathology and genetics of tumours of soft tissue and bone. Lyon (France): IARC Press; 2002. p. 262–3.

55. Unni KK, Inwards CY, Bridge JA, et al. Atlas of tumor pathology: tumors of the bones and joints. Washington, DC: Armed Forces Institute of Pathology; 2005.

56. Lucas D. Osteoblastoma. Arch Pathol Lab Med 2010;134(10):1460–6.

57. Lucas DR, Unni KK, McLeod RA, et al. Osteoblastoma: clinicopathologic study of 306 cases. Hum Pathol 1994;25(2):117–34.

58. McLeod RA, Dahlin DC, Beabout JW. The spectrum of osteoblastoma. AJR Am J Roentgenol 1976; 126(2):321–5.

59. Deyrup AT, Montag AG. Epithelioid and epithelial neoplasms of bone. Arch Pathol Lab Med 2007; 131(2):205–16.

60. Dorfman HD, Czerniak B. Bone tumors. St Louis (MO): Mosby; 1998.

61. Bahk WJ, Mirra JM. Pseudoanaplastic tumors of bone. Skeletal Radiol 2004;33(11):641–8.

62. Bertoni F, Unni KK, Lucas DR, et al. Osteoblastoma with cartilaginous matrix. An unusual morphologic presentation in 18 cases. Am J Surg Pathol 1993; 17(1):69–74.

63. Dorfman HD, Weiss SW. Borderline osteoblastic tumors: problems in the differential diagnosis of aggressive osteoblastoma and low-grade osteosarcoma. Semin Diagn Pathol 1984;1(3):215–34.

64. Oliveira CR, Mendonca BB, Camargo OP, et al. Classical osteoblastoma, atypical osteoblastoma, and osteosarcoma: a comparative study based on clinical, histological, and biological parameters. Clinics (Sao Paulo) 2007;62(2):167–74.

65. Bertoni F, Bacchini P, Donati D, et al. Osteoblastoma-like osteosarcoma. The Rizzoli Institute experience. Mod Pathol 1993;6(6):707–16.

66. Bertoni F, Unni KK, McLeod RA, et al. Osteosarcoma resembling osteoblastoma. Cancer 1985; 55(2):416–26.

67. Hosono A, Yamaguchi U, Makimoto A, et al. Utility of immunohistochemical analysis for cyclo-oxygenase 2 in the differential diagnosis of osteoblastoma and osteosarcoma. J Clin Pathol 2007;60(4):410–4.

68. Baruffi MR, Volpon JB, Neto JB, et al. Osteoid osteomas with chromosome alterations involving 22q. Cancer Genet Cytogenet 2001;124(2):127–31.

69. Carsi B, Rock MG. Primary osteosarcoma in adults older than 40 years. Clin Orthop Relat Res 2002; 397:53–61.

70. Sergi C, Zwerschke W. Osteogenic sarcoma (osteosarcoma) in the elderly: tumor delineation and predisposing conditions. Exp Gerontol 2008; 43(12):1039–43.

71. Salas S, de Pinieux G, Gomez-Brouchet A, et al. Ezrin immunohistochemical expression in cartilaginous tumours: a useful tool for differential diagnosis between chondroblastic osteosarcoma and chondrosarcoma. Virchows Arch 2009;454(1):81–7.

72. Gomez-Brouchet A, Mourcin F, Gourault PA, et al. Galectin-1 is a powerful marker to distinguish chondroblastic osteosarcoma and conventional chondrosarcoma. Hum Pathol 2010;41(9):1220–30.

73. Huvos AG, Heilweil M, Bretsky SS. The pathology of malignant fibrous histiocytoma of bone. A study of 130 patients. Am J Surg Pathol 1985;9(12):853–71.

74. Jeon DG, Song WS, Kong CB, et al. MFH of bone and osteosarcoma show similar survival and chemosensitivity. Clin Orthop Relat Res 2011;469(2): 584–90.

75. Naka T, Fukuda T, Shinohara N, et al. Osteosarcoma versus malignant fibrous histiocytoma of bone in patients older than 40 years. A clinicopathologic and immunohistochemical analysis with special reference to malignant fibrous histiocytoma-like osteosarcoma. Cancer 1995;76(6):972–84.

76. Adelani M, Schultenover S, Holt G, et al. Primary leiomyosarcoma of extragnathic bone: clinicopathologic features and reevaluation of prognosis. Arch Pathol Lab Med 2009;133(9):1448–56.

77. Matsuno T, Okada K, Knuutila S. Telangiectatic osteosarcoma. In: Fletcher CD, Unni KK, Mertens F, editors. World Health Organization classification of tumours: pathology and genetics of tumours of soft tissue and bone. Lyon (France): IARC Press; 2002. p. 271–2.

78. Raymond AK, Jaffe N. Conditions that mimic osteosarcoma. Cancer Treat Res 2010;152:85–121.

79. Oliveira AM, Hsi BL, Weremowicz S, et al. USP6 (Tre2) fusion oncogenes in aneurysmal bone cyst. Cancer Res 2004;64(6):1920–3.

80. Oliveira AM, Perez-Atayde AR, Inwards CY, et al. USP6 and CDH11 oncogenes identify the neoplastic cell in primary aneurysmal bone cysts and are absent in so-called secondary aneurysmal bone cysts. Am J Pathol 2004;165(5):1773–80.

81. Kalil R, Bridge JA. Small cell osteosarcoma. In: Fletcher CD, Unni KK, Mertens F, editors. World Health Organization classification of tumours: pathology and genetics of tumours of soft tissue and bone. Lyon (France): IARC Press; 2002. p. 273–4.

82. Li S, Siegal GP. Small cell tumors of bone. Adv Anat Pathol 2010;17(1):1–11.

83. Machado I, Alberghini M, Giner F, et al. Histopathological characterization of small cell osteosarcoma with immunohistochemistry and molecular genetic support. A study of 10 cases. Histopathology 2010;57:162–7.

84. Bishop JA, Shum CH, Sheth S, et al. Small cell osteosarcoma: cytopathologic characteristics and differential diagnosis. Am J Clin Pathol 2010; 133(5):756–61.

85. Ayala AG, Ro JY, Raymond AK, et al. Small cell osteosarcoma—a clinicopathologic study of 27 cases. Cancer 1989;64(10):2162–73.

86. Ariizumi T, Ogose A, Kawashima H, et al. Expression of podoplanin in human bone and bone tumors: new marker of osteogenic and chondrogenic bone tumors. Pathol Int 2010;60(3):193–202.

87. Unni KK, Dahlin DC, McLeod RA, et al. Intraosseous well-differentiated osteosarcoma. Cancer 1977;40(3):1337–47.

88. Kurt AM, Unni KK, McLeod RA, et al. Low-grade intraosseous osteosarcoma. Cancer 1990;65(6):1418–28.

89. Bertoni F, Bacchini P, Fabbri N, et al. Osteosarcoma: low-grade intraosseous-type osteosarcoma, histologically resembling parosteal osteosarcoma, fibrous dysplasia, and desmoplastic fibroma. Cancer 1993;71(2):338–45.

90. Ragazzini P, Gamberi G, Benassi MS, et al. Analysis of SAS gene and CDK4 and MDM2 proteins in low-grade osteosarcoma. Cancer Detect Prev 1999;23(2):129–36.

91. Yoshida A, Ushiku T, Motoi T, et al. Immuno-histochemical analysis of MDM2 and CDK4 distinguishes low-grade osteosarcoma from benign mimics. Mod Pathol 2010;23(9):1279–88.

92. Bathurst N, Sanerkin N, Watt I. Osteoclast-rich osteosarcoma. Br J Radiol 1986;59(703):667–73.

93. Horvai A, Unni KK. Premalignant conditions of bone. J Orthop Sci 2006;11(4):412–23.

94. Raymond AK. Surface osteosarcoma. Clin Orthop Relat Res 1991;(270):140–8.

95. Ayala AG, Raymond AK, Czerniak B, et al. Periosteal osteosarcoma. In: Fletcher CD, Unni KK, Mertens F, editors. World Health Organization classification of tumours: pathology and genetics of tumours of soft tissue and bone. Lyon (France): IARC Press; 2002. p. 282–3.

96. Wold L, McCarthy EF, Knuutila S. High-grade surface osteosarcoma. In: Fletcher CD, Unni KK, Mertens F, editors. World Health Organization classification of tumours: pathology and genetics of tumours of soft tissue and bone. Lyon (France): IARC Press; 2002. p. 284–5.

97. Mejia-Guerrero S, Quejada M, Gokgoz N, et al. Characterization of the 12q15 MDM2 and 12q13-14 CDK4 amplicons and clinical correlations in osteosarcoma. Genes Chromosomes Cancer 2010; 49(6):518–25.

98. Gamberi G, Ragazzini P, Benassi MS, et al. Analysis of 12q13-15 genes in parosteal osteosarcoma. Clin Orthop Relat Res 2000;377:195–204.

99. Nielsen GP, Rosenberg AE. Update on bone forming tumors of the head and neck. Head Neck Pathol 2007;1(1):87–93.

100. Greenspan A. Benign bone-forming lesions: osteoma, osteoid osteoma, and osteoblastoma. Clinical, imaging, pathologic, and differential considerations. Skeletal Radiol 1993;22(7):485–500.

101. Okada K, Unni KK, Swee RG, et al. High grade surface osteosarcoma: a clinicopathologic study of 46 cases. Cancer 1999;85(5):1044–54.

102. Bertoni F, Bacchini P, Staals EL, et al. Dedifferentiated parosteal osteosarcoma: the experience of the Rizzoli Institute. Cancer 2005;103(11):2372–82.

103. Sheth DS, Yasko AW, Raymond AK, et al. Conventional and dedifferentiated parosteal osteosarcoma. Diagnosis, treatment, and outcome. Cancer 1996; 78(10):2136–45.

104. Wold LE, Unni KK, Beabout JW, et al. Dedifferentiated parosteal osteosarcoma. J Bone Joint Surg Am 1984;66(1):53–9.

105. Bertoni F, Boriani S, Laus M, et al. Periosteal chondrosarcoma and periosteal osteosarcoma. Two distinct entities. J Bone Joint Surg Br 1982;64(3): 370–6.

WELL-DIFFERENTIATED CENTRAL CARTILAGE TUMORS OF BONE: AN OVERVIEW

Lizette Vila Duckworth, MD[a], John D. Reith, MD[a,b],*

KEYWORDS

• Chondroma • Enchondroma • Chondrosarcoma • Cartilage • Pathology • Radiology

ABSTRACT

Well-differentiated hyaline cartilage tumors are among the most common tumors encountered in the skeleton; their radiographic and pathologic classification and clinical management can be challenging. Pathologists find cartilage tumors difficult because their precise classification is as dependent on the clinical and radiographic findings as the histologic features; the distinction between benign and malignant cartilage neoplasms demands good communication and teamwork between pathologists, orthopedic surgeons, and radiologists. This review focuses on the necessary clinical, radiographic, and pathologic features that allow distinction between enchondroma and low-grade central chondrosarcoma and interpretation of lesions encountered in the enchondromatosis syndromes.

OVERVIEW

As a group, well-differentiated cartilage tumors represent the most common primary bone tumors.[1] In its classification of cartilage tumors, the World Health Organization recognizes 3 entities that are composed of mature hyaline cartilage: osteochondroma, chondroma (which includes enchondroma, periosteal chondroma, and the multiple chondromatosis syndromes), and chondrosarcoma (including central chondrosarcoma, both primary and secondary, and peripheral chondrosarcoma).[2] Cartilage lesions can also be divided into those that arise within the medullary cavity—enchondroma and central chondrosarcoma—and those that arise on the surface of the bone—osteochondroma, periosteal chondroma, and peripheral chondrosarcoma. Whether located within the medullary cavity or on the surface of the bone, the well-differentiated chondrosarcomas (grade 1) can occur as primary lesions or arise secondary to an underlying lesion, such as an enchondroma or osteochondroma.[3]

Unlike tumors in many other organ systems, the distinction between the various benign and malignant cartilage tumors, in particular those composed of relatively mature hyaline cartilage, is difficult based on histologic grounds alone. The key principles to consider when trying to distinguish an enchondroma from a low-grade chondrosarcoma are:[4]

1. Growth—established clinically by the presence of pain or radiographically by evidence of change, particularly over serial radiographs
2. Invasion—implied by certain radiographic features or identified histologically.

The diagnosis of enchondroma or chondrosarcoma is often evident on the basis of clinical and radiographic findings alone. In the event that a well-differentiated cartilage tumor is biopsied, however, good communication between the pathologist, radiologist, and orthopedic surgeon

[a] Department of Pathology, Immunology, and Laboratory Medicine, University of Florida College of Medicine, Gainesville, FL, USA
[b] Department of Orthopaedics and Rehabilitation, University of Florida College of Medicine, Gainesville, FL, USA
* Corresponding author. Department of Pathology, Immunology, and Laboratory Medicine, University of Florida College of Medicine, PO Box 100275, Gainesville, FL 32610-0275.
E-mail address: Reith@pathology.ufl.edu

Surgical Pathology 5 (2012) 147–161
doi:10.1016/j.path.2011.12.001
1875-9181/12/$ – see front matter © 2012 Elsevier Inc. All rights reserved.

is vital to arrive at the proper diagnosis. The difficulty in interpreting the histologic findings is magnified in the multiple enchondroma syndromes (Ollier disease and Maffucci syndrome).

This article reviews the clinical, radiographic, and histologic features that help distinguish the well-differentiated cartilage tumors identified centrally within bone and reviews several diagnostic pitfalls.

CENTRAL CARTILAGE TUMORS: ENCHONDROMA VERSUS LOW-GRADE CHONDROSARCOMA

CLINICAL FINDINGS

When considering the well-differentiated cartilage tumors that arise within the medullary cavity, it is important to be aware of the patient's age, the specific site of the lesion, and the patient's clinical presentation. Enchondromas are common benign cartilage tumors that affect patients over a wide age distribution and may be seen in both children and adults. They arise most frequently in the small tubular bones of the hands and feet. In the long tubular bones, the proximal humerus and femur are the most commonly affected sites. Enchondromas seldom occur in flat bones, such as the skull, pelvis, or spine.[1–3] The symptoms related to enchondromas and the manner in which these tumors are discovered clinically vary somewhat depending on the location of the lesion. Enchondromas of the small bones of the hands and feet may cause pathologic fractures, and those arising in long bones are often discovered during bone scans for the evaluation of metastatic carcinoma, during the work-up for internal derangement of the knee or a rotator cuff tear, or incidentally on radiographs obtained for arthritis or fractures.[5,6] Enchondromas are asymptomatic unless complicated by a pathologic fracture, and significant

	Pathologic Key Features ENCHONDROMA AND CHONDROSARCOMA	
	Enchondroma	**Low-Grade Chondrosarcoma**
Clinical	Painless lesions unless complicated by a pathologic fracture. Pain may result from an arthritic joint or other painful musculoskeletal condition (torn rotator cuff, tendinitis, etc.).	Growing lesions in skeletally mature patients which often cause pain.
Radiology	Typically well-defined lesions with stippled or ring-and-arc calcifications. Important is what is NOT identified, particularly in long bone lesions— significant bone destruction surrounding an area of mineralization; endosteal scalloping in the presence of a thickened cortex; periosteal reaction; soft tissue mass. In short tubular bones, some expansile remodeling may be seen with larger lesions.	Growing lesions in skeletally mature patients. Significantly more bone destruction than is seen with enchondromas, often associated with deep endosteal scalloping, thickened cortex, periosteal reaction, and a soft tissue mass.
Pathology	Lobules of well-differentiated hyaline cartilage with peripheral encasement by woven or lamellar bone (enchondroma encasement pattern). Important is what is NOT identified—there should not be any evidence of invasion of the medullary cavity, cortex, or adjacent soft tissue. Cytologic features are not reliable in distinguishing enchondroma from low-grade chondrosarcoma.	Diagnosis is established by demonstrating invasion (chondrosarcoma permeation pattern). Entrapment of cancellous bone, permeation of the haversian system, and extension into adjacent soft tissue are all features diagnostic of chondrosarcoma. Cytologic features are not reliable in distinguishing enchondroma from low-grade chondrosarcoma.

pain that can be attributed directly to a well-differentiated cartilage tumor arising in the medullary cavity (and not a torn rotator cuff, tendinitis, or arthritis in an adjacent joint) should raise the possibility of chondrosarcoma.[5–7] Because enchondromas are derived from portions of the growth plate,[8] their growth should cease at approximately the time of skeletal maturity, hence should not cause pain in a patient who is skeletally mature.

Chondrosarcoma is the second most common primary bone sarcoma.[3] Low-grade chondrosarcomas, in contrast to enchondromas, are seldom encountered in children and typically affect patients who are skeletally mature, most often in the sixth decade and later.[9] They arise with similar frequency in the pelvis and long bones, in particular the femur and humerus, but are uncommon in the small bones of the hands and feet,[10,11] the spine, and the craniofacial bones. Low-grade chondrosarcomas are actively growing neoplasms that typically induce pain. Therefore, the presence of pain, when directly attributable to the lesion, is a strong indicator of clinical growth and, therefore, malignancy in a hyaline cartilage tumor.[4,5]

RADIOLOGY TO EVALUATE CARTILAGINOUS LESIONS

Radiology is perhaps the single most important parameter used in the evaluation of cartilaginous lesions and, to accurately categorize cartilage tumors, pathologists must be familiar with the spectrum of radiographic findings that may be encountered.[12] Plain radiographs and CT scans are excellent modalities for evaluating patterns of mineralization, bone destruction, and the integrity of the cortex. In long bones, enchondromas typically arise in the metaphysis or diaphysis and may appear radiolucent, partially mineralized, or heavily mineralized.[5] Epiphyseal enchrondromas are seldom encountered. The pattern of mineralization in enchondromas is characteristic and includes a combination of rings or arcs and stippled radiodensities (**Fig. 1**). The radiographic finding of rings and arcs is the result of the radiolucent lobules of cartilage being surrounded by a radiodense rim of bone, and the stippled radiodensities result from necrosis and subsequent dystrophic calcification in the central areas of the cartilage nodules. Enchondromas are typically centrally located within long bones, and larger lesions may cause a mild degree of endosteal scalloping, which is accompanied by thinning of the overlying cortex, particularly in the metaphysis where cortical bone is thin. However, associated periosteal reaction and a soft tissue mass are

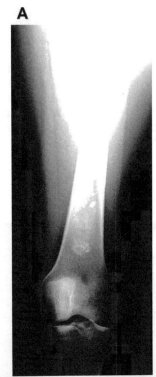

A

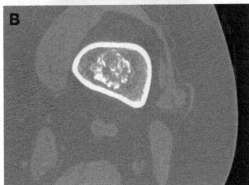

B

Fig. 1. (*A*) Plain radiograph showing the typical appearance of a large enchondroma in the distal femur. The lesion is sharply circumscribed, heavily mineralized, with no cortical changes, periosteal reaction, or soft tissue mass present. (*B*) Axial CT scan of the same lesion highlighting the typical appearance of cartilaginous matrix, including stippled calcifications, rings, and arcs.

absent.[13] Serial radiographs or CT scans demonstrating lack of growth may also be used to support a diagnosis of enchondroma if there is uncertainty regarding the biologic potential of a given cartilage tumor.[4,5]

Enchondromas arising in the small tubular bones of the hands and feet often show aggressive radiographic features and must be evaluated using different criteria than those applied to long bone lesions. Enchondromas of the hands and feet may be purely radiolucent or heavily mineralized and can occasionally cause marked expansile remodeling of the cortex, a finding that raises suspicion for malignancy in a long bone (**Fig. 2**). Therefore, to recognize a hyaline cartilage tumor in a small tubular bone as malignant, there must be frank cortical destruction and formation of a soft tissue mass.[4,10,14]

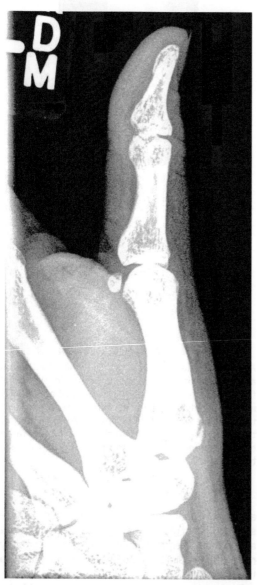

Fig. 2. Plain radiograph of an enchondroma in the thumb metacarpal. The lesion is radiolucent with calcifications and fills the entire medullary cavity.

In contrast to enchondromas, low-grade central chondrosarcomas typically show significantly more destructive properties (**Figs. 3–5**). Whereas enchondromas typically have discrete, well-defined borders, chondrosarcomas are characterized by ill-defined areas of bone destruction. Most low-grade chondrosarcomas contain areas of mineralization, although these areas are often accompanied by a surrounding, ill-defined zone of radiolucency. Important radiographic features of low-grade chondrosarcomas that are not seen with enchondromas include endosteal scalloping in the presence of cortical thickening, cortical destruction with a soft tissue mass, and periosteal reaction in the absence of a fracture.[4,12,15–17] All of these features are indicative of either growth or invasion. Cortical thickening, in particular, represents a response to tumor invasion of the haversian system of the cortex.

Some cartilage tumors may have clinical or radiographic features which are borderline or indeterminate with respect to their biologic potential. In such instances, limited biopsies are unlikely to reliably distinguish enchondroma from low-grade chondrosarcoma. One helpful strategy for borderline cases is to monitor the lesion with serial radiographic studies in regular intervals (3 to 6 months).[4,17] Any interval growth of the lesion, provided a patient is skeletally mature, is indicative of low-grade chondrosarcoma (**Fig. 6**). Lack of any interval change in a borderline lesion, however, particularly in an asymptomatic patient, suggests a nonaggressive process, and the patient can continue to be followed clinically/radiographically without being subject to biopsy.

The usefulness of other imaging modalities in the diagnosis of cartilage tumors and their ability to distinguish benign from malignant lesions has also been investigated. MRI is useful in characterizing bone tumors as cartilaginous on the basis of their high water content, resulting in lesions of low signal intensity on T1-weighted MRI and high signal intensity on T2-weighted images.[5] Therefore, MRI is useful in directing the extent of surgical excision for low-grade chondrosarcomas. MRI is less useful, however, in helping to distinguish enchondromas from low-grade chondrosarcomas when a lesion is confined to the medullary cavity.[18] The detection of a soft tissue component on MRI scan confirms the diagnosis of chondrosarcoma. It has also been shown that early and exponential enhancement on fast contrast-enhanced MRI is a feature of chondrosarcomas but not enchondromas.[19] The usefulness of [18]FDG-PET has also been studied in cartilage tumors, with mixed results.[20–22]

Fig. 3. Plain radiograph of grade 1 chondrosarcoma in the proximal humerus. The lesion contains typical matrix calcifications distally, exhibits deep endosteal scalloping, and extends through the lateral cortex into the soft tissue where there is an associated periosteal reaction.

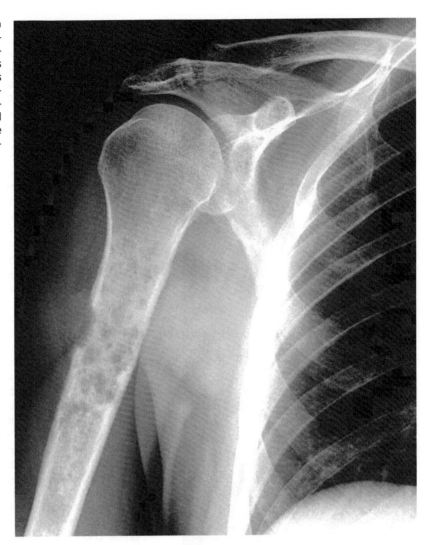

GROSS AND MICROSCOPIC PATHOLOGY

Because most enchondromas are either observed or curetted, it is uncommon to encounter these lesions intact. Therefore, most enchondromas consist of fragments of gray, translucent tissue with foci of calcification and ossification. Intact enchondromas are sharply circumscribed from the adjacent cancellous bone and frequently multinodular with individual nodules separated by normal bone marrow or cancellous bone (**Fig. 7**).

Low-grade chondrosarcomas also have a translucent, gray cut surface with foci of calcification on gross examination. They are far more destructive than enchondromas and typically cause prominent endosteal scalloping with associated thickening of the cortex. Deep penetration into the cortex may result in the formation of a periosteal reaction, and the presence of a soft tissue extension is a finding never encountered with an enchondroma (**Fig. 8**).

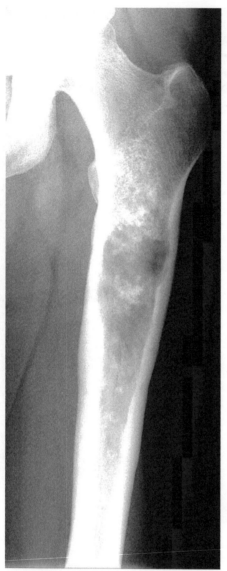

Fig. 4. Grade 1 chondrosarcoma of the proximal femur. Centrally the lesion is radiolucent and associated with endosteal scalloping and cortical thickening; the remainder of the lesion has stippled calcifications and rings typical of cartilaginous matrix.

Microscopically, enchondromas are composed of mature hyaline cartilage lacking invasive properties, features that are best appreciated by low-power examination. Intact enchondromas often contain lobules of cartilage separated by normal bone marrow and cancellous bone (Fig. 9), and many of the lobules are either partially or completely encompassed by a shell of bone (enchondroma encasement) (Fig. 10).[23–25] These important diagnostic features may be difficult to identify on limited biopsy or curettage material. Foci of dystrophic calcification are common in enchondromas, and small foci of myxoid change are also occasionally identified. At higher magnification, enchondromas are highly variable in cellularity depending on whether a patient has an enchondromatosis syndrome (Ollier disease or Maffucci syndrome) and the specific location of the lesion. Lesions arising in the setting of enchondromatosis, those occurring in children, or those located in the small bones of the hands and feet may be extremely cellular and appear proliferative. Most enchondromas are low in cellularity, however, and the chondrocyte nuclei are pyknotic, hyperchromatic, and lacking nuclear detail (Fig. 11). The presence of binucleate chondrocytes or multiple chondrocytes occupying a single lacuna may be identified in both enchondromas and low-grade chondrosarcomas; therefore, cytologic features alone cannot reliably distinguish between the two.

Low-grade chondrosarcomas have similar features to enchondromas, making their distinction difficult on histologic grounds alone. Because of the considerable overlap in the high-magnification appearance of these two lesions, the single most important microscopic feature required to diagnose a low-grade chondrosarcoma is infiltration (chondrosarcoma permeation).[24] At low-magnification, low-grade chondrosarcomas frequently show confluent lobules of mature cartilage, separated only by thin fibrous bands (Fig. 12). The cartilaginous nodules in a low-grade chondrosarcoma have invasive properties and permeate bone and marrow, overrunning the marrow and entrapping fragments of cancellous bone, which is frequently necrotic (Fig. 13). The cartilage may infiltrate the haversian system, and the finding of an extraosseous soft tissue mass is never encountered in an enchondroma in the absence of a pathologic fracture. Cytologically, low-grade chondrosarcomas often have larger nuclei with open chromatin, and nuclear detail, such as nucleoli, may be identified (Fig. 14). These features may also be encountered, however, in some enchondromas, and cytologic features alone should not be used to distinguish low-grade chondrosarcoma from enchondroma.

DIFFERENTIAL DIAGNOSIS

In most instances, the clinical, radiographic, and pathologic features point to a well-differentiated cartilage tumor, with a main differential diagnosis

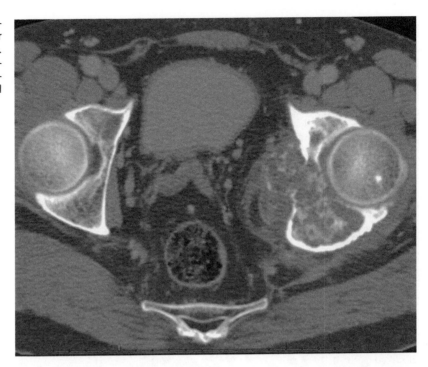

Fig. 5. Axial CT scan depicting a large periacetabular grade 1 chondrosarcoma. The lesion is highly destructive and contains matrix mineralization typical of a cartilaginous lesion.

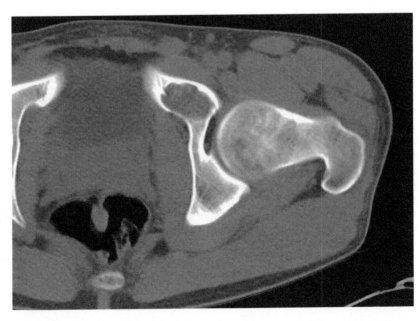

Fig. 6. Some cartilaginous lesions may have borderline radiographic features. This axial CT scan depicts a radiolucent lesion in the pubis with faint calcifications and mild endosteal scalloping. The initial radiographic diagnosis included various benign conditions such as fibrous dysplasia; however, the patient had progressive pain, and serial CT scans showed interval growth of the lesion, which was eventually excised and proved to be a grade 1 chondrosarcoma.

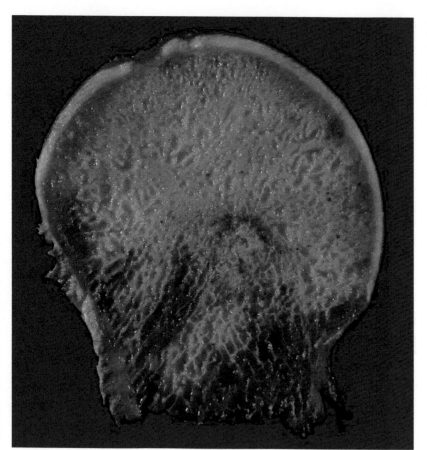

Fig. 7. Gross photograph of an incidentally discovered enchondroma in a femoral head removed after a fracture. Note the typical pearly, gray appearance of the cartilage.

of enchondroma versus low-grade chondrosarcoma. Other processes may mimic a well-differentiated cartilage tumor, including bone infarcts, osteoblastic metastases, and fibrous dysplasia with cartilaginous differentiation. Bone infarcts and metastatic disease are often included in the radiographic differential diagnosis of enchondroma and low-grade chondrosarcoma but are easily separated from cartilage tumors on the basis of their histologic features. Fibrous dysplasia with cartilaginous differentiation, or fibrocartilaginous dysplasia, can be a tricky pitfall, particularly when the cartilaginous component is the dominant finding. Furthermore, the cartilaginous areas may be quite cellular microscopically and contain chondrocyte atypia, raising the possibility of a low-grade chondrosarcoma. The most important feature that separates fibrocartilaginous dysplasia from both enchondroma and low-grade chondrosarcoma is the identification and recognition of the benign fibro-osseous component (**Fig. 15**).[26] Additionally, most patients with fibrocartilaginous dysplasia are in their teens or 20s, and most of these cases occur in the typical sites for fibrous dysplasia, including the intertrochanteric region of the proximal femur. Therefore, careful radiographic correlation and consideration of the clinical presentation are also important in distinguishing fibrocartilaginous dysplasia from enchondroma and low-grade chondrosarcoma.

Fig. 8. Gross photograph of the grade 1 chondrosarcoma seen in Fig. 3. The lesion has the typical gray appearance of cartilage with foci of calcification. Marked endosteal scalloping can be seen in the right side of the photograph, whereas soft tissue extension and elevation of the periosteum can be seen on the opposite side.

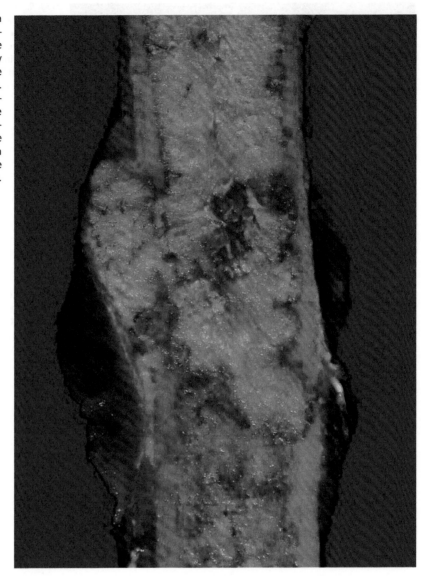

TREATMENT AND PROGNOSIS

Enchondromas of long bones can safely be followed clinically and radiographically, whereas those in the hands and feet may be managed with curettage when symptomatic.[5] The incidence of local recurrence for enchondromas is low after surgery. The most appropriate surgical management of low-grade chondrosarcomas has been debated, and some investigators advocate en bloc surgical resection whereas others suggest that curettage with an adjuvant agent is sufficient given the risk of local recurrence, very low risk for the development of metastases, and risk of dedifferentiation.[27–29]

Diagnostic Pitfalls
CARTILAGE TUMORS

! Interpreting the pathology of a cartilage tumor without the aid of clinical and radiographic information is fraught with danger and inevitably leads to either overdiagnosis or underdiagnosis.

! Fibrocartilaginous dysplasia may easily be confused with a cartilage tumor; however, careful consideration of the clinical scenario and radiographic findings, as well as a diligent search for the fibro-osseous component, should allow distinction from a cartilaginous lesion.

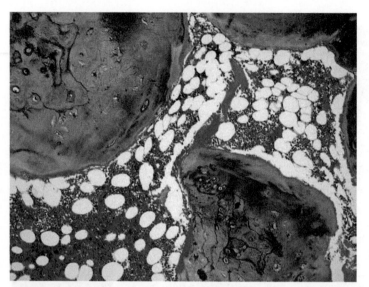

Fig. 9. Low-power photomicrograph of an enchondroma. The tumor is composed of discontinuous islands of mature hyaline cartilage partially encased in a thin shell of bone and separated by islands of normal hematopoietic marrow.

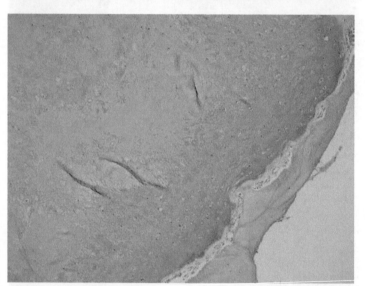

Fig. 10. Low-power photomicrograph of an enchondroma showing encasement of a lobule of tumor by a complete rim of bone.

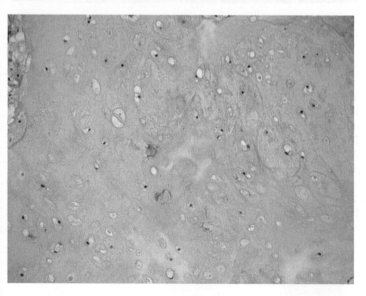

Fig. 11. High-power photomicrograph of an enchondroma. The chondrocyte nuclei within enchondromas are typically pyknotic and dark and lack detail.

Fig. 12. Low-power photomicrograph of a grade 1 chondrosarcoma showing confluent lobules of tumor separated by only thin fibrous bands.

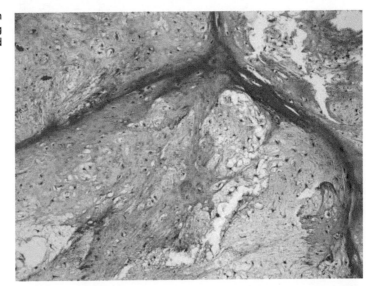

Fig. 13. Low-power photomicrograph of a grade 1 chondrosarcoma showing the characteristic entrapment of partially necrotic cancellous bone by cartilage lobules. This finding is diagnostic of chondrosarcoma and is not seen in enchondromas.

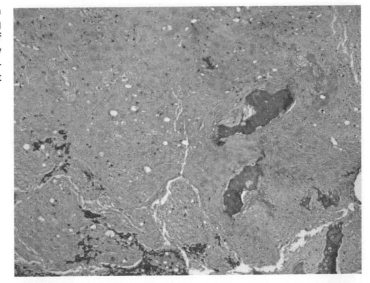

Fig. 14. High-power photomicrograph of a grade 1 chondrosarcoma. The lesion is slightly more cellular than an enchondroma, and the chondrocyte nuclei are slightly enlarged and more vesicular than those typically seen in an enchondroma. These findings should not be overinterpreted, however, and may be seen in enchondromas in the hands or feet and in the setting of enchondromatosis. When trying to distinguish enchondroma from low-grade chondrosarcoma, the low-power growth pattern is far more important than the cytologic features.

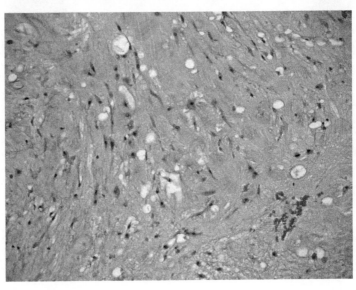

158

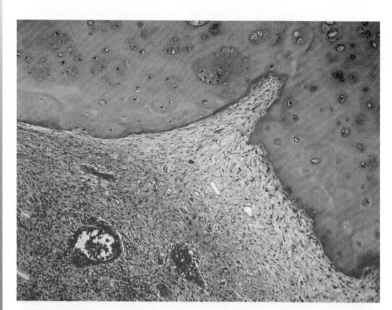

Fig. 15. The cartilaginous component may predominate in a case of fibrocartilaginous dysplasia, and careful radiographic correlation and identification of the fibro-osseous component are keys to the recognition of this entity.

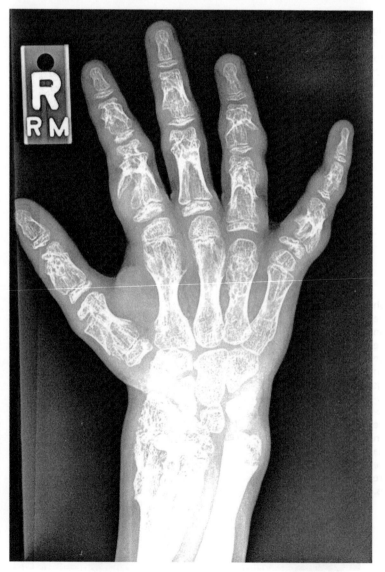

Fig. 16. Plain radiograph of the hand in a patient with Ollier disease. Note the enchondromas in nearly every bone, including the distal radius and ulna.

Fig. 17. Maffucci syndrome is characterized by multiple enchondromas and soft tissue hemagiomas, which are evident as calcified phleboliths within the soft tissues in this plain radiograph of the hand.

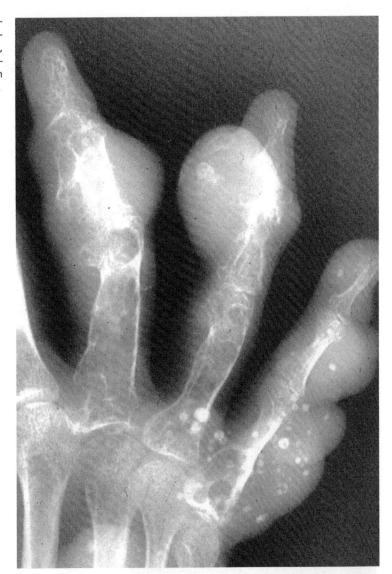

Fig. 18. The enchondromas of Ollier disease and Maffucci syndrome are often highly cellular and have cytologic atypia, making the distinction from a chondrosarcoma difficult.

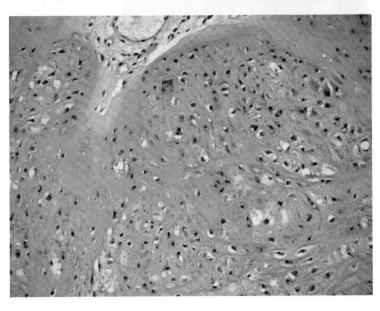

ENCHONDROMATOSIS

Ollier disease and Maffucci syndrome are un-common, nonheritable disorders characterized by multiple enchondromas and periosteal chondro-mas.[1] In addition to multiple enchondromas, patients with Maffucci syndrome have vascular tumors of the skin and soft tissue as well as a variety of nonchon-droid and nonvascular tumors.[30,31] Both disorders carry a significant risk for the development of chon-drosarcoma, although the exact risk is unclear.

The presence of an underlying enchondromato-sis syndrome can pose significant diagnostic chal-lenges in interpreting cartilage tumors from these

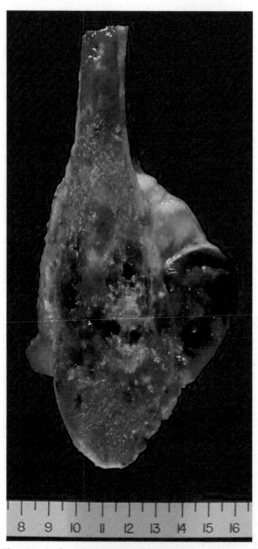

Fig. 19. A chondrosarcoma arising in the setting of Ollier disease. The chondrosarcomatous component has a gelatinous appearance, whereas the underlying enchondromas have a more firm, gray appearance.

patients. The enchondromas in these syndromes can appear aggressive radiographically and histologically, depending on the site of origin. Radiographically, the deformities of the bones involved can range from mild to severe, and lesions can occur both centrally and beneath the periosteum (Fig. 16). The lesions in Ollier disease and Maffucci syndrome may be limited to a single limb or widespread in distribution. In long bones and the pelvis, columns of radiolu-cent cartilage alternate with interspersed radio-dense bone, creating a characteristic fan-like appearance.[3] Lesions in the hands and feet can cause marked deformities. The vascular tumors in patients with Maffucci syndrome are often evident on plain radiographs as calcified phlebo-liths within soft tissue (Fig. 17).

Histologically, the enchondromas encountered in these disorders are often highly cellular with cytologic atypia, frequently raising concern for chondrosarcoma (Fig. 18). Sarcomatous transfor-mation should be suspected based primarily on clinical and radiographic findings, in particular sudden, rapid lesional growth after skeletal matu-rity and frank cortical destruction with soft tissue involvement (Fig. 19).[30,32]

REFERENCES

1. Unni KK, Inwards CY, Bridge JA, et al. AFIP atlas of tumor pathology series 4. Tumors of the bones and joints. Washington, DC: American Registry of Pathology; 2005. p. 37–118.
2. Fletcher CD, Unni KK, Mertens F, editors. World Health Organization classification of tumours. pathology and genetics. Tumours of soft tissue and bone. Lyon (France): IARC Press; 2002. p. 225–6.
3. Dorfman HD, Czerniak B. Bone tumors. St Louis (MO): Mosby; 1998. p. 253–440.
4. McCarthy EF, Tyler WK. Distinguishing enchondroma from low-grade central chondrosarcoma. Pathol Case Rev 2001;6:8–13.
5. Scarborough MT, Moreau G. Benign cartilage tumors. Orthop Clin North Am 1996;27:583–9.
6. Levy JC, Temple HT, Mollabashy A, et al. The causes of pain in benign solitary enchondromas of the prox-imal humerus. Clin Orthop 2005;431:181–6.
7. Marco RA, Gitleis S, Brabach GT, et al. Cartilage tumors: evaluation and treatment. J Am Acad Orthop Surg 2000;8:292–304.
8. Milgram JW. The origins of osteochondromas and enchondromas. A histopathologic study. Clin Orthop 1983;174:264–84.
9. Huvos AG, Marcove RC. Chondrosarcoma in the young. A clinicopathologic analysis of 79 patients younger than 21 years of age. Am J Surg Pathol 1987;11:930–42.

10. Bovee JV, van der Heul R, Taminiau AH, et al. Chondrosarcoma of the phalanx: a locally aggressive lesion with minimal metastatic potential. Cancer 1999;86:1724–32.

11. Ogose A, Unni KK, Swee RG, et al. Chondrosarcoma of small bones of the hands and feet. Cancer 1997;80:50–9.

12. Greenspan A. Tumors of cartilage origin. Orthop Clin North Am 1989;20:347–66.

13. Bui KL, Ilaslan H, Bauer TW, et al. Cortical scalloping and cortical penetration by small eccentric chondroid lesions in the long tubular bones: not a sign of malignancy? Skeletal Radiol 2009;38:791–6.

14. Cawte TG, Steiner GC, Beltran J, et al. Chondrosarcoma of the short tubular bones of the hands and feet. Skeletal Radiol 1998;27:625–32.

15. Flemming DJ, Murphey MD. Enchondroma and chondrosarcoma. Semin Musculoskelet Radiol 2000;4: 59–71.

16. Murphey MD, Flemming DJ, Boyea SR, et al. Enchondroma versus chondrosarcoma in the appendicular skeleton: differentiating features. Radiographics 1998;18:1213–37.

17. Soldatos T, McMarthy EF, Attar S, et al. Imaging features of chondrosarcoma. J Comput Assist Tomogr 2011;35:504–11.

18. De Beuckeleer LH, De Schepper AM, Ramon F, et al. Magnetic resonance imaging of cartilaginous tumors: a retrospective study of 79 patients. Eur J Radiol 1995;21:34–40.

19. Geirnaerdt MJ, Hogendoorn PC, Bloem JL, et al. Cartilaginous tumors: fast contrast-enhanced MR imaging. Radiology 2000;214:539–46.

20. Brenner W, Conrad EU, Eary JF. FDG PET imaging for grading and prediction of outcome in chondrosarcoma patients. Eur J Nucl Med Mol Imaging 2004;31:189–95.

21. Feldman F, Van Heertum R, Saxena C, et al. 18FDG-PET applications for cartilage neoplasms. Skeletal Radiol 2005;34:367–74.

22. Lee FY, Yu J, Chang S, et al. Diagnostic value and limitations of fluorine-18 fluorodeoxyglucose positron emission tomography for cartilaginous tumors of bone. J Bone Joint Surg Am 2004;86:2677–85.

23. Brien EW, Mirra JM, Kerr R. Benign and malignant cartilage tumors of bone and joint: their anatomic and theoretical basis with an emphasis on radiology, pathology, and clinical biology. I. The intramedullary tumors. Skeletal Radiol 1997;26:325–53.

24. Mirra JM, Gold R, Downs J, et al. A new histologic approach to the differentiation of enchondroma and chondrosarcoma of the bones. A clinicopathologic analysis of 51 cases. Clin Orthop 1985;201: 214–37.

25. Schiller AL. Diagnosis of borderline cartilage lesions of bone. Semin Diagn Pathol 1985;2:42–62.

26. Ishida T, Dorfman HD. Massive chondroid differentiation in fibrous dysplasia of bone (fibrocartilaginous dysplasia). Am J Surg Pathol 1993;17:924–30.

27. Donati D, Colangeli S, Colangeli M, et al. Surgical treatment of grade 1 central chondrosarcoma. Clin Orthop Relat Res 2010;468:581–9.

28. Mohler DG, Chiu R, McCall DA, et al. Curettage and cryosurgery for low-grade cartilage tumors is associated with low recurrence and high function. Clin Orthop Relat Res 2010;468:2765–73.

29. Hanna SA, Whittingham-Jones P, Sewell MD, et al. Outcome of intralesional curettage for low-grade chondrosarcoma of long bones. Eur J Surg Oncol 2009;35:1343–7.

30. Pansuriya TC, Kroon HM, Bovee JV. Enchondromatosis: insights on the different subtypes. Int J Clin Exp Pathol 2010;3:557–69.

31. Fanburg JC, Meis-Kindblom JM, Rosenberg AE. Multiple enchondromas associated with spindle-cell hemangioendotheliomas. An overlooked variant of Maffucci's syndrome. Am J Surg Pathol 1995;19: 1029–38.

32. Silve C, Juppner H. Ollier disease. Orphanet J Rare Dis 2006;1:37.

CHONDROSARCOMA VARIANTS

Scott E. Kilpatrick, MD

KEYWORDS

- Chondrosarcoma • Dedifferentiated • Mesenchymal • Myxoid • Clear cell • Cartilage

ABSTRACT

This article presents a review of chondrosarcoma variants, with a focus on the extraordinarily rare variants of chondrosarcoma in which hyaline cartilage is not the dominant feature. Discussed are the differential diagnoses for these neoplasms, radiologic studies, gross and microscopic features, and prognosis. Summaries are provided of the key features for the major variants.

OVERVIEW

In addition to classical intramedullary localization, conventional chondrosarcoma of bone rarely may arise from other anatomic sites, including periosteum and synovium. Although criteria for separating benign from malignant chondroid lesions necessarily vary depending on their anatomic site, all share the fact that they are virtually exclusively composed of hyaline cartilage. In this article, the focus is on the extraordinarily rare variants of chondrosarcoma in which hyaline cartilage is not the dominant feature and, in fact, in most cases of myxoid chondrosarcoma (chordoid sarcoma), is absent. Although hyaline cartilage usually does not predominate in these tumors, its presence is essential to establish the diagnosis, the exception being chordoid sarcoma. Dedifferentiated chondrosarcoma, mesenchymal chondrosarcoma, clear cell chondrosarcoma, and chordoid sarcoma generally are easily recognizable (and diagnosable), provided the pathologist is familiar with and/or has encountered them previously. Small biopsy specimens, such as core or fine-needle aspiration biopsies, are especially problematic, as the hyaline cartilage may not be sampled, requiring careful attention to clinicopathologic features and judicious use of ancillary studies to establish a correct diagnosis. Not surprisingly, the differential diagnoses for these neoplasms tend to be related to the dominant cell type but not other cartilaginous neoplasms. For example, the differential diagnosis of dedifferentiated chondrosarcoma usually includes other spindle cell, noncartilaginous pleomorphic sarcomas, whereas mesenchymal chondrosarcoma is more apt to be confused with Ewing sarcoma.

DEDIFFERENTIATED CHONDROSARCOMA

OVERVIEW

Dedifferentiated chondrosarcoma represents approximately 10% of all reported cases of chondrosarcomas. Strictly defined, dedifferentiated chondrosarcoma requires the presence of a high-grade, nonchondrosarcomatous sarcoma usually sharply juxtaposed to a low-grade chondrosarcoma. Although most examples arise from intramedullary, central chondrosarcomas, it also may rarely originate from a preexisting osteochondroma or periosteal chondrosarcoma (peripheral chondrosarcoma).[1,2]

Most patients are older than 50 years at diagnosis. Common anatomic sites include the pelvic bones, femur, and humerus. The most common presenting complaint is pain, often associated with a soft tissue mass.[3,4] Radiologically, the low-grade cartilaginous component shows the typical mineralization of a cartilage tumor, whereas the dedifferentiated portion appears ill-defined,

Disclosure statement: The author has nothing to disclose.
Pathologists Diagnostic Services, Forsyth Medical Center, 3333 Silas Creek Parkway, Winston-Salem, NC 27104, USA
E-mail address: sekilpatrick@novanthealth.org

Surgical Pathology 5 (2012) 163–181
doi:10.1016/j.path.2011.10.002
1875-9181/12/$ – see front matter © 2012 Elsevier Inc. All rights reserved.

permeative, lytic, and associated with extraosseous extension. In many cases, the dedifferentiated component completely dwarfs the smaller, low-grade cartilaginous portion (Fig. 1).

GROSS FEATURES

In most circumstances, the 2 components, blue-gray cartilaginous lesion and the fleshy, hemorrhagic to necrotic component, juxtapose one another, with the latter generally dwarfing (in size) the former (Fig. 2). For the more common intramedullary form, the cartilaginous component is within bone (central), whereas the dedifferentiated

portion extends through the bony cortex, forming a large, extraosseous mass.

MICROSCOPIC FEATURES

In en bloc or resected specimens, the diagnosis of dedifferentiated chondrosarcoma is relatively straightforward if the low-grade cartilaginous component is recognized as malignant. The histologic hallmark is the finding of an abrupt transition between a low-grade chondrosarcoma and a high-grade, often spindle cell, sarcoma, giving the appearance of 2 separate neoplasms (Fig. 3); however, focal areas may show a more gradual transition between the 2 components (Fig. 4). The

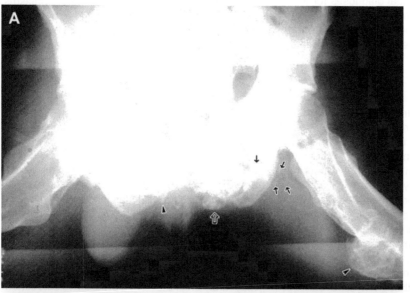

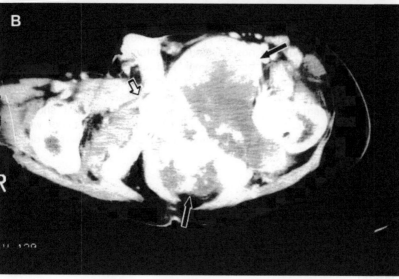

Fig. 1. Dedifferentiated chondrosarcoma arising in a patient with multiple osteochondromatosis. (A) An anteroposterior radiograph of the pelvis shows multiple osteochondromas (arrowheads). A large soft tissue mass is accompanied by multiple, irregular calcifications at the left pubic ramus (arrows). (B) An axial computed tomographic scan shows the extension of soft tissue mass anterior (dark arrow) and posterior to the left pubic rami. The mass is heterogeneous, probably secondary to necrosis, and calcifications are noted. An osteochondroma (open arrow) arises from the right pubic ramus.

high-grade dedifferentiated component is most frequently represented as a nonmatrix-producing, spindle cell pleomorphic sarcoma, resembling so-called malignant fibrous histiocytoma.[3,4] As is in dedifferentiated liposarcoma, however, the dedifferentiated component may show divergent differentiation, resembling osteosarcoma, leiomyosarcoma, or rhabdomyosarcoma (**Fig. 5**).[4–6]

Among smaller biopsy specimens, sampling is a bigger issue and may result in considerable difficulty in establishing the diagnosis. In the author's experience, core needle biopsy and fine-needle aspiration biopsy preferentially sample the larger, higher-grade dedifferentiated component. The resulting diagnosis is most often simply high-grade pleomorphic sarcoma, not otherwise specified.[7] To establish the diagnosis in this circumstance requires radiologic correlation and a high suspicion for an "unsampled," concomitant low-grade chondrosarcomatous component.

Immunohistochemistry is not generally helpful for the diagnosis of dedifferentiated chondrosarcoma. Cytogenetic analysis has revealed no reproducible, specific chromosomal aberrations or translocations in dedifferentiated chondrosarcoma. A variety of structural and numerical aberrations have been reported, probably reflecting the wide histologic diversity of the dedifferentiated component.[8]

DIFFERENTIAL DIAGNOSIS

Because the high-grade, nonchondromatous component usually is dominant (compared with the low-grade cartilaginous portion) and thus is more likely to be sampled, the differential diagnosis mainly includes other noncartilage-producing spindle cell and pleomorphic sarcomas, especially so-called malignant fibrous histiocytoma. In addition, as the dedifferentiated component may show divergent differentiation, other more specific histologic subtypes, such as osteosarcoma or rhabdomyosarcoma, must also be considered. In the final analysis, only the

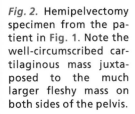

Fig. 2. Hemipelvectomy specimen from the patient in Fig. 1. Note the well-circumscribed cartilaginous mass juxtaposed to the much larger fleshy mass on both sides of the pelvis.

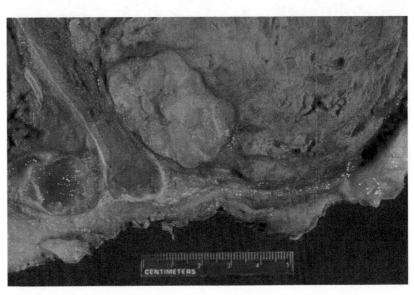

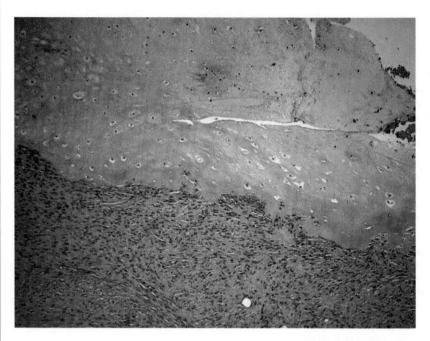

Fig. 3. Dedifferentiated chondrosarcoma characterized most commonly by sharp juxtaposition of the low-grade cartilaginous component and the non-cartilaginous, high-grade sarcomatous component (Hemotoxylin-eosin [H&E], original magnification ×40).

recognition of the concomitant low-grade cartilaginous component permits distinction from these other high-grade sarcomas. Attention to clinicoradiologic details and judicious use of immunohistochemistry allows separation of dedifferentiated chondrosarcoma from metastatic spindle cell or sarcomatoid carcinomas.

PROGNOSIS

Unfortunately, the prognosis of patients with dedifferentiated chondrosarcoma is uniformly poor, regardless of the form of therapy used. Most patients die of distant metastases within 1 year of the initial diagnosis.[3,9]

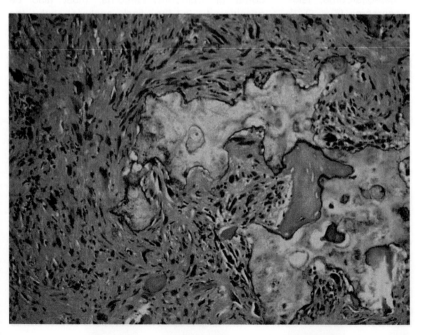

Fig. 4. Rarely, dedifferentiated chondrosarcoma shows a gradual, more intermingled transition between the 2 components (H&E, original magnification ×200).

Fig. 5. The high-grade component most frequently represents a high-grade, spindled pleomorphic sarcoma, resembling so-called malignant fibrous histiocytoma (*A*); however, divergent differentiation may occur, with leiomyosarcomatous, rhabdomyosarcomatous, or even osteosarcomatous (*B*) elements (H&E, original magnification x200).

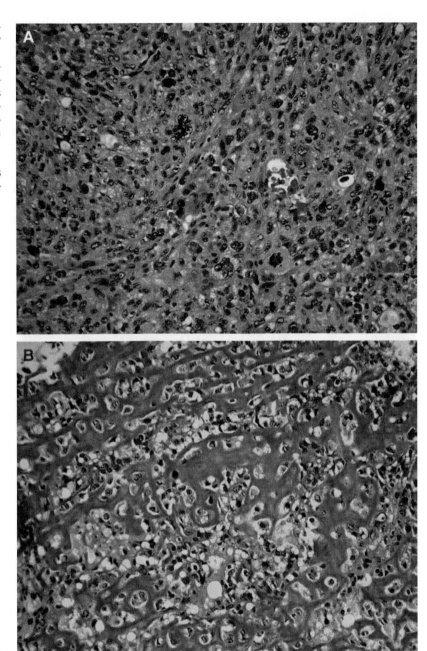

MESENCHYMAL CHONDROSARCOMA

OVERVIEW

Mesenchymal chondrosarcoma is a rare, high-grade, bimorphic sarcoma composed of undifferentiated small round cells and variable amounts of well-differentiated hyaline cartilage. Similar to skeletal osteosarcoma, most afflict patients between 10 and 30 years, but it may arise at any age.[10,11] Males and females appear equally affected. It is most commonly a primary bone neoplasm but will rarely arise in extraosseous soft tissues. When mesenchymal chondrosarcoma arises in children, however, it is more likely to be extraosseous.[12] Common skeletal sites include the skull and craniofacial region (especially the mandible), ribs, spine, and pelvis and lower extremities. In extraskeletal soft tissues, mesenchymal chondrosarcoma most often involves the meninges followed by the lower extremities and soft tissues of the head and neck.[10] Localized pain is a common symptom, often accompanied by soft tissue swelling or mass effect, and such symptoms may have been present for several years before diagnosis.

Radiologically, most skeletal examples are permeative and lytic with ill-defined borders and usually contain calcifications. Cortical destruction with extraskeletal soft tissue extension is common in primary bone lesions. In contrast to Ewing sarcoma, periosteal reaction occurs less frequently. Pathologic fracture also is less commonly observed.[10] Mesenchymal chondrosarcomas arising in extraskeletal sites almost always form a nonspecific soft tissue mass that, like its skeletal counterpart, exhibits stippled to flocculent calcified densities (Fig. 6).[10]

GROSS FEATURES

The tumors may appear deceptively circumscribed, fleshy gray to gray-white with randomly distributed areas of mineralization and/or blue-gray cartilage deposits. Hemorrhage and necrosis are sometimes seen. As in the radiographs, resected bony lesions typically show bone destruction with soft tissue extension.

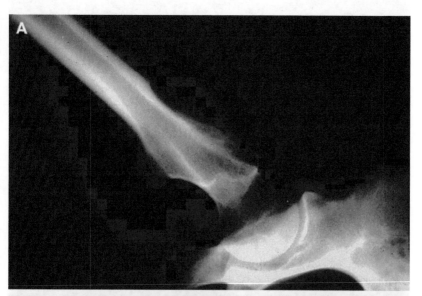

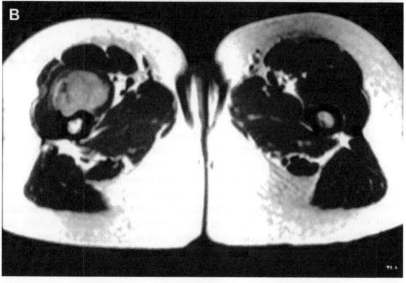

Fig. 6. (A) Lateral radiograph of the proximal femur reveals an erosion of the anterior femoral cortex with irregular, flocculent soft tissue calcifications. (B) A proton-density magnetic resonance image shows a large soft tissue mass adjacent the anterior proximal femur.

MICROSCOPIC FEATURES

Mesenchymal chondrosarcoma has a characteristic bimorphic pattern consisting of nests and sheets of undifferentiated small tumor cells, resembling Ewing sarcoma, alternating with areas of cartilaginous differentiation, with a benign to low-grade appearance (Fig. 7).[13] The latter is usually very distinctly separated from the round cell component but occasionally may blend imperceptibly. In the more cellular regions, the undifferentiated small cells may be arranged in sheets and alveolar patterns, and a background hemangiopericytomalike vascular pattern, characterized by angulated to staghornlike blood vessels, is common (Fig. 8). Occasionally, spindling of the tumor cells represents the dominant pattern. In less-cellular zones, the stroma may become hyalinized to myxoid, with tumor cells arranged in cords and single-file growth patterns (Fig. 9). Eosinophilic material, resembling osteoid, and bone formation may mimic small cell osteosarcoma (Fig. 10)[10]; however, lacelike pericellular osteoid deposition should be absent. Rarely, especially in small biopsy specimens, the volume of cartilage may be so extensive as to mask the undifferentiated small cell component (Fig. 11). Extensive necrosis is usually not seen in primary untreated tumors. Cytologically, the small tumor cells are mostly uniform, round to ovoid, with high nuclear to cytoplasmic ratios, hyperchromasia, and scant amounts of clear to slightly eosinophilic cytoplasm cytoplasm (Fig. 12). Mitotic activity often is paradoxically low, averaging fewer than 1 mitotic figure per 10 high power fields.[10,13]

Similar to dedifferentiated chondrosarcoma, small biopsies, such as core needle biopsy and fine-needle aspiration, usually sample only the undifferentiated cellular portion, leaving the concomitant cartilaginous component behind. It is doubtful that the cellular portion of mesenchymal chondrosarcoma can be diagnosed by H&E alone, but judicious use of ancillary studies may allow a more specific diagnosis. Immunohistochemically, the "small blue cell" component of mesenchymal chondrosarcoma is positive for vimentin and frequently shows a divergent phenotype. A strong and diffuse, membranous reactivity for CD99 is observed in more than 75% of cases.[14,15] Consequently, the undifferentiated small cell component of mesenchymal chondrosarcoma cannot be distinguished from Ewing sarcoma based solely on CD99 immunoreactivity. I should also point out that CD99 positivity also has been documented in small cell osteosarcoma.[16] Neuron-specific enolase and desmin often are expressed, but keratins, epithelial membrane antigen (EMA), and smooth muscle actin generally are negative.[15,17] Not unexpectedly, S-100 protein is expressed in the cartilaginous component of the tumor but rarely is observed in the more cellular, undifferentiated portion.

No definite and reliable cytogenetic abnormality has been observed in mesenchymal chondrosarcoma. Recently, Naumann and colleagues[18]

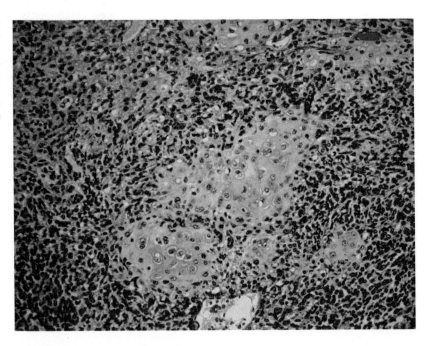

Fig. 7. Mesenchymal chondrosarcoma with classic bimorphic appearance with nodules of well-differentiated chondrosarcoma arising within a background small round cell tumor population (H&E, original magnification ×100).

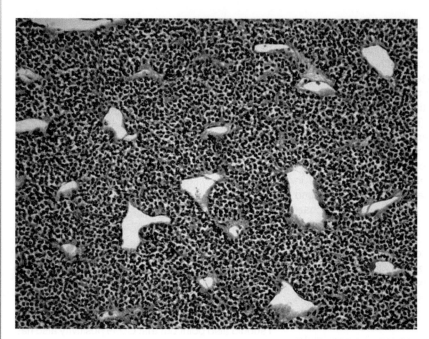

Fig. 8. A background hemangiopericytomalike vascular pattern is frequently observed in the small cell component (H&E, original magnification ×100).

described 2 tumors with an identical Robertsonian translocation involving chromosomes 13 and 21 [der(13;21)(q10;q10)]. Rare examples have also been described harboring the t(11;22)(q24;q12), usually associated with Ewing sarcoma.[19]

DIFFERENTIAL DIAGNOSIS

In the vast majority of cases, the differential diagnosis includes other small round cell neoplasms, primarily Ewing sarcoma and small cell osteosarcoma, in skeletal lesions. Meticulous attention to clinical and radiologic features and generous sampling usually allow for distinction between these entities; however, smaller biopsy specimens may be problematic, and, as previously mentioned, immunohistochemistry (eg, CD99) does not allow reliable distinction among mesenchymal chondrosarcoma, small cell osteosarcoma, and Ewing sarcoma. Although rare examples of mesenchymal chondrosarcoma have been reported with the t(11;22), the vast majority do not show the specific translocations and fusion types seen in Ewing sarcoma. The presence of lacelike osteoid in a small cell tumor of bone helps establish the diagnosis of small cell osteosarcoma.

△△ **Differential Diagnosis**
MESENCHYMAL CHONDROSARCOMA

1. When both the cartilaginous and small cell components are present, the diagnosis of mesenchymal chondrosarcoma is not problematic.

2. In the absence of the low-grade cartilaginous component, the "small cells" of mesenchymal chondrosarcoma are indistinguishable from Ewing sarcoma and small cell osteosarcoma.

3. The presence of CD99 positivity is not usually helpful, as it is often expressed in both mesenchymal chondrosarcoma and Ewing sarcoma and, less commonly, in small cell osteosarcoma.

4. It will sometimes be impossible, especially in small biopsy specimens, to separate Ewing sarcoma from mesenchymal chondrosarcoma. In such a circumstance, treating an osseous small round cell sarcoma with multimodality therapy, similar to what is done with Ewing sarcoma, would be preferable, as no specific therapy exists for mesenchymal chondrosarcoma.

Fig. 9. Mesenchymal chondrosarcoma with an infiltration pattern of single cells and cords within a myxohyalinized stroma (H&E, original magnification ×100).

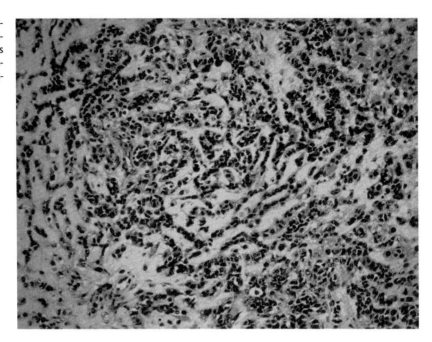

PROGNOSIS

The prognosis of mesenchymal chondrosarcoma generally is poor, with 5-year survival rates ranging between 40% and 55% and 10-year survival rates of approximately 27% to 29%.[10,11] Mesenchymal chondrosarcoma involving the jaw bones appears to have a better prognosis than those occurring in extragnathic sites, with 5-year and 10-year

Fig. 10. Osteoid/woven bone formation may be present in mesenchymal chondrosarcoma (H&E, original magnification ×200).

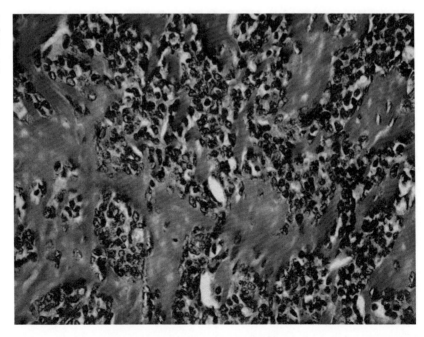

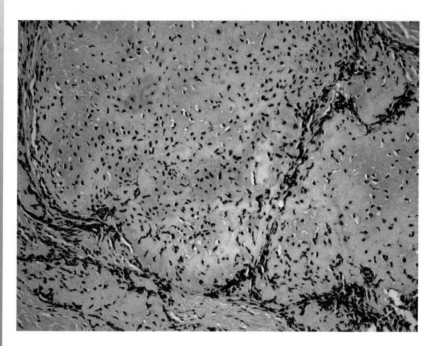

Fig. 11. In occasional examples, the nodules of well-differentiated cartilage may predominate, obscuring the underlying small round cell component (H&E, original magnification ×100).

survival rates of 82% and 56%, respectively.[12] The mainstay of treatment is radical surgery, but the role of radiation therapy and chemotherapy is unclear. As mesenchymal chondrosarcoma clearly represents a high-grade sarcoma, some have advocated a combined modality treatment, similar to that of osteosarcoma.[11] At the author's institutions, mesenchymal chondrosarcoma typically has been treated similar to Ewing sarcoma or osteosarcoma.

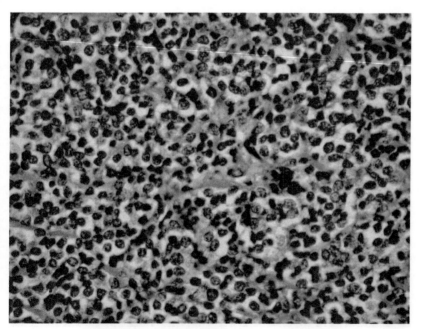

Fig. 12. Individual tumor cells in mesenchymal chondrosarcoma are generally uniform, small, round to ovoid, with vesicular nuclei, small to inconspicuous nucleoli, resembling Ewing sarcoma (H&E, original magnification ×400).

CLEAR CELL CHONDROSARCOMA

OVERVIEW

Clear cell chondrosarcoma is a very rare variant of low-grade chondrosarcoma with a predilection for long bone epiphyses. Most patients are young to middle-aged adults, and men are more often afflicted than women. Although any bone may potentially be affected, including the larynx, most reported examples have occurred in the humeral and femoral head epiphyses.[20–22] Most patients complain of localized pain, often of long duration. Radiographically, it generally forms sharply demarcated, lytic lesions of a long bone end, often associated with a sclerotic rim (Fig. 13). Cortical destruction, extraosseous extension, and periosteal new bone formation are not typically present, except in lesions arising within the axial skeleton.[23] Such radiographic features may be indistinguishable from chondroblastoma.

GROSS FEATURES

Most examples appear gray-white to brown with firm, gritty areas of mineralization, ranging up to 13 cm in greatest dimension. Obvious blue-gray hyaline cartilage is not a feature typically observed grossly.

MICROSCOPIC FEATURES

The characteristic "clear cells" occur as lobules and sheets infiltrating bone. Cytologically, these cells appear large, round to polygonal, with a large, round to ovoid nucleus, inconspicuous to small nucleoli, and abundant clear cytoplasm (Fig. 14). Occasional cells may have a more eosinophilic cytoplasm, resembling chondroblasts (Fig. 15). Osteoclast-type giant cells are randomly distributed throughout the lesion. Mitotic figures are never prominent. The presence of osteoid and bony trabeculae may cause confusion with osteoblastoma. Variable amounts of hyaline cartilage, resembling low-grade conventional chondrosarcoma, may be present (Fig. 16).[20,21]

Immunohistochemistry is not generally needed to establish the diagnosis. Individual tumor cells appear positive for vimentin and S100 protein but negative for EMA and keratins. No specific molecular or cytogenetic abnormalities have been documented, although the actual number of reported cases is very small. Extra copies of chromosome 20 and loss or rearrangements of 9p appear to be recurrent.[24]

DIFFERENTIAL DIAGNOSIS

The most important differential diagnosis, especially given the location, is chondroblastoma. Chondroblastoma generally occurs in the long bone epiphyses of skeletally immature patients, age younger than 20 years. The clear cells typical of most cases of clear cell chondrosarcoma are not present in chondroblastoma. Soder and colleagues[25] have shown that in difficult cases,

---

Key Points
CLEAR CELL CHONDROSARCOMA

1. Clear cell chondrosarcoma is a rare chondrosarcoma variant typically involving the end of long bones (epiphysis).

2. Most examples occur in young to middle-aged adults.

3. Radiologically, the neoplasm may have a benign appearance, lytic with a sclerotic rim. As such, it can be indistinguishable from chondroblastoma.

4. The diagnostic clear cells are usually arranged in sheets infiltrating bone. Lesions may be significantly ossified, and variable amounts of low-grade–appearing hyaline cartilage is present.

△△ Differential Diagnosis
CLEAR CELL CHONDROSARCOMA

1. The differential diagnosis of clear cell chondrosarcoma mainly represents chondroblastoma and metastatic renal cell carcinoma.

2. Both chondroblastoma and metastatic renal cell carcinoma are significantly more common than clear cell chondrosarcoma.

3. Chondroblastoma occurs in the epiphysis of long bones of skeletally immature patients (eg, children/adolescents). The dominant cell type is eosinophilic (not clear cell), uniform, and often exhibits round to kidney-bean–shaped nuclei. Nodules of pink chondroid are more typical than hyaline cartilage.

4. Metastatic renal cell carcinoma may exhibit similar-appearing clear cells; however, it is not associated with hyaline cartilage production and ossification does not occur. Difficult cases may benefit from immunohistochemical analysis.

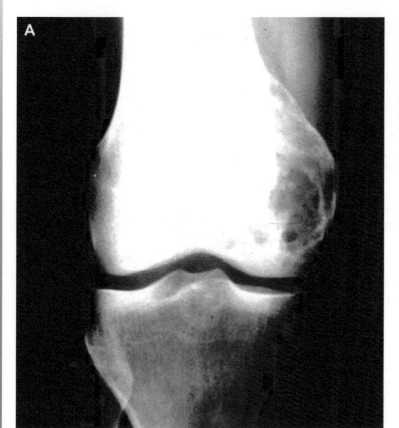

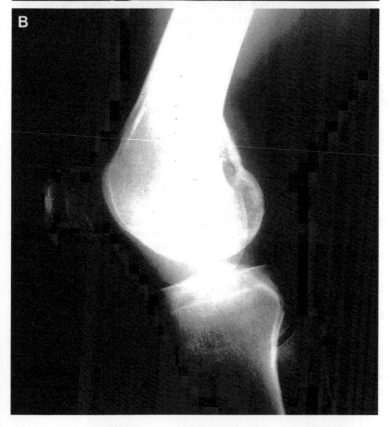

Fig. 13. Anteroposterior (*A*) and lateral (*B*) radiographs of the knee show a lytic lesion in the medial aspect of the distal femoral epimetaphysis. In contrast to giant cell tumor of bone, clear cell chondrosarcoma does not typically extend to subchondral bone.

Fig. 14. (*A*) On low power, the permeating cells of clear cell chondrosarcoma are associated with new bone and hyaline cartilage formation (H&E, original magnification ×40). (*B*) At higher power, these polygonal-shaped tumor cells appear mostly uniform with round to ovoid nuclei and abundant pale cytoplasm (H&E, original magnification ×400).

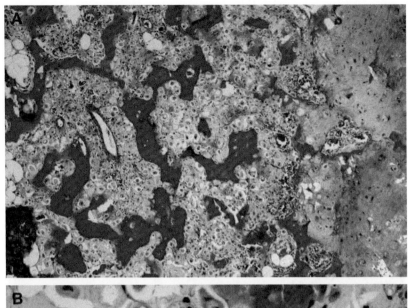

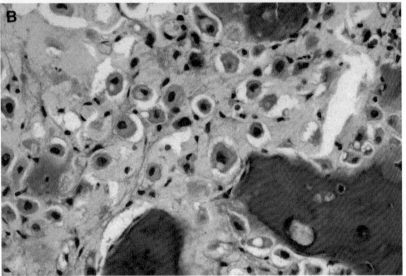

Fig. 15. Occasional examples of clear cell chondrosarcoma reveal cells resembling chondroblastoma, often arranged in cords and nests (H&E, original magnification ×100).

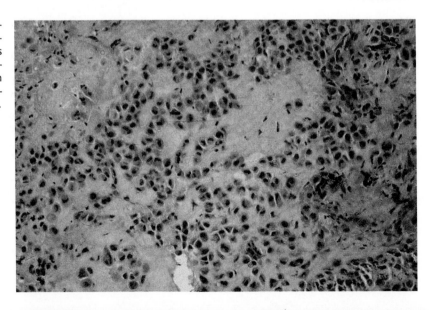

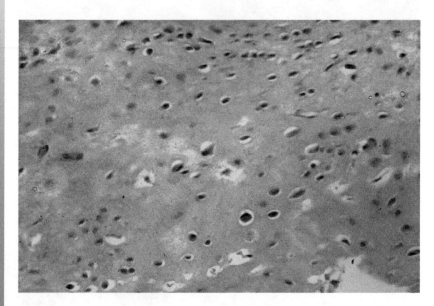

Fig. 16. The hyaline cartilage formation in clear cell chondrosarcoma is indistinguishable from conventional low-grade chondrosarcoma (H&E, original magnification ×100).

the presence of type II collagen in the extracellular tumor matrix significantly supports the diagnosis of clear cell chondrosarcoma, as it is not seen in chondroblastoma. When the tumor is heavily ossified, a resemblance to osteoblastoma may be seen; however, osteoblastoma shows prominent osteoblastic rimming with intertrabecular, hypovascular spaces. In adult patients, metastatic clear cell carcinoma of the kidney may mimic clear cell chondrosarcoma. Clear cell renal cell carcinomas do not produce hyaline cartilage. For difficult cases or small biopsies, clinicoradiologic correlation and judicious use of immunohistochemistry should help establish the diagnosis.

PROGNOSIS

Clear cell chondrosarcoma is a curable tumor, provided that it is correctly diagnosed and treated. En bloc resection with negative margins is the treatment of choice; local recurrence invariably occurs after curettage or incomplete resection. Pulmonary and skeletal metastases have been documented among inadequately treated cases.[26] High-grade dedifferentiated clear cell chondrosarcoma has been documented in a few cases.[27]

"EXTRASKELETAL" MYXOID CHONDROSARCOMA (CHORDOID SARCOMA)

OVERVIEW

Extraskeletal myxoid chondrosarcoma is a rare sarcoma usually arising in older adults and more

commonly affecting men.[28] As the nomenclature implies, the overwhelming majority arise in the deep soft tissues of the lower extremities (usually proximal) and, less frequently, the trunk. Most patients complain of an enlarging but painless soft tissue mass. Rare primary skeletal cases have been reported (**Fig. 17**).[29] As expected, it is difficult to describe such primary osseous tumors using the nomenclature for essentially identical neoplasms in soft tissues. It probably is more appropriate to label such neoplasms as "chordoid

Key Points
CHORDOID SARCOMA

1. Chordoid sarcoma, also known as extraskeletal myxoid chondrosarcoma, usually manifests as an extremity soft tissue mass. Rare examples have been described in bone.

2. Morphologically, the tumor appears multilobulated and distinctly myxoid, containing a uniform round to spindled cell population often arranged in cords, loops, and chains.

3. Cytoplasmic vacuolation may be present, raising the possibility of chondroma. Physaliferous cells are distinctly absent.

4. Immunohistochemically, chordoid sarcoma frequently expresses vimentin, synaptophysin, and S100 protein. Less often, EMA also is positive; however, cytokeratin is negative.

Fig. 17. Myxoid chondrosarcoma of bone. (*A*) Oblique view of the knee shows an ill-defined lytic lesion in the supracondylar portion of the distal femur. Cortical destruction along the medial femoral cortex is associated with periosteal new bone formation. (*B*) Magnetic resonance imaging reveals an ill-defined, permeative, and destructive lesion within the distal femur with an associated soft tissue mass. These features are consistent with osseous origin.

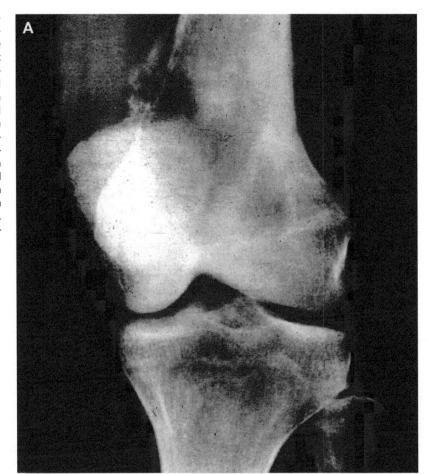

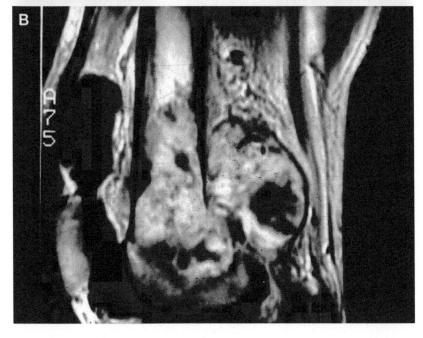

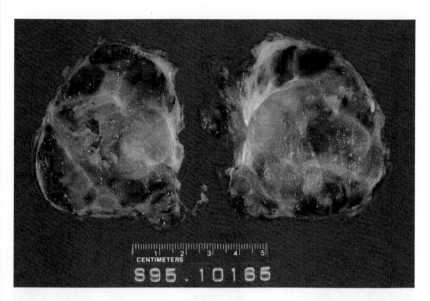

Fig. 18. Myxoid chondro-sarcoma grossly shows distinctly myxoid, variably sized lobules separated by whitish tissue septa.

sarcoma" to avoid confusion with conventional skeletal chondrosarcoma with myxoid change.

GROSS FEATURES

Chordoid sarcomas typically form large masses (up to 25 cm), appearing lobulated but well demarcated. The cut surface is shiny gray to brown, multinodular, and gelatinous to mucinous (**Fig. 18**). Areas of hemorrhage and cystic change may be apparent. More cellular lesions appear less myxoid and fleshier.

MICROSCOPIC FEATURES

Morphologically, chordoid sarcoma is abundantly myxoid and multilobular, with individual lobules frequently traversed by fibrous tissue septa (**Fig. 19**). Cellularity ranges from moderate to marked, with a tendency in some nodules toward increased cellularity at the periphery. Compared with other myxoid sarcomas, chordoid sarcomas are considerably less vascular. The tumor cells are classically arranged in anastomosing strands, rings, and nests and appear uniform, round to

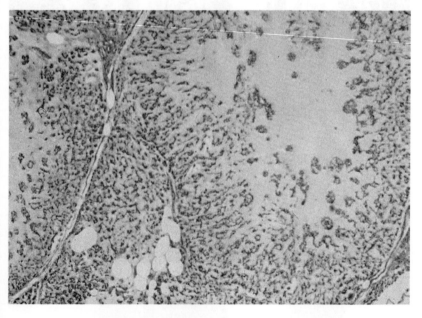

Fig. 19. Myxoid chondro-sarcoma at low power with classic multinodular appearance, often exhibiting increased cellularity at the periphery of the myxoid nodules (H&E, original magnification ×20).

slightly spindled with hyperchromatic nuclei, inconspicuous nucleoli, and surrounded by clear, vacuolated to eosinophilic cytoplasm (Fig. 20).[28] Epithelioid cells with vesicular nuclei and abundant eosinophilic cytoplasm (rhabdoid features) are occasionally observed (Fig. 21). Mitotic activity tends to be fewer than 1 to 2 mitoses per 10 high power fields. More cellular foci lacking the characteristic myxoid stroma may exhibit greater mitotic activity. Hyaline cartilage is rarely seen.

Immunohistochemistry is not usually required to establish the diagnosis. Chordoid sarcomas typically express vimentin, neuron-specific enolase, and synaptophysin.[30,31] S-100 protein positivity is observed in approximately 50% of cases. Epithelial membrane antigen is expressed less frequently. Desmin, actin, smooth muscle actin, and cytokeratin are almost always negative. Cytogenetic analysis in most cases reveals t(9;22)(q22–31;q11–12) with the EWS-CHN (TEC) gene fusion product.[32]

DIFFERENTIAL DIAGNOSIS

Based solely on microscopic features, distinction between chordoid sarcoma and chordoma may

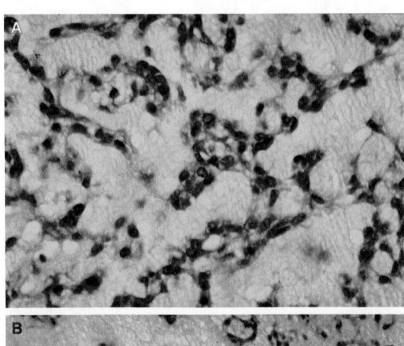
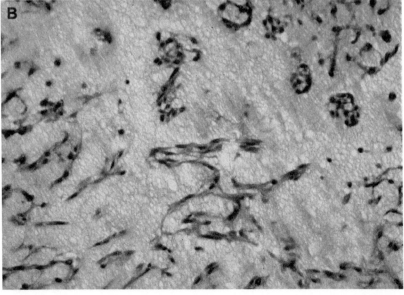

Fig. 20. (*A, B*) At higher power, individual tumor cells appear round to spindled, often arranged in ill-defined nests, cords, and strands (H&E, original magnification *A*, ×200; *B*, ×100).

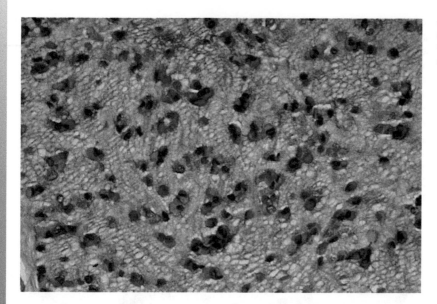

Fig. 21. Occasionally, myxoid chondrosarcomas show "rhabdoid" features (H&E, original magnification ×200).

be difficult. Diagnostic physaliferous cells are absent in chordoid sarcoma and the cytoplasmic vacuolation, when present, tends to be focal rather than diffuse. Although S100 protein may be expressed in both, keratin positivity is characteristic of chordoma. The differential diagnosis also includes metastatic mucinous adenocarcinoma. As with other variants of chondrosarcoma, a thorough clinical examination and meticulous attention to pathologic features will avoid this misdiagnosis.

PROGNOSIS

Although classically considered low grade, more recent evidence with long-term follow-up suggests local recurrence and metastatic rates approaching 50%.[28] Adverse prognostic indicators include older age of the patient, large tumor size (larger than 10 cm), and localization in the proximal extremities or limb girdle. Whether tumor grade and high cellularity are correlated with clinical outcome is unclear, as reports have produced conflicting data.[28,30] Wide surgical resection with negative margins is recommended. The role of chemotherapy and radiation therapy is uncertain. The prognosis of skeletal examples is very limited but preliminary data also suggest more aggressive behavior, especially compared with conventional chondrosarcoma.[29] In the meantime, the author would propose therapeutic guidelines similar to what is offered for primary extraskeletal tumors, as mentioned in this section.

REFERENCES

1. Mitchell A, Rudan JR, Fenton PV. Juxtacortical dedifferentiated chondrosarcoma from a primary periosteal chondrosarcoma. Mod Pathol 1996;9:279–83.
2. Kilpatrick SE, Pike EJ, Ward WG, et al. Dedifferentiated chondrosarcoma in patients with multiple osteochondromatosis: report of a case and review of the literature. Skeletal Radiol 1997;26:370–4.
3. Dahlin DC, Beabout JW. Dedifferentiation of low-grade chondrosarcomas. Cancer 1971;28:461–6.
4. Johnson S, Tetu B, Ayala AG, et al. Chondrosarcoma with additional mesenchymal component (dedifferentiated chondrosarcoma): a clinicopathologic study of 26 cases. Cancer 1986;58:278–86.
5. Reith JD, Bauer TW, Fischler DF, et al. Dedifferentiated chondrosarcoma with rhabdomyosarcomatous differentiation. Am J Surg Pathol 1996;20:293–8.
6. Akahane T, Shimizu T, Isobe K, et al. Dedifferentiated chondrosarcoma arising in a solitary osteochondroma with leiomyosarcomatous component: a case report. Arch Orthop Trauma Surg 2008;128:951–3.
7. Rinas AC, Ward WG, Kilpatrick SE. Potential sampling error in the fine needle aspiration biopsy of dedifferentiated chondrosarcoma. Acta Cytol 2005;49:554–9.
8. O'Malley DP, Opheim KE, Barry TS, et al. Chromosomal changes in dedifferentiated chondrosarcoma: a case report and review of the literature. Cancer Genet Cytogenet 2001;124:105–11.
9. Grimer RJ, Gosheger G, Taminiau A, et al. Dedifferentiated chondrosarcoma: prognostic factors and

outcome from a European group. Eur J Cancer 2007;43:2060–5.

10. Nakashima Y, Unni KK, Shives TC, et al. Mesenchymal chondrosarcoma of bone and soft tissue: a review of 111 cases. Cancer 1986;57:2444–53.

11. Huvos AG, Rosen G, Dabska M, et al. Mesenchymal chondrosarcoma: a clinicopathologic analysis of 35 patients with emphasis on treatment. Cancer 1983; 51:1230–7.

12. Dantonello TM, Int-Veen C, Leuschner I, et al. Mesenchymal chondrosarcoma of soft tissues and bone in children, adolescents, and young adults: experiences of the CWS and COSS study groups. Cancer 2008;112:2424–31.

13. Vencio EF, Reeve CM, Unni KK, et al. Mesenchymal chondrosarcoma of the jaw bones: clinicopathologic study of 19 cases. Cancer 1998;82:2350–5.

14. Granter SR, Renshaw AA, Fletcher CD, et al. CD99 reactivity in mesenchymal chondrosarcoma. Hum Pathol 1996;27:1273–6.

15. Hoang MP, Suarez PA, Donner LR, et al. Mesenchymal chondrosarcoma: a small cell neoplasm with polyphenotypic differentiation. Int J Surg Pathol 2000;8:291–301.

16. Stevenson AJ, Chatten J, Bertoni F, et al. CD99 (p30/32mic) neuroectodermal/Ewing's sarcoma antigen as an immunohistochemical marker. Review of more than 600 tumors and the literature experience. Appl Immunohistochem 1994;2:231–40.

17. Fanburg-Smith JC, Auerbach A, Marwaha JS, et al. Immunoprofile of mesenchymal chondrosarcoma: aberrant desmin and EMA expression, retention of INI1, and negative estrogen receptor in 22 female-predominant central nervous system and musculoskeletal cases. Ann Diagn Pathol 2010;14:8–14.

18. Naumann S, Krallman PA, Unni KK, et al. Translocation der(13;21)(q10;q10) in skeletal and extraskeletal mesenchymal chondrosarcoma. Mod Pathol 2002;15:572–6.

19. Sainati L, Scapinello A, Montaldi A, et al. A mesenchymal chondrosarcoma of a child with the reciprocal translocation (11;22)(q24;q12). Cancer Genet Cytogenet 1993;71:144–7.

20. Unni KK, Dahlin DC, Beabout JW, et al. Chondrosarcoma: clear-cell variant. A report of sixteen cases. J Bone Joint Surg Am 1976;58:676–83.

21. Bjornsson J, Unni KK, Dahlin DC, et al. Clear cell chondrosarcoma of bone: observations in 47 cases. Am J Surg Pathol 1984;8:223–30.

22. Kleist B, Poetsch M, Lang C, et al. Clear cell chondrosarcoma of the larynx: a case report of a rare histologic variant in an uncommon location. Am J Surg Pathol 2002;26(3):386–92.

23. Collins MS, Koyama T, Swee RG, et al. Clear cell chondrosarcoma: radiographic, computed tomographic, and magnetic resonance findings in 34 patients with pathologic correlation. Skeletal Radiol 2003;32:687–94.

24. Nishio J, Reith JD, Ogose A, et al. Cytogenetic findings in clear cell chondrosarcoma. Cancer Genet Cytogenet 2005;162:74–7.

25. Soder S, Oliveira AM, Inwards CY, et al. Type II collagen, but not aggrecan expression, distinguishes clear cell chondrosarcoma and chondroblastoma. Pathology 2006;38:35–8.

26. Itala A, Leerapun T, Inwards C, et al. An institutional review of clear cell chondrosarcoma. Clin Orthop Relat Res 2005;440:209–12.

27. Kalil RK, Inwards CY, Unni KK, et al. Dedifferentiated clear cell chondrosarcoma. Am J Surg Pathol 2000; 24:1079–86.

28. Meis-Kindblom JM, Bergh P, Gunterberg B, et al. Extraskeletal myxoid chondrosarcoma: a reappraisal of its morphologic spectrum and prognostic factors based on 117 cases. Am J Surg Pathol 1999;23:636–50.

29. Kilpatrick SE, Inwards CY, Fletcher CD, et al. Myxoid chondrosarcoma (chordoid sarcoma) of bone: a report of two cases and review of the literature. Cancer 1997;79:1903–10.

30. Oliveira AM, Sebo TJ, McGrory JE, et al. Extraskeletal myxoid chondrosarcoma: a clinicopathologic, immunohistochemical, and ploidy analysis of 23 cases. Mod Pathol 2000;13:900–8.

31. Goh YW, Spagnolo DV, Platten M, et al. Extraskeletal myxoid chondrosarcoma: a light microscopic, immunohistochemical, ultrastructural and immuno-ultrastructural study indicating neuroendocrine differentiation. Histopathology 2001;39:514–24.

32. Antonescu C, Argani P, Erlandson R, et al. Skeletal and extraskeletal myxoid chondrosarcoma: a comparative clinicopathologic, ultrastructural, and molecular study. Cancer 1998;83:1504–21.

GIANT CELL TUMOR OF BONE

David R. Lucas, MD

KEYWORDS

● Giant cell tumor ● Bone remodeling ● Anti–RANK-ligand therapy ● Cytokine-mediated pathways

ABSTRACT

This article provides an overview of giant cell tumor, including the typical clinical, radiographic, and pathologic findings, as well as some unusual features, such as multifocality and metastases. The article addresses recent advances in the molecular biology of giant cell tumor, particularly receptor activator of nuclear factor kappa B (RANK)-ligand signaling, in addition to novel anti–RANK-ligand therapy, the use of which seems promising for unresectable and metastatic tumors.

OVERVIEW

Recent developments in understanding its pathogenesis and consequent emergence of a novel form of targeted therapy (anti–receptor activator of nuclear factor kappa B [RANK]-ligand) have placed giant cell tumor (GCT) of bone in the limelight.[1] Although the histogenesis of GCT has been a subject of debate over the years, with some investigators proposing a mesenchymal origin and others a monocytic origin, current compelling evidence favors mesenchymal derivation. The neoplastic stromal cells seem to have molecular biologic properties similar to osteoblasts, in particular their ability to recruit and activate osteoclasts by cytokine-mediated pathways associated with bone remodeling; especially via RANK-ligand production.[2–6] In general, GCT is regarded as a benign tumor, albeit with a very low metastatic potential, especially to the lungs. Rare examples of multifocal GCT have also been reported. In addition, GCT can rarely transform into a malignant tumor, especially following radiation.

GCT, like most primary bone tumors, is uncommon, accounting for approximately 5% of all bone tumors and 20% of benign bone tumors.[7] It classically affects skeletally mature individuals, usually during the third and fourth decades of life, and has a slight female predilection. The age spectrum, however, is broad and includes elderly patients as well as rare cases of children. GCT can occur in association with Paget disease. GCT has a wide skeletal distribution and occurs in both tubular and flat bones. It most often occurs at the end of a long bone, with the 3 most common sites being distal femur (26%), proximal tibia (20%), and distal radius (11%). The sacrum is the fourth most common site (9%) and the most common flat bone. GCT can occur in the small bones of hands and feet, spine, and craniofacial

> ### Key Points
> #### GIANT CELL TUMOR OF BONE
>
> - Cytologic features of the mononuclear stromal cells of GCT is the basis of diagnosis.
> - Osteoclastic giant cells are common to many bone tumors, both benign and malignant.
> - The characteristic radiographic appearance of GCT as a long bone tumor in a skeletally mature individual is an eccentric, osteolytic tumor involving the epimetaphyseal area.
> - GCT occurs in both tubular and flat bones.
> - GCT has a high propensity for local recurrence, especially following simple curettage and bone grafting.

Disclosures: The author has nothing to disclose.
Department of Pathology, University of Michigan, 2G 332 UH, 1500 Catherine Street, Ann Arbor, MI 48109-0054, USA
E-mail address: drlucas@umich.edu

Surgical Pathology 5 (2012) 183–200
doi:10.1016/j.path.2011.07.012
1875-9181/12/$ – see front matter © 2012 Elsevier Inc. All rights reserved.

bones. It is exceedingly rare in the jaws.[8] It also occurs as a primary soft tissue tumor.[9]

RADIOGRAPHIC FEATURES OF GIANT CELL TUMOR OF BONE

When presenting as a long bone tumor in a skeletally mature individual, GCT has a characteristic radiographic appearance. It forms an eccentric, osteolytic tumor involving the epimetaphyseal area extending to the subchondral bone at the articular surface (Figs. 1–3). Only rare examples of nonepiphyseal GCT have been reported, usually in children with open growth plates.[10] Long bone GCT is usually expansile, well-marginated without peripheral sclerosis, and frequently shows at least focal cortical destruction. Intralesional mineralization and periosteal reaction are usually absent. In flat bones, GCT has a nonspecific radiographic appearance (Figs. 4 and 5). The level of aggression in GCT varies from marginated tumors with surrounding sclerosis limited to the medullary cavity to large, highly destructive tumors with extensive

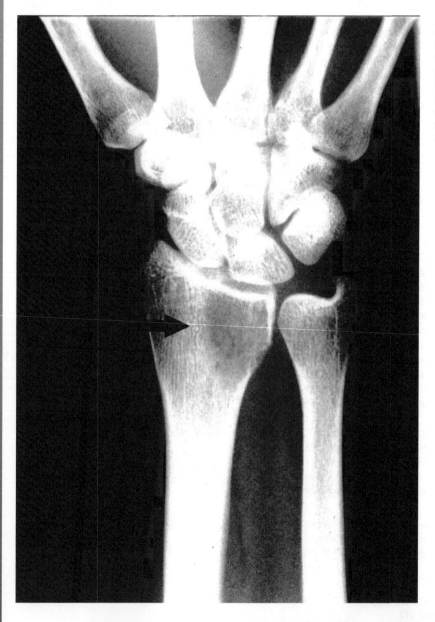

Fig. 1. GCT typically occurs at the end of a long bone in a skeletally mature person. This radiograph depicts a radiolucent bone tumor in the distal radius (*arrow*) of a 29-year-old woman. The tumor is well marginated but lacks a sclerotic border.

Fig. 2. Distal femur is the most common site of GCT. This composite radiograph and magnetic resonance image (MRI) illustrates an eccentric, osteolytic tumor at the end of the bone with destruction of the lateral cortex (*arrow*). The MRI (*right*) shows heterogeneous signaling within the mass.

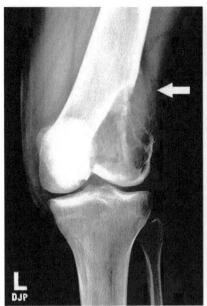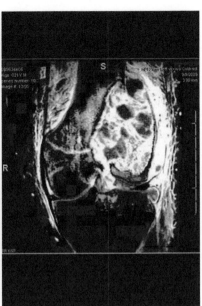

osteolysis and soft tissue invasion. Spinal GCT is typically centered within the vertebral body as opposed to the dorsal elements (**Fig. 6**). Around 10% of GCTs present with a pathologic fracture.

GROSS FEATURES OF GIANT CELL TUMOR OF BONE

GCTs are usually red-brown and friable with hemorrhagic and cystic areas (**Figs. 7** and **8**). Some tumors are white and fleshy (**Fig. 9**). Yellow areas indicate sheets of lipid-filled macrophages (xanthoma cells). Indolent tumors remain confined within the medulla, whereas advanced tumors destroy bone and invade soft tissue. Soft tissue recurrent tumors are often encased by a shell of bone (**Fig. 10**).

MICROSCOPIC FEATURES OF GIANT CELL TUMOR OF BONE

GCT is comprised of a mixture of mononuclear stromal cells and osteoclastic giant cells. The giant cells are usually distributed evenly throughout the tumor (**Figs. 11** and **12**) and sometimes are very large, with up to 100 nuclei (**Fig. 13**). The mononuclear stromal cells typically have oval to reniform nuclei, abundant cytoplasm, and ill-defined cell borders (see **Fig. 12**; **Fig. 14**). Nuclei can be spindle shaped, especially in storiform areas. Mitotic figures may be frequent, but atypical mitotic figures are not seen. Although historically the nuclei of the mononuclear stromal and giant cells were thought to be identical, this is not always the case. In fact, this assumption was largely based on the thought that the giant cells represented fused mononuclear cells, which is probably not true.

Cytologic atypia, including tumors with mild nuclear pleomorphism and hyperchromasia and brisk mitotic activity, can be seen in GCT. However, histologic grading has not been shown to have prognostic value. GCT often has an infiltrative growth pattern entrapping bone and invading marrow and soft tissue (**Fig. 15**). Vascular invasion in the form of tumor thrombi within venous channels at the periphery of the tumor (**Fig. 16**) is common in GCT. Vascular invasion does not seem to indicate more aggressive behavior. In rare instances, GCT can form large thrombi within muscular veins.

The histologic appearance of GCT is highly variable, primarily because of the secondary alterations, which can obscure the diagnostic areas. Common secondary alterations include fibrohistiocytic (**Fig. 17**) and xanthomatous (**Fig. 18**) patterns, fibrosis and hemosiderosis, coagulation

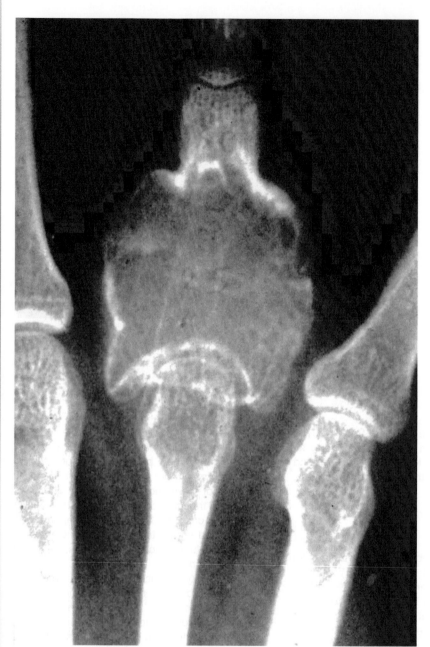

Fig. 3. GCT is rare in the acral extremities. This radiograph depicts a destructive, osteolytic bone tumor at the proximal end of the proximal third phalange of the hand. It differs from giant cell reparative granuloma, which usually does not involve the end of the bone and is less aggressive.

necrosis (**Fig. 19**), secondary aneurysmal bone cyst formation (**Fig. 20**), abundant woven bone, and rarely cartilage formation (**Fig. 21**). In addition, some tumors or areas within a tumor lack giant cells altogether (see **Fig. 14**). In such cases, the diagnosis is rendered based on cytologic features of the stromal cells along with clinical and radiographic correlations.

TUMOR BIOLOGY

GCT shows a wide spectrum of cytogenetic abnormalities with both clonal and random chromosomal aberrations. Telomeric associations are the most frequent cytogenetic finding. These associations represent end-to-end fusions of whole,

Fig. 4. GCT occurs in flat bones exemplified by this large radiolucent bone tumor (*arrow*) in the left ilium of a 35-year-old man.

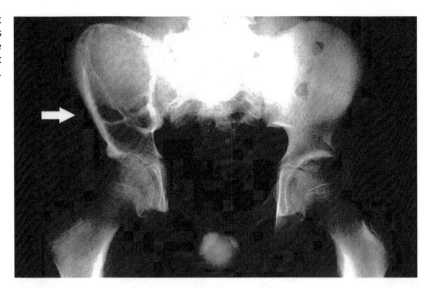

Fig. 5. GCT is very rare in the craniofacial bones. This computed tomography image depicts a destructive tumor involving the sphenoid bone (*arrow*). True GCT of bone almost never occurs in the jaw bones; most giant cell–rich jaw tumors represent giant cell reparative granulomas.

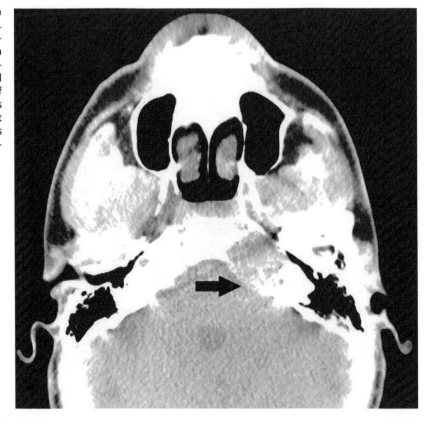

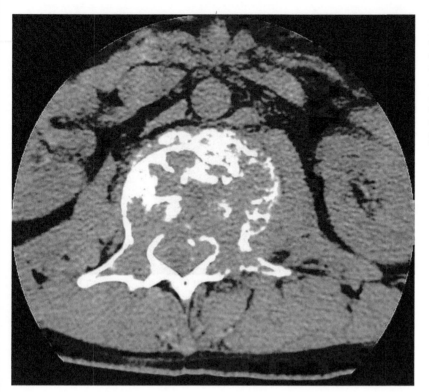

Fig. 6. Unlike aneurysmal bone cyst and osteoblastoma, spinal GCT is distinctive in that it affects the vertebral body as opposed to the dorsal elements, exemplified by this destructive thoracic vertebral tumor in a 40-year-old man.

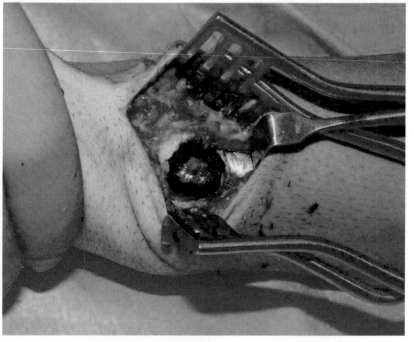

Fig. 7. Because GCT is frequently hemorrhagic, it often dark-red, demonstrated in this intraoperative image of the surface of a proximal fibular tumor.

Fig. 8. This gross specimen shows the cut surface of a distal femoral GCT depicting its classic red-brown color, friable consistency, and extension to the end of the bone.

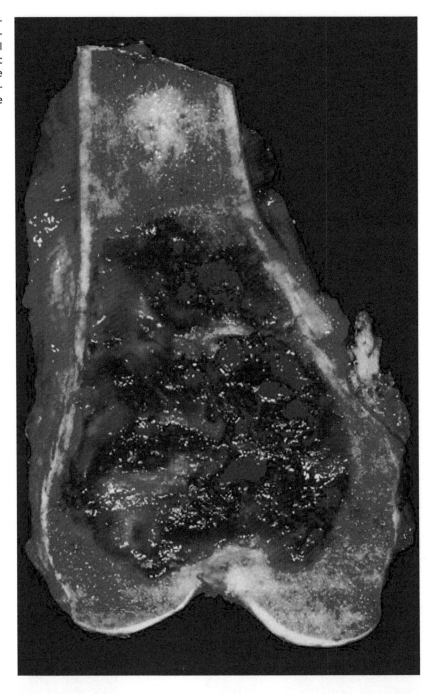

intact chromosomes, which result in the reduction in telomere lengths. Various chromosomes can be affected, especially chromosome 11p, which is frequently altered.[11] High levels of telomeric fusions are thought to initiate chromosomal instability and be responsible for tumorigenesis.[12] Tumors with clonal cytogenetic aberrations are thought to be more aggressive than those without.[11]

Enzymatic bone lysis is an important mechanism in the pathogenesis of GCT, and several enzymes have been implicated, especially matrix metalloproteinases.[13] Current evidence suggests that a subset of mononuclear stromal cells

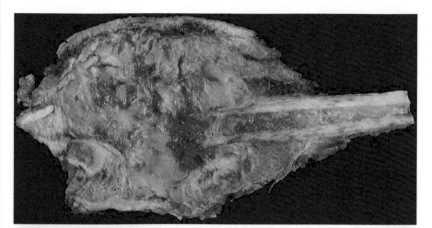

Fig. 9. Some GCTs are white-tan and fleshy, such as this destructive distal radial bone tumor in a 32-year-old man.

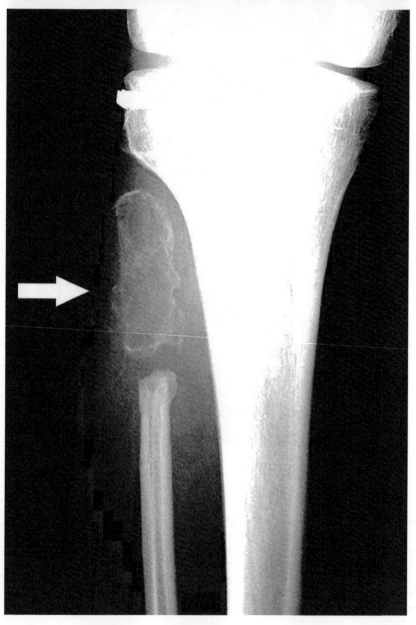

Fig. 10. Soft tissue recurrences of GCT are typically encased by an osseous rim (*arrow*) demonstrated by this radiograph of this previously resected fibular tumor from a 45-year-old woman.

Fig. 11. GCT is typically comprised of numerous, evenly distributed osteoclastic giant cells and mononuclear stromal cells.

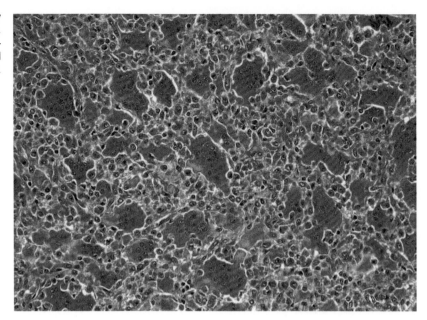

represents the neoplastic element of GCT. These cells seem to have an osteoblastic phenotype and stimulate the formation and activation of osteoclasts via a RANK ligand-dependent process. Identical to what occurs during normal bone remodeling, this mechanism seems integral to the pathogenesis of GCT[3–5] and serves as the basis for a clinical trial using a monoclonal antibody against RANK-ligand to control unresectable or metastatic disease.[1]

Fig. 12. The mononuclear stromal cells consist of spindle or polygonal cells with oval to reniform nuclei and abundant cytoplasm with indistinct cell borders. Intralesional hemorrhage is common as shown.

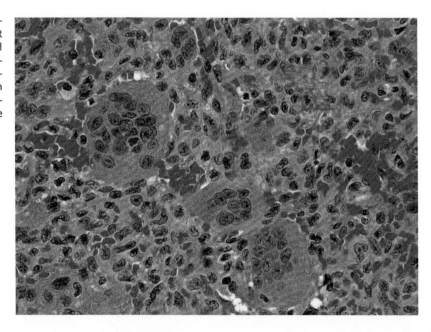

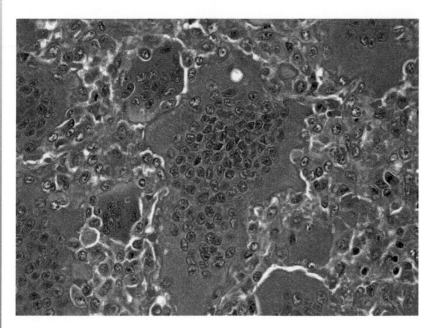

Fig. 13. Occasionally GCTs have very large osteoclastic giant cells, including some with more than 100 nuclei.

DIAGNOSIS OF GIANT CELL TUMOR OF BONE

Although most tumors are densely populated with osteoclastic giant cells, GCT is diagnosed based on the cytologic features of the mononuclear stromal cells. This point is important because various other bone tumors can be giant cell–rich, ranging from non-neoplastic reactive lesions to malignant tumors. In addition, as noted, some GCTs are giant cell–poor. In such cases, clinicoradiological correlation may be essential for arriving at the correct diagnosis.

DIFFERENTIAL DIAGNOSIS OF GIANT CELL TUMOR OF BONE

Osteoclastic giant cells are common to many bone tumors, both benign and malignant. They may be abundant and such tumors are regarded as being giant cell–rich. Careful microscopic assessment in

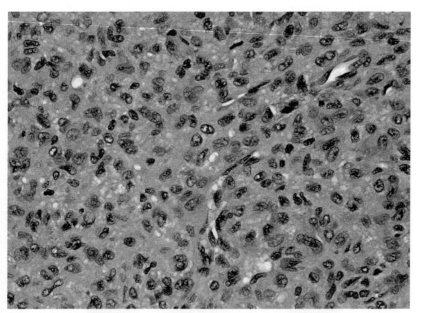

Fig. 14. It is common to find large areas within GCT that lack osteoclastic giant cells. In such cases, the diagnosis depends on identifying classic cytologic features of the mononuclear stromal cells, such as oval and reniform nuclei and ill-defined cytoplasm. Clinicoradiological correlation may be required.

Fig. 15. GCT tends to have an invasive growth pattern depicted by destructive invasion of bone (*left*), infiltration into marrow (*center*), and soft tissue invasion (*right*).

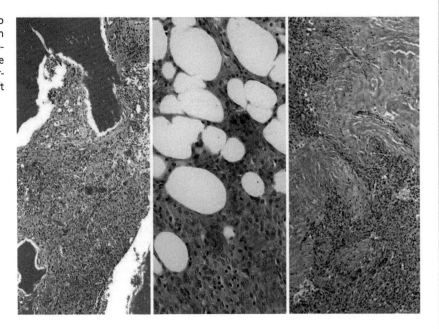

conjunction with clinical and imaging features, especially patient age, anatomic location, specific site within the bone, and radiographic appearance, lead to the correct diagnosis in most cases. The most common giant cell–rich bone tumors are listed later and differential diagnostic features are summarized in the "*Differential diagnosis table*: *giant cell tumor of bone*."

- Giant cell reparative granuloma
- Brown tumor of hyperparathyroidism
- Giant cell–rich osteosarcoma
- Nonossifying fibroma
- Aneurysmal bone cyst
- Chondroblastoma
- Osteoblastoma.

Fig. 16. Vascular invasion is common in GCT as depicted by this large intravenous tumor thrombus at the periphery of a tumor. It has not been shown to have prognostic value.

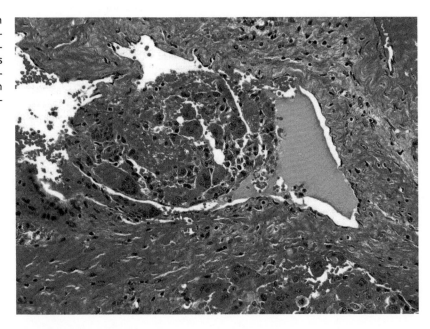

Differential Diagnosis
TABLE GIANT CELL TUMOR OF BONE

Diagnosis	Location	Radiographic Appearance	Histologic Architecture	Cytologic Features	Comment
Giant cell reparative granuloma (GCRG)	• Small tubular bones of hands and feet • Jaw bones	• Radiolucent • Expansile • Well demarcated	• Numerous giant cells in clusters • Loosely textured fibrous stroma • Osteoid/woven bone	Fibroblastic spindle cells	• In small tubular bones usually does not go to the end of bone • GCT very rare in jaw bones
Brown tumor of primary hyperparathyroidism	Multiple sites: digits, pubis, clavicle, vertebra, and so forth	Diffuse osteopenia and radiolucent tumors	• Similar to GCRG • Marked osteoclastic resorption (tunneling)	Similar to GCRG	• Parathyroid adenoma • Hypercalcemia and marked PTH elevation • Rare GCTs can be multifocal
Giant cell–rich osteosarcoma	• Long bones • Proximal skeleton	Destructive osteolytic bone tumor	Numerous osteoclastic giant cells admixed with malignant stromal cells and lacelike osteoid	• Hyperchromatic, pleomorphic stromal cells • Atypical mitotic figures	Benign giant cells may obscure underling malignant features
Nonossifying fibroma	Metaphyseal, intracortical long bone, especially tibia, femur, fibula	• Eccentric • Expansile • Radiolucent • Trabeculated • Sclerotic margin	• Storiform • Giant cell clusters • Hemosiderin	Benign fibrohistiocytic spindle cells and xanthoma cells	GCT can have fibro histiocytic areas identical to NOF
Aneurysmal bone cyst	• Metaphyseal long bones or flat bones • Dorsal elements of vertebrae	• Markedly expansile • Radiolucent • Fluid-fluid levels on magnetic resonance imaging	• Blood-filled cysts • Trabeculae and solid areas • Fibromyxoid stroma • Clustered giant cells • Osteoid and spiculated calcifications	• Benign myofibroblastic spindle cells • Frequent mitoses	GCT can have secondary ABC change
Chondroblastoma	• Epiphyses of long bones • Flat bones of pelvis • Small bones of feet	Well-demarcated with sclerotic rim and frequent intralesional calcifications	• Sheets of epithelioid cells admixed with multinucleated giant cells • Geographic areas of chondroid matrix • Calcifications	• Abundant eosinophilic or clear cytoplasm with sharp cell borders • Eccentric nuclei with grooves	Although located in epiphysis, cytologic features distinguish it from GCT
Osteoblastoma	Any bone, but predilection for spine and sacrum	Variable, but usually expansile with intralesional ossification	Interconnecting trabeculae of osteoid and woven bone with osteoblastic rimming and osteoclasts	Osteoblasts with abundant cytoplasm with perinuclear clearing and eccentric vesicular nuclei	GCT can sometimes have extensive ossification and fibrosis to mimic osteoblastoma

Fig. 17. Fibrohistiocytic or fibroxanthomatous change is common in GCT and is generally regarded as a secondary or degenerative alteration. Because it may compose a large portion of a given tumor, distinguishing it from nonossifying fibroma can be challenging in the absence of proper clinicoradiologic correlation. This pattern is characterized by storiform arrays of fibroblastic spindle cells and foamy macrophages (xanthoma cells).

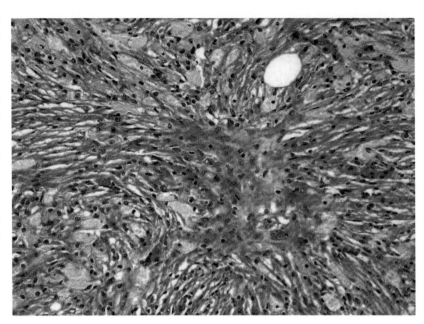

Fig. 18. Some GCTs have extensive xanthomatous change consisting of sheets of foamy macrophages (*left*) that impart a golden-yellow color to the tissue (*right*).

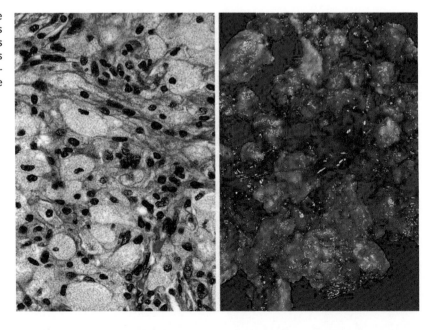

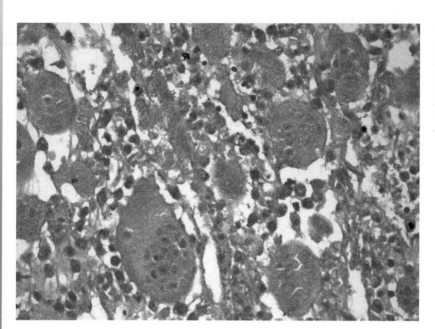

Fig. 19. Infarction is common in GCT, especially following pathologic fracture. Note the ghostlike remnants of giant cells and stromal cells in this femoral tumor from a 12-year-old girl that fractured.

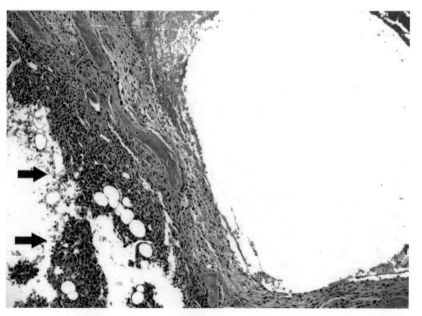

Fig. 20. Extensive intralesional hemorrhage is common in GCT. Sometimes large cystic hemorrhage spaces or secondary aneurysmal bone cyst (ABC) develop as shown. Distinguishing GCT with secondary ABC from primary ABC can be challenging. In addition to clinicoradiological correlation, careful search for more compact areas of conventional GCT morphology (*arrows*) is required to establish the diagnosis.

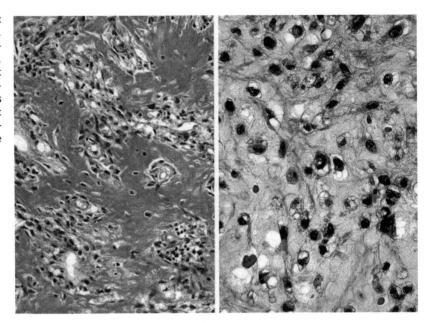

Fig. 21. Osseous matrix (*left*) is common in GCT. It usually presents as trabeculae of woven bone, is more prominent at the periphery of the tumor, and can sometimes be so extensive as to mimic osteoblastoma. Cartilaginous matrix (*right*) is rare in GCT.

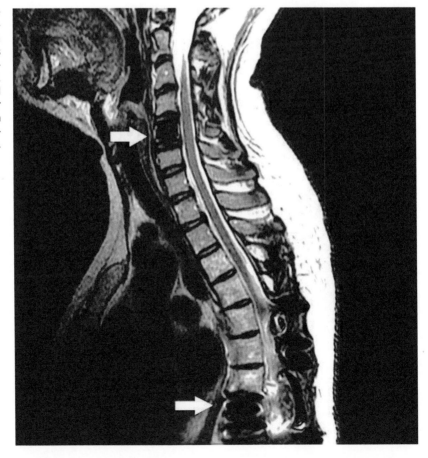

Fig. 22. Rarely GCT can be multifocal. This 35-year-old man presented with multiple vertebral tumors (*arrows*) with typical morphologic features of GCT. Distinguishing multifocal GCT from brown tumor of hyperparathyroidism requires clinical correlation and laboratory analysis.

BEHAVIOR AND PROGNOSIS OF GIANT CELL TUMOR OF BONE

GCT has a high propensity for local recurrence, especially following simple curettage and bone grafting whereby it approaches 50%. Modern surgical techniques, including application of chemical or thermal adjuvants and polymethyl methacrylate bone cementation, have significantly improved on this.

Multicentric involvement (**Fig. 22**) by primary GCT is a rare event occurring in less than 1% of cases.[14] Patients with multifocal skeletal involvement by giant cell lesions should be evaluated for hyperparathyroidism because brown tumors of hyperparathyroidism can mimic GCT.

Metastases occur in only around 2% of cases[15] and most are pulmonary (**Fig. 23**). However, various other sites of metastasis have been reported, including bone, brain, kidney, adrenal gland, gastrointestinal tract, and skin. Patients with metastatic disease often have a long, indolent course. However, the prognosis is unpredictable, with 25% dying of disease.[15] There are rare reports of spontaneous regression of metastases.[15,16]

Malignant transformation in GCT is rare (**Fig. 24**). It can be a primary event characterized by juxtaposition of GCT and sarcoma within the tumor or more often a secondary event characterized by sarcoma arising in the site of a previously excised GCT. Secondary malignancy in GCT often follows radiotherapy. The phenotype of the sarcomatous component can be either an osteosarcoma or a nonosteogenic spindle cell sarcoma.

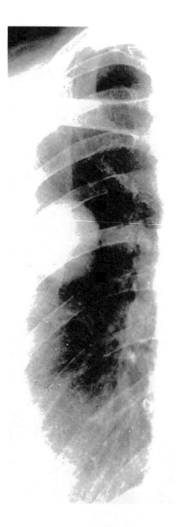
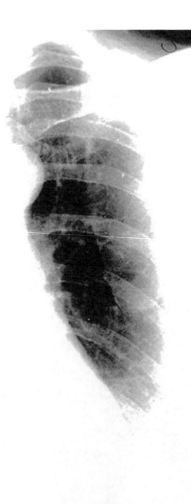

Fig. 23. Metastases develop from otherwise typical GCT in 1% to 3% of cases. Most of these cases are preceded by prior surgical manipulation of the primary site. Pulmonary metastases are most common as shown; however, GCT can also metastasize to other sites. Many, but not all, cases of metastatic GCT pursue a protracted course.

Fig. 24. Malignant GCT is defined as sarcoma arising at the site of an established GCT. It may be primary, presenting at the time of diagnosis, but is more often secondary, occurring years later following initial treatment. It is often radiation associated. This gross resection specimen of the distal radius and carpal bones from a 42-year-old man discloses an osteo-blastic osteosarcoma with sunburst osseous spiculation (*arrow*) arising adjacent to a plug of methyl methacrylate bone cement (*asterisk*) that was used to treat his GCT 7 years earlier.

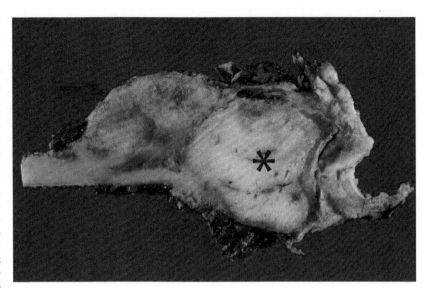

SUMMARY: GIANT CELL TUMOR OF BONE

GCT is enigmatic in terms of its histogenesis and its behavior. Based on a better understanding of the cellular mechanisms involved in bone remodeling and a greater understanding of the biology of GCT itself, a mesenchymal osteoblastlike derivation seems more plausible than a monocytic one. An early report on the effectiveness of anti–RANK-ligand therapy, which targets a key cytokine in bone remodeling, certainly supports this conclusion.[1] Behaviorwise, GCT continues to be enigmatic. It straddles the boundary between benign and malignant. Although most tumors remain localized, albeit with a high propensity for recurrence and locally aggressive behavior, there are rare tumors that metastasize, are multifocal, or transform into fully malignant tumors. To date, histology and other biologic markers have not been shown to reliably predict prognosis in the clinical setting.

REFERENCES

1. Thomas D, Henshaw R, Skubitz K, et al. Denosumab in patients with giant-cell tumour of bone: an open-label, phase 2 study. Lancet Oncol 2010;11(3): 275–80.
2. Nishimura M, Yuasa K, Mori K, et al. Cytological properties of stromal cells derived from giant cell tumor of bone (GCTSC) which can induce osteoclast formation of human blood monocytes without cell to cell contact. J Orthop Res 2005;23(5):979–87.
3. Murata A, Fujita T, Kawahara N, et al. Osteoblast lineage properties in giant cell tumors of bone. J Orthop Sci 2005;10(6):581–8.
4. Ghert M, Simunovic N, Cowan RW, et al. Properties of the stromal cell in giant cell tumor of bone. Clin Orthop Relat Res 2007;459:8–13.
5. Morgan T, Atkins GJ, Trivett MK, et al. Molecular profiling of giant cell tumor of bone and the osteo-clastic localization of ligand for receptor activator of nuclear factor kappa B. Am J Pathol 2005; 167(1):117–28.
6. Atkins GJ, Kostakis P, Vincent C, et al. RANK Expression as a cell surface marker of human osteoclast precursors in peripheral blood, bone marrow, and giant cell tumors of bone. J Bone Miner Res 2006;21(9):1339–49.
7. Fechner RE, Mills SE, Armed Forces Institute of Pathology (U.S.), Universities Associated for Research and Education in Pathology. Tumors of the bones and joints. Washington, DC: Armed Forces Institute of Pathology: Available from the American Registry of Pathology Armed Forces Institute of Pathology; 1993.
8. Unni KK, Inwards CY, Bridge JA, et al. Tumors of the bone and joints, vol. 4. Silver Spring (MD): American registry of pathology; 2005.
9. Oliveira AM, Dei Tos AP, Fletcher CD, et al. Primary giant cell tumor of soft tissues: a study of 22 cases. Am J Surg Pathol 2000;24(2):248–56.
10. Fain JS, Unni KK, Beabout JW, et al. Nonepiphyseal giant cell tumor of the long bones. Clinical, radiologic, and pathologic study. Cancer 1993;71(11):3514–9.

11. Bridge JA, Neff JR, Bhatia PS, et al. Cytogenetic findings and biologic behavior of giant cell tumors of bone. Cancer 1990;65(12):2697–703.

12. Schwartz HS, Juliao SF, Sciadini MF, et al. Telomerase activity and oncogenesis in giant cell tumor of bone. Cancer 1995;75(5):1094–9.

13. Si AI, Huang L, Xu J, et al. Expression and localization of extracellular matrix metalloproteinase inducer in giant cell tumor of bone. J Cell Biochem 2003; 89(6):1154–63.

14. Dahlin DC, Cupps RE, Johnson EW Jr. Giant-cell tumor: a study of 195 cases. Cancer 1970;25(5): 1061–70.

15. Rock MG, Pritchard DJ, Unni KK. Metastases from histologically benign giant-cell tumor of bone. J Bone Joint Surg Am 1984;66(2):269–74.

16. Kay RM, Eckardt JJ, Seeger LL, et al. Pulmonary metastasis of benign giant cell tumor of bone. Six histologically confirmed cases, including one of spontaneous regression. Clin Orthop Relat Res 1994;(302):219–30.

FIBRO-OSSEOUS LESIONS

Jacquelyn A. Knapik, MD

KEYWORDS

- Fibrous dysplasia • Osteofibrous dysplasia • Adamantinoma of long bones
- McCune-albright syndrome • Mauzabraud syndrome

ABSTRACT

This article describes the clinical, radiographic, gross, microscopic, and histologic features; differential diagnosis; molecular pathology; treatment; and prognosis of fibrous dysplasia, osteofibrous dysplasia, and adamantinoma of long bones.

FIBROUS DYSPLASIA

OVERVIEW

Fibrous dysplasia is a benign, intramedullary, dysplastic process of bone-forming mesenchymal tissue that commonly involves the long bones, ribs, pelvis, and craniofacial bones. The disease that Lichtenstein described in 1938 as polyostotic fibrous dysplasia[1] had previously been reported in the literature under a variety of titles, such as "osteo-dystrophia fibrosa unilateralis," "unilateral polyostotic osteitis fibrosa," "focal osteitis fibrosa," "osteitis fibrosa in multiple foci," "osteitis fibrosa with formation of hyaline cartilage," "osteitis fibrosa disseminata," and so forth.[1,2] This process was further described by Lichtenstein and Jaffe in 1942 when it was recoined as fibrous dysplasia when referring to the solitary form of the disease.[3]

Fibrous dysplasia represents approximately 5% to 7% of benign bone tumors.[4,5] It can affect one bone as a solitary lesion (monostotic) or multiple bones with multiple lesions (polyostotic), and can be associated with other conditions. The monostotic form is more common, occurring in 75% to 80% of the cases diagnosed.[6] It typically involves the proximal femur, tibia, ribs, and craniofacial bones. The polyostotic form has 2 variants: monomelic and polymelic. The monomelic variant affects the lower extremity and ipsilateral pelvis. The polymelic variant is more severe and involves both of the extremities, the trunk, and craniofacial bones.

CLINICAL FEATURES OF FIBROUS DYSPLASIA

Fibrous dysplasia can occur at any age, but most cases present clinically within the first 3 decades of life. The polyostotic form often manifests itself at a younger age than the monostotic form.[7] Patients with monostotic fibrous dysplasia typically present between 5 to 20 years of age, whereas those with polyostotic fibrous dysplasia usually present before the age of 10. The lesions grow with the child until puberty, at which time the lesions stabilize. Gender and racial predilection has not been clearly established for this disease process.

Lesions of fibrous dysplasia are often asymptomatic and discovered incidentally on radiographs taken for other reasons. When patients are symptomatic, they usually present with localized bone pain and pathologic fractures. Lesions in the medial aspect of the femoral neck are more prone to fractures, as a result of the high level of stress

Key Features
FIBROUS DYSPLASIA

- Ground glass appearance on plain radiographs
- Computed tomography is best mode of imaging
- Delicate trabeculae of immature bone with no osteoblastic rimming
- Background of bland dysplastic fibrous stroma
- Chinese characters or alphabet soup

Department of Pathology, University of Florida, 1600 South West Archer Road, Gainesville, FL 32610, USA
E-mail address: knapik@pathology.ufl.edu

Surgical Pathology 5 (2012) 201–229
doi:10.1016/j.path.2011.07.013
1875-9181/12/$ – see front matter © 2012 Elsevier Inc. All rights reserved.

that occurs in this weight-bearing region of the bone.[8] Female patients affected by the disease may have pain during their menstrual cycle or during pregnancy because of the presence of estrogen receptors located in the bony lesions.[9]

Bone deformities can occur in patients with either monostotic or polyostotic fibrous dysplasia. The age of the patient, site of the lesion, and size of the lesion all have bearing on the extent of deformation. Patients with diffuse polyostotic fibrous dysplasia in the weight-bearing bones are more prone to bowing deformities even after skeletal maturity. The classic deformity is a lateral bowing of the proximal femur that is known as the "shepherd's crook deformity" (**Fig. 1**). Other deformities reported include scoliosis[10] and craniofacial deformities of the maxilla, zygomatic, and ethmoid bones.[11]

RADIOGRAPHIC FEATURES OF FIBROUS DYSPLASIA

Plain radiographs reveal a radiolucent lesion within the medullary canal of the metaphysis or diaphysis of the bone with expansion of the contour and thinning of the cortex (**Fig. 2**). As normal bony trabeculae are replaced by fibrous tissue and dysplastic woven bone, the lesion takes on a homogeneous "ground glass" or hazy appearance. A distinct rim of reactive bone forms around this expansile mass, whereas slow resorption of the cortex leads to endosteal scalloping. Focal areas of cartilage may be present in these lesions and can calcify, resulting in dense, punctate foci on radiographs.[12,13]

Radionuclide bone scintography is a sensitive but nonspecific imaging modality. Actively forming lesions have increased isotope uptake, which reveals the extent of the lesion and correlates closely with the extent of the lesion seen on plain radiographs. As the lesion matures, uptake decreases and the image becomes less intense.[12] Bone scintography can be used to exclude the polyostotic form of the disease.

Computed tomography (CT) accurately delineates the extent of the lesion and is the best technique for demonstrating the radiographic features of fibrous dysplasia (**Fig. 3**). The thickness of the cortex, endosteal scalloping, and reactive periosteal bone are visualized with more detail than radiographs or magnetic resonance imaging (MRI). In addition, contrast media can be used to enhance the lesion because of its high vascularity.[12]

MRI has the added advantage of providing coronal and sagittal evaluation of the lesion.[13] T1-weighted and T2-weighted images are dependent on the amount of fibrous tissue, bony trabeculae, and secondary changes present in the lesion.[12] T1-weighted images of highly fibrous lesions have low signal intensity, whereas T2-weighted intensity is variable. Secondary changes, such as cystic degeneration, hemorrhage, or the presence of a cartilaginous component results in heterogeneity on MRI studies. Cystic changes often have high signal intensity on T2-weighted images because of the high water content.[13]

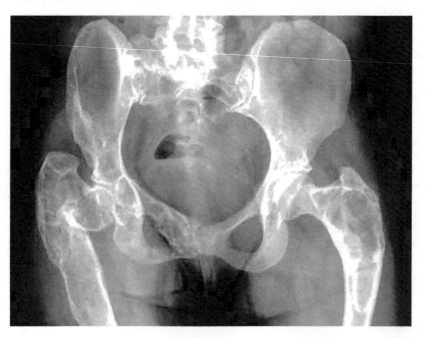

Fig. 1. Fibrous dysplasia. Radiographic features. An anteroposterior (AP) view of the pelvis demonstrating the so-called "shepherd's crook deformity" with bowing of the proximal femurs.

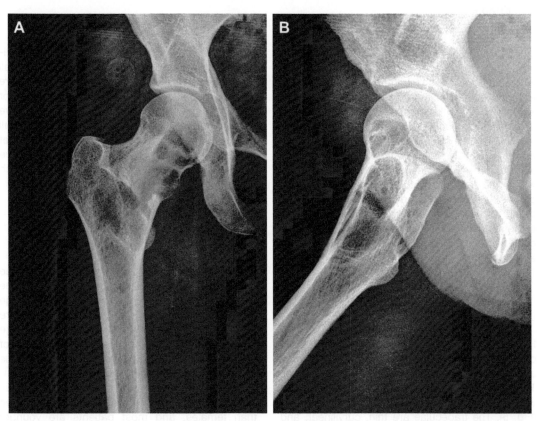

Fig. 2. Fibrous dysplasia. Radiographic features. (*A*) An AP view of the proximal femur shows a lucent lesion with a "ground glass" appearance. (*B*) An oblique view of the femur shows the lesion is well demarcated by a thick rim of sclerotic reactive bone.

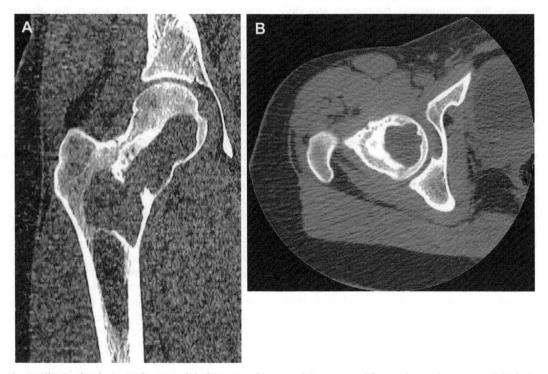

Fig. 3. Fibrous dysplasia. CT features. (*A*) This coronal image of the proximal femur shows the extent of the lesion and thickness of the cortex. (*B*) The axial image shows an intramedullary lesion with endosteal scalloping and a rim of sclerotic reactive bone.

GROSS FEATURES OF FIBROUS DYSPLASIA

Fibrous dysplasia is an intramedullary process that expands and thins the surrounding cortex. The lesion has sharp borders and is surrounded by a thin rim of reactive bone, which allows easy removal with blunt dissection or curettage.[12] The tissue is usually yellow-white and has a gritty texture from the presence of bony trabeculae within the lesion. Fractures through the lesion before curettage can lead to hemorrhagic tissue owing to the high concentration of small vessels in the neoplastic tissue. In addition, these lesions can become cystic, leaving little tissue for examination.

MICROSCOPIC FEATURES OF FIBROUS DYSPLASIA

Histologic examination of fibrous dysplasia reveals cytologically bland spindle cells in a fibrous stroma arranged in a whorled or storiform pattern (Fig. 4). The stroma encases trabeculae of immature woven bone that have no osteoblastic rimming (Fig. 5). The trabeculae are thin, curvilinear, and focally anastomosing structures that are described as resembling Chinese characters (Fig. 6). Under polarized light, the woven bone displays the characteristic haphazard arrangement of immature matrix (Fig. 7). Abnormal mitotic figures, cytologic atypia, and necrosis are usually not present.

Lesions of fibrous dysplasia typically are well circumscribed with varying proportions of fibrous stroma and trabeculae. In patients with multiple lesions, some are rich in stroma with few trabeculae, whereas other lesions have an abundant bony component. Proportions of each can vary within an individual lesion as well. Mineralized matrix that forms concentrically laminated calcifications, or "cementoid bodies," can occasionally be found in lesions that have a heavy trabecular component (Fig. 8). Cementoid bodies, however, tend to be more prevalent in fibrous dysplasia of the craniofacial bones.

As lesions age, they can develop secondary changes that may complicate the diagnostic picture. Lesions can become cystic and filled with yellow-tinged serous fluid, often leaving little lesional tissue for evaluation (Fig. 9). Pathologic fractures through the lesion can result in hemorrhage and multinucleated giant cells in curettage specimens, raising the question of an aneurysmal bone cyst. As the fracture begins to heal, reactive bone with osteoblastic rimming appears in the lesion, which contradicts the usual finding of

trabeculae without osteoblastic rimming. In addition, foamy macrophages may be present in small clusters or as a dense infiltrate and may obscure other diagnostic features (Fig. 10). Mature or aging lesions of fibrous dysplasia tend to have a more extensive fibrous component. With all the possibilities discussed, it is imperative that adequate clinical history and imaging studies are available for review when trying to establish a diagnosis.

FIBROUS DYSPLASIA WITH FOCI OF CARTILAGINOUS DIFFERENTIATION (FIBROCARTILAGINOUS DYSPLASIA)

Occasionally, nodules of hyaline cartilage can be found in lesions of fibrous dysplasia.[14,15] The amount of cartilage seen is variable and can range from microscopic foci to large areas that are grossly visible. When there is abundant cartilage present, some prefer to use the terminology of "fibrocartilaginous dysplasia," rather than fibrous dysplasia with foci of cartilaginous differentiation.[15]

Fibrous dysplasia with foci of cartilaginous differentiation is slightly more prevalent in males than females, and most patients are younger than 30 years. The most common site of occurrence is the femur,[15,16] and it rarely involves the craniofacial bones.[15] When there is a significant amount of cartilage in the lesion, the affected bone is often severely deformed. This process can occur in patients with either monostotic or polyostotic fibrous dysplasia, but is more common in the polyostotic form and can be present in one or multiple lesions.[15]

The radiographic appearance is similar to fibrous dysplasia but with lucent areas where the cartilage nodules are present in the lesion. When the cartilage nodules become calcified, they appear as ringlike or punctate foci that can be small and scattered through the lesion or can be exuberant, resembling a primary cartilaginous neoplasm (Fig. 11).[15]

Histologically, the typical features of fibrous dysplasia are present with irregularly shaped trabeculae of immature bone with no osteoblastic rimming within a fibrous stroma. Nodules of hyaline cartilage are scattered among the trabeculae within the fibrous stroma (Fig. 12). Some of the nodules may have a rim of woven bone, and less frequently lamellar bone, around the periphery. Chondrocytes within the nodules usually lack atypia and are evenly distributed through the cartilage or arranged in small clusters.[15]

This entity is distinct from "focal fibrocartilaginous dysplasia," which involves the pes anserinus and causes tibia vara in young children.[15] Focal

Fig. 4. Fibrous dysplasia. Microscopic features. The fibrous stroma is composed of bland spindle cells arranged in a vaguely whorled or storiform pattern (hematoxylin and eosin [H&E], original magnification ×10).

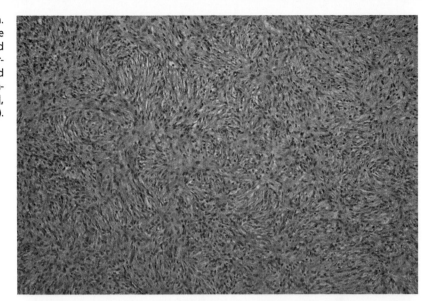

Fig. 5. Fibrous dysplasia. Microscopic features. Anastomosing trabeculae of immature woven bone without osteoblastic rimming (H&E, original magnification ×10).

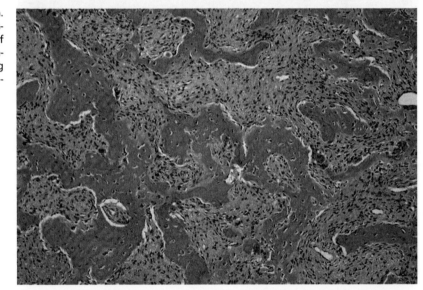

Fig. 6. Fibrous dysplasia. Microscopic features. Curvilinear trabeculae often described as resembling "Chinese characters" (H&E, original magnification ×20).

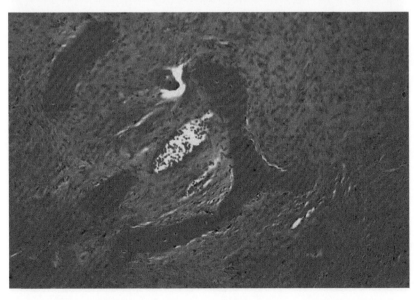

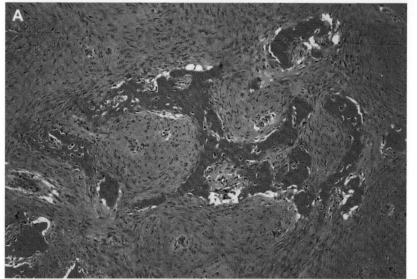

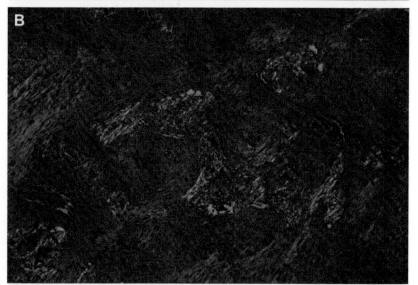

Fig. 7. Fibrous dysplasia. Microscopic features. (*A*) Irregularly shaped trabeculae of woven bone without osteoblastic rimming set in a bland fibrous stroma (H&E, original magnification ×20). (*B*) Appearance of immature trabeculae under polarized light demonstrates the haphazard arrangement of woven bone (polarized H&E, original magnification ×20).

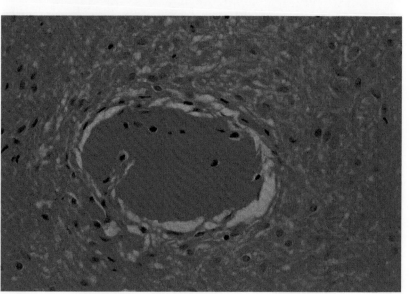

Fig. 8. Fibrous dysplasia. Microscopic features. Immature trabeculae with concentric laminated calcifications demonstrating cementum-like features (cementoid bodies) (H&E, original magnification ×40).

Fig. 9. Fibrous dysplasia. Microscopic features. Cystic change can occur in a lesion of fibrous dysplasia and may be confused with an anuerysmal bone cyst (H&E, original magnification ×4).

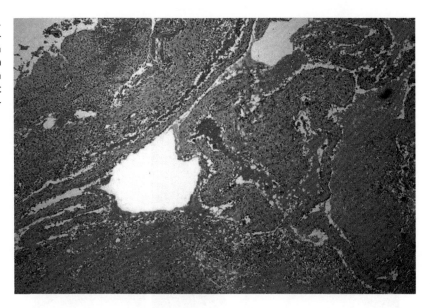

fibrocartilaginous dysplasia has dense fibrous tissue that resembles a tendon in structure and arrangement, and foci where fibroblasts lay in lacunae, creating an appearance similar to fibrocartilage. No hyaline cartilage is present in the lesion. The lesions have a close relationship to the insertion site of the pes anserinus.[17]

Fibrocartilaginous mesenchymoma is another fibrous bone lesion with a cartilage component that is considered by some to be synonymous with fibrocartilaginous dysplasia; however, this is controversial.[15,16,18,19] Because this lesion is locally aggressive, it should be distinguished from fibrocartilaginous dysplasia.[15,16]

Fig. 10. Fibrous dysplasia. Microscopic features. Foamy macrophages may be present in small clusters or as a dense infiltrate (H&E, original magnification ×10).

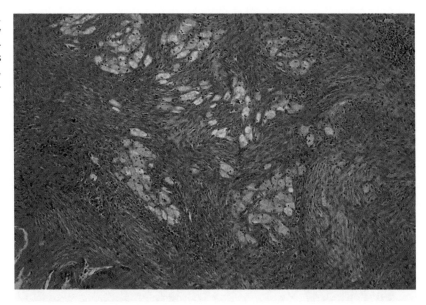

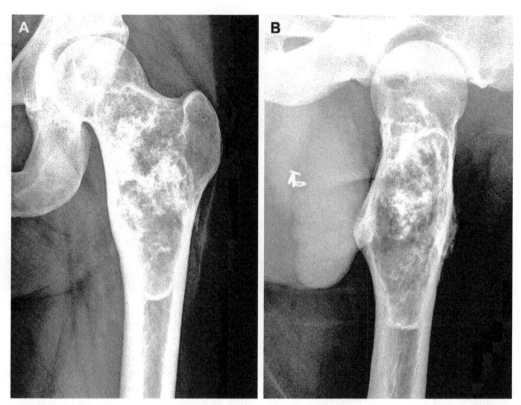

Fig. 11. Fibrous dysplasia with foci of cartilaginous differentiation. Radiographic features. (*A*) AP and (*B*) oblique views show the proximal femur lesion is well demarcated and has stippled or ringlike foci where nodules of cartilage have calcified.

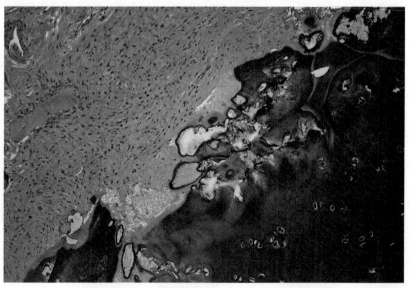

Fig. 12. Fibrous dysplasia with foci of cartilaginous differentiation. Microscopic features. Nodules of hyaline cartilage are scattered through the typical bland stroma of fibrous dysplasia (H&E, original magnification ×10).

DIFFERENTIAL DIAGNOSIS OF FIBROUS DYSPLASIA

The radiographic differential diagnosis of fibrous dysplasia includes simple (unicameral) bone cyst, desmoplastic fibroma, and low-grade intramedullary osteosarcoma. All are intramedullary lytic lesions that can involve the metaphyseal region of long bones in a young population. They are well-marginated lesions with sharp borders, except for osteosarcomas, which have a more aggressive appearance with infiltrative borders that often erode through the cortex.

Simple bone cysts are well marginated but produce a radiolucent lesion that tends to be larger and more lucent than fibrous dysplasia. They also have a rim of reactive bone that is usually thinner. Fibrous stroma with trabeculae of immature bone lacking osteoblastic rimming are absent in simple bone cysts but thin fibrous membranes are present.

Desmoplastic fibroma has dense, uniformly collagenized, tissue that lacks trabeculae of immature bone but infiltrates and entraps remnants of bone with osteoclastic resorption or trabeculae of reactive bone with osteoblastic rimming.

The histologic differential diagnosis includes osteofibrous dysplasia (OFD), nonossifying fibroma (metaphyseal fibrous defect), and adamantinoma. OFD is a rare lytic lesion of bone that occurs in the tibia or fibula and affects children younger than 10 years, slightly younger than the age group affected by fibrous dysplasia. It also differs from fibrous dysplasia in its intracortical location, as opposed to intramedullary location. Microscopically, it is composed of fibrous stroma and bony trabeculae but osteoblastic rimming is present.

Adamantinomas occur in the tibia of individuals younger than 20 years. It is an intracortical lytic lesion but can extend into the medullary cavity. This lesion is composed of fibrous stroma with immature trabeculae of bone, such as that seen in fibrous dysplasia; however, osteoblastic

Pitfalls
FIBROUS DYSPLASIA

! Secondary changes may lead to incorrect diagnosis:

! reparative changes in fracture site may be confused with OFD

! cartilaginous component may be confused with chondroid neoplasm

! cystic change with hemorrhage and giant cells may be confused with aneurysmal bone cyst

rimming is present. In addition, adamantinomas have an epithelial component that is not seen in fibrous dysplasia.

Nonossifying fibroma is a sharply circumscribed intracortical lytic lesion that occurs in the metaphyseal region of the bone. It is composed of fibrous tissue in a haphazard arrangement with trabeculae of reactive bone that have osteoblastic rimming. Fibrous dysplasia, on the other hand, is a lytic intramedullary lesion that has fibrous stroma with a storiform pattern and trabeculae of immature bone without osteoblastic rimming.

MOLECULAR PATHOLOGY OF FIBROUS DYSPLASIA

The etiology of fibrous dysplasia has been linked to a somatic mutation in the Gs alpha subunit (Gsα) gene (*GNAS1*) located at 20q13.2 to 13.3. The mutation occurs in a mosaic distribution early in embryogenesis. It was first identified in the development of endocrinopathies of patients with McCune-Albright syndrome and in the associated dysplastic bone lesions.[12,20,21]

Virtually all cell types express the Gsα subunit, which is a member of the G family of proteins involved with cell signal transduction pathways. Alteration of the pathways results in disruption of the tissue differentiation process.[20] Gsα proteins bind guanine nucleotides and transmit signals from cell surface receptors to intracellular enzymes that generate second messengers, such as cyclic AMP. Single nucleotide mutations involving exon 8 of the Gsα gene lead to a substitution of histidine, cysteine, or serine for arginine at position 201. The mutations disrupt the guanosine triphosphate activity of the alpha chain, lead to increased stimulation of adenylyl cyclase, and result in overproduction of intracellular cAMP.[20–22]

Differential Diagnosis
FIBROUS DYSPLASIA

- Simple bone cyst
- Osteofibrous dysplasia
- Nonossifying fibroma
- Low-grade intramedullary osteosarcoma
- Desmoplastic fibroma

> ### Key Features
> ##### MOLECULAR PATHOLOGY FIBROUS DYSPLASIA
>
> - Gsα mutation (GNAS1)
> - Increased cAMP and IL-6
> - Overproduction of *c-fos* and *c-jun*

Chronic transcriptional activation by mutations of Gsα protein can result in increased levels of *c-fos* and *c-jun*.[20] These proto-oncogenes play a role in controlling the proliferation and differentiation of bone cells, and have been associated with the development of benign and malignant bone tumors.[13] Increased expression of cAMP induces *c-fos*, which leads to increased cell proliferation and inappropriate cell differentiation with abnormal osteoblasts.[23,24] Mutated cells are morphologically altered, resulting in overproduction of a disorganized fibrotic bone matrix.[24–26] The abnormal osteoblasts produce an excess amount of interleukin 6 (IL-6), which enhances osteoclastic activity. This results in expanding osteolytic lesions within the fibrous tissue and the surrounding normal bone.[26–28] For fibro-osseous lesions that are diagnostically challenging, the identification of the Gsα mutation may be of help in distinguishing fibrous dysplasia from well-differentiated fibroblastic osteosarcoma.[20]

In patients with McCune-Albright syndrome, activating Gsα mutations produces elevated levels of cAMP. The increased production of cAMP stimulates both cell proliferation and hormone secretion in many endocrine glands, resulting in multiple endocrinopathies.[21,22] Gsα mutations and increased levels of cAMP also appear to be responsible for café-au-lait spots. A study by Kim and colleagues[29] suggests that the skin pigmentation results from the activating mutation of Gsα in melanocytes and involves the c-AMP-mediated tyrosinase gene activation.

The clinical manifestations observed in each patient are primarily determined by the extent and specific distribution of the mutated cells.[20–22] Genetic testing is available, but the somatic nature of the disease may lead to a false negative result because of testing of unaffected tissue.

FIBROUS DYSPLASIA IN DIFFERENT ANATOMIC SITES

Fibrous dysplasia can occur in many different anatomic sites and, dependent on the site, the differential diagnosis, clinical presentation, and treatment will vary.[16] The most common site of involvement by solitary fibrous dysplasia is the craniofacial bones, with the maxilla being affected most frequently, followed by the mandible.[30,31] Overall, craniofacial involvement is more prevalent in patients with the polyostotic form of the disease (50%) as compared with patients with the monostotic form (27%).[30,32] Females are affected more often than males.[30,31] The term "craniofacial fibrous dysplasia" is typically used when the only site of involvement is the craniofacial bones.[25] These lesions present clinically as facial asymmetry or firm, painless swelling.[11,33]

Craniofacial fibrous dysplasia was previously classified as *leontiasis ossea* or, incorrectly, as *cherubism*.[20] Leontiasis ossea is a form of facial swelling described with fibrous dysplasia that occurs because of maxillary expansion with loss of the nasomaxillary angle, resulting in a feline facial appearance.[33]

Other potential sites of involvement are the ribs, flat bones (pelvis and scapula), and rarely the short tubular bones of the hands and feet. The flat bones and short tubular bones are affected more frequently in polyostotic fibrous dysplasia than monostotic.[16]

McCUNE-ALBRIGHT AND MAZABRAUD SYNDROMES

Fibrous dysplasia can be associated with extraskeletal abnormalities. In 1937, McCune and Albright described an association between café-au-lait spots, precocious puberty, and polyostotic fibrous dysplasia.[34,35] The original clinical triad has since been revised to include nonendocrine, as well as several additional endocrine abnormalities, such as Cushing syndrome, hyperthyroidism, excess growth hormone, and renal phosphate wasting, to name a few.[36]

McCune-Albright syndrome, as it is now known, is a rare disorder with an estimated prevalence between 1 of 100,000 and 1 of 1,000,000.[16,36] Precocious puberty is far more common in affected females than in males; however, other manifestations of the syndrome probably occur equally in both sexes and all races. Clinical manifestations can occur at any time during childhood, including during infancy. Patients with McCune-Albright syndrome may come to medical attention by presenting with symptoms and workup for an endocrinopathy rather than the lesions of fibrous dysplasia.

Somatic mutations that occur in the *GNAS* gene during early development result in a mosaic of normal and mutant-bearing cells. The extent and distribution of abnormal cells determines the clinical presentation of each individual.[22] Genetic testing is possible, but because of the somatic nature of the disease, a negative test result does not exclude the presence of the mutation.[36]

Another rare disorder was described by Mazabraud and colleagues[37] in 1967. Mazabraud syndrome is the association between fibrous dysplasia and benign intramuscular soft tissue myxomas. The lower extremity is the most frequent site to be involved and a soft tissue mass is usually present years before the diagnosis of fibrous dysplasia. In patients with Mazabraud syndrome, fibrous dysplasia is usually polyostotic. The lesions more commonly occur in the femur and in the myxomas the lesions more commonly occur in the quadriceps muscle. In more than 70% of the cases, there are multiple myxomas identified. Although there is no continuity between the lesions of fibrous dysplasia and the myxoma, there is a strong correlation between the location of the dysplastic bone and the soft tissue mass.[38]

Mazabraud syndrome has a strong gender predilection with the syndrome, affecting twice as many females as it does males. Several hypotheses have been proposed, but the etiology of this syndrome is still unclear[38]; however, there have been sporadic reports of *GNAS* mutation involving intramuscular myxomas.[21]

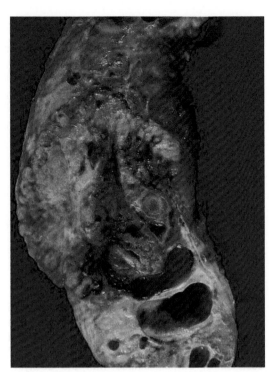

Fig. 13. Fibrous dysplasia. Gross features of sarcoma arising in fibrous dysplasia.

TREATMENT OF FIBROUS DYSPLASIA

Fibrous dysplasia often comes to attention when a patient has imaging studies performed for other reasons. Radiographic features are very characteristic for fibrous dysplasia. If the classic features are present, a tissue diagnosis is seldom necessary. Clinical observation with repeat imaging studies every 6 months is considered sufficient, if no progression of the lesion has occurred. Patients with impending fracture or progressive deformity may require surgical intervention with curettage of the lesion and bone grafting, with or without cryosurgery.[39,40] Internal fixation may be necessary for lesions in the proximal part of the femur to provide greater mechanical strength.[12]

Some clinicians use intravenous bisphosphonates in patients with polyostotic disease to inhibit bone resorption and decrease bone turnover. Patients report a decrease in bone pain, and radiographically, the lesions become ossified and the corticies thickened.[27,39–41]

PROGNOSIS OF FIBROUS DYSPLASIA

The prognosis for patients with monostotic fibrous dysplasia is generally good and may require

clinical observation only. Patients with polyostotic disease, however, have a variably worse outcome depending on the extent of the disease,[13] complications, and association with other clinical conditions.

Malignant transformation of fibrous dysplasia is rare but can occur.[42–44] The reported range of prevalence is from 0.4% to 4.0%[12] and is slightly more prevalent in patients with monostotic disease versus polyostotic disease. Radiation exposure may play a role in malignant transformation of the tumor in those patients reported to have received radiation therapy. The most common malignancies reported were osteosarcoma, fibrosarcoma, and chondrosarcoma (**Fig. 13**). The craniofacial region was the most common site for transformation, followed by the femur and tibia.[42,43] The prognosis tends to be worse for patients with malignant transformation than it is for those with a similar primary sarcoma not associated with fibrous dysplasia.[12]

OSTEOFIBROUS DYSPLASIA

OVERVIEW OF OSTEOFIBROUS DYSPLASIA

OFD is a rare, benign, intracortical, fibro-osseous proliferation that occurs in children. It was first

Key Features

OSTEOFIBROUS DYSPLASIA

- Localization to the tibia, usually anterior, mid shaft, or fibula

- Immature trabeculae with osteoblastic rimming

- Myxoid to fibrous stroma

- Zonal pattern of architecture:
  - sparse, thin, immature trabeculae near the center of the lesion
  - abundant, wider, and more mature trabeculae at the periphery

described by Frangenheim in 1921 under the name of "congenital osteitis fibrosa."[45–47] In 1966, Kempson described the same entity and called it an "ossifying fibroma of long bones" because of the similarities with the ossifying fibroma of the jaw.[48] The lesion has also been described by a variety of other terms such as congenital fibrous dysplasia,[49] and intracortical fibrous dysplasia.[50] The terminology used today was coined by Campanacci in 1976,[51] after noting the lesion was similar yet differentiated from fibrous dysplasia by the clinical, radiographic, and histologic features.

The distinctive feature of this lesion is its predilection for the anterior cortex of the tibia, most often affecting the mid-diaphyseal portion. Occasionally, it involves the ipsilateral fibula and has been reported in other long bones, such as the radius and ulna.[52] The incidence of OFD is low, accounting for less than 1% of all long bone tumors.[16] It is believed to be a self-limited process, with the lesion evolving until puberty, at which time it stabilizes or begins to regress with skeletal maturation.[46,52–55]

CLINICAL FEATURES OF OSTEOFIBROUS DYSPLASIA

OFD presents during the first 2 decades of life and can also have a congenital presentation.[56–58] No definitive gender predilection has been established, although a slight male predominance is most frequently reported.[46] Patients present with swelling or bowing of the anterior tibia that may be associated with pain. Approximately one-third of the cases are discovered incidentally when imaging studies are performed for other reasons.

On rare occasions, a pathologic fracture through the lesion brings the patient to medical attention.

RADIOGRAPHIC FEATURES OF OSTEOFIBROUS DYSPLASIA

Radiographically, OFD is a cortically based, lytic lesion with a distinct predilection for the anterior diaphysis of the tibia (**Fig. 14**). Cortical expansion with anterior bowing may be present. The lesion is longitudinally oriented and fairly well marginated with peripheral sclerosis. It is often multiloculated with intervening sclerotic septations.[46,52] Synchronous lesions can occur in the proximal and/or distal ends of the tibia, and less commonly in the fibula.[16] Radiographic progression of the lesion stops when the patient reaches skeletal maturity.[46,53]

Increased isotope uptake is observed and the lesion appears hot on bone scans.[59,60] CT and MRI demonstrate details of the multiloculated lesions with cortical expansion.[16] CT imaging delineates the cortical epicenter with the zone of sclerosis separating the lesion from the outer soft tissues and intramedullary canal (**Fig. 15**A: CT & B: MRI). T1-weighted and fat-suppressed images on MRI show mixed signals, whereas T2-weighted images show high-intensity signals.[59]

GROSS FEATURES OF OSTEOFIBROUS DYSPLASIA

Resected segments of bone reveal a thin cortex with expansion by a well-demarcated, multiloculated lesion. The tissue is white-yellow, gritty, fibrotic, and surrounded by a rim of sclerosis. Cortical disruption and extraosseous involvement are usually not present.[16]

MICROSCOPIC FEATURES OF OSTEOFIBROUS DYSPLASIA

Microscopically, the lesion is composed of fibrous stroma with bony trabeculae that have prominent osteoblastic rimming (**Fig. 16**). The stroma has bland spindle cells that are often arranged in a storiform pattern and matrix that varies from myxoid to moderately fibrous. A distinct zonal pattern of architecture is demonstrated with sparse, thin trabeculae of immature bone situated in a prominent fibrous stroma at the center of the lesion, and numerous wider, more mature trabeculae situated toward the periphery of the lesion.[46,52,61] Mitotic figures are rarely present.[59]

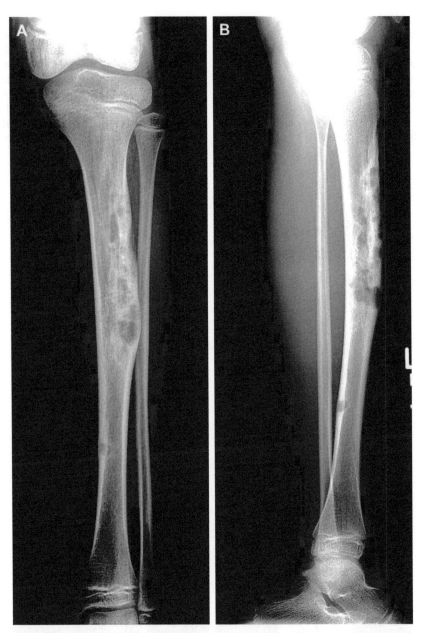

Fig. 14. Osteofibrous dysplasia. Radiographic features. (*A*) AP and (*B*) lateral views show a lytic diaphyseal lesion of the anterior tibia with a mild bowing deformity.

IMMUNOHISTOCHEMISTRY OF OSTEOFIBROUS DYSPLASIA

Occasionally, scattered individual cytokeratin-positive cells are present that are identified only by using immunohistochemical studies (**Fig. 17**). The fibrous stromal cells are Vimentin positive,[59,60] and occasionally show reactivity to S-100 and Leu7.[59]

DIAGNOSIS AND DIFFERENTIAL DIAGNOSIS OF OSTEOFIBROUS DYSPLASIA

The radiographic differential diagnosis for cortically based lesions includes osteoid osteoma, osteoblastoma, Brodie abscess, eosinophilic granuloma, and adamantinoma.[52] After histologic examination of a tissue biopsy, the first 4 diagnoses can be readily excluded from the differential diagnosis.

Histologically, the differential diagnosis includes fibrous dysplasia and adamantinoma. Fibrous dysplasia is composed of bland fibrous stroma with trabeculae of immature woven bone. The bony trabeculae, however, do not have osteoblastic rimming, which is present around the trabeculae in OFD. The fibrous stroma is typically less cellular in OFD[60] and individual cytokeratin positive cells may be present.[60,61] In addition, OFD displays a zonal phenomenon that is not seen in fibrous dysplasia.[52] Radiographically, fibrous dysplasia is an intramedullary process that can occur in many different bones, whereas OFD is an intracortical process that typically involves the anterior tibia. On a molecular level, there is no recurring cytogenetic abnormality in fibrous dysplasia, except for mutations of the GNAS1 gene, which is absent in cases of OFD.[62]

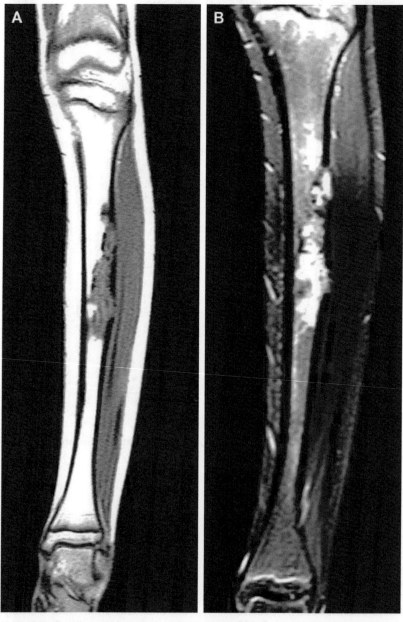

Fig. 15. Osteofibrous dysplasia. Imaging studies. (*A*) CT and (*B*) MRI demonstrate a cortically based multiloculated lytic lesion with sclerotic septations.

Fig. 16. Osteofibrous dysplasia. Microscopic features. Irregularly shaped trabeculae of woven bone with osteoblastic rimming set in a bland fibrous stroma (H&E, original magnification ×10).

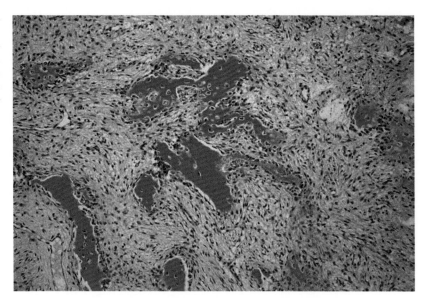

Overexpression of *c-fos* and *c-jun*, however, has been demonstrated in both tumors.[63]

Adamantinoma is the main neoplasm in the clinical, radiographic, and histologic differential diagnosis of osteofibrous dyplasia. It is an intracortical lesion that also typically involves the anterior tibia. Two subtypes of adamantinoma have been described: differentiated or OFD-like adamantinoma and classic adamantinoma. Of the 2, differentiated adamantinomas are the most problematic and difficult to discern from OFD. This tumor affects children in the first 2 decades of life and is limited to the cortex. Classic adamantinomas, on the other hand, affect individuals between 20 and 50 years of age and are often more extensive, involving the medullary cavity and/or extraosseous soft tissues (unlike OFD).

Histologically, differentiated adamantinomas resemble OFD, with immature trabeculae rimmed by prominent osteoblasts. They are arranged in a zonal pattern within bland fibrous stroma. An epithelial component is present that consists of individual tumor cells or small nests that can usually be identified on routine hematoxylin and eosin (H&E) staining, whereas OFD may or may not have rare cytokeratin-positive cells that are identified only with the use of immunohistochemistry.

Cytogenetic studies have demonstrated the presence of chromosomal abnormalities in cases of OFD. Similar chromosomal findings were identified in cases of adamantinoma,[64] as well as the same proto-ocogenes.[65] With all the common features that exist between OFD and differentiated adamantinoma, some believe that a relationship exists between the 2 entities; however, the topic remains highly controversial.

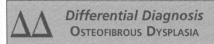

Differential Diagnosis
OSTEOFIBROUS DYSPLASIA

- OFD-like adamantinoma
- Classic adamantinoma
- Fibrous dysplasia

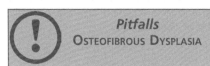

Pitfalls
OSTEOFIBROUS DYSPLASIA

! Single cytokeratin-positive cells should not lead to diagnosis of adamantinoma.

! Thorough sampling required to exclude diagnosis of adamantinoma.

! OFD has pathologic and radiologic similarities to OFD-like adamantinoma and classic adamantinoma.

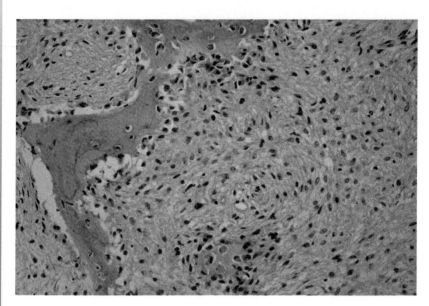

Fig. 17. Osteofibrous dysplasia. Microscopic features. Individual cytokeratin-positive cells are occasionally present that are identified only by using immunohistochemical studies (AE1/AE3, original magnification ×20).

MOLECULAR PATHOLOGY OF OSTEOFIBROUS DYSPLASIA

The few cytogenetic studies on OFD published in the literature report recurring chromosomal abnormalities. Studies by Bridge and colleagues[66] using cytogenetic analysis and fluorescence in situ hybridization demonstrated trisomies of chromosomes 7, 8, 12, and 22. Another study by Parham and colleagues,[62] demonstrated trisomies of chromosomes 7, 8, 12, 21 and 22. These repeated findings support the use of cytogenetic studies for ancillary testing of fibro-osseous lesions of bone.

In other studies using immunohistochemistry, Maki and Athanasou[65] and Sakamoto and colleagues[63] demonstrated immunoreactivity for proto-oncogenes *c-fos* and *c-jun* in the spindled stromal cells. The products of *c-fos* and *c-jun* have been associated with control of bone cell proliferation and differentiation and the potential development of bone tumors.[63,67,68]

TREATMENT AND PROGNOSIS OF OSTEOFIBROUS DYSPLASIA

A biopsy to confirm the diagnosis should be performed even in the face of classic radiographic features.[46] Once confirmed, conservative management by observation without surgical intervention is recommended for small lesions.[46,61] Surgery should be reserved for larger lesions, or those with severe deformity, risk of fracture, or pseudoarthrosis. Removal of the lesion or curettage should be avoided during the proliferative phase, before puberty or before skeletal maturation, as this frequently leads to recurrence of the lesion.[49] If surgery is necessary, it is recommended that it be delayed until after puberty.[52,54,69]

OFD is a self-limited process. Lesions grow slowly until skeletal maturity, at which time they stabilize.[49] Smaller lesions may undergo spontaneous regression and larger lesions may become sclerotic. Therefore, surgical removal of the lesion is not recommended unless complications necessitate intervention.[16,49] See **Table 1** for comparison of fibrous dysplasia and OFD.

ADAMANTINOMA OF LONG BONES

OVERVIEW OF ADAMANTINOMA

Adamantinoma of the long bones is a rare low-grade malignancy that occurs primarily in the mid shaft of the tibia. Two main categories have been described: 1) classic adamantinoma and 2) differentiated adamantinoma, also known as "regressing," "juvenile intracortical," or "OFD-like" adamantinoma. Although similar to the odontogenic adamantinoma of the jawbones (now referred to as ameloblastoma), there is no evidence to support that the 2 neoplasms are from the same histopathogenetic origin.[16] In addition, similarities that exist between the adamantinoma and OFD have

Table 1
Fibrous dsyplasia versus osteofibrous dysplasia

	Fibrous Dysplasia	Osteofibrous Dysplasia
Age	All ages	Infancy to childhood
Sex distribution	Equal	Men>Women
Osteoblastic rimming	No	Yes
Epicenter	Medullary	Cortex
Molecular	Gsα mutation c-fos/c-jun present	No Gsα mutation c-fos/c-jun present
Location	Jaw, long bones, ribs, skull	Anterior tibia
Syndromic association	McCune-Albright / Mazabraud	None

resulted in significant controversy over the possible relationship between the 2 neoplasms and a potential spectrum of disease with transition from one form to the other.[52,70,71]

CLINICAL FEATURES OF ADAMANTINOMA

Classic adamantinoma typically affects patients between 20 and 50 years of age, although younger and older patients have been reported. It is slightly more common in men than women.[72] The tumor typically occurs in the diaphysis of the tibia, and may or may not involve the ipsilateral fibula. Infrequently, it involves other long bones. Initially, the clinical course is slow and indolent with nonspecific symptoms. Patients often present with swelling and a bowing deformity of the tibia that may be associated with pain. In most cases, there is a history of trauma, and occasionally, a pathologic fracture is identified in the affected bone.[52]

Differentiated adamantinomas, on the other hand, arise in the first 2 decades of life. Patients typically present with a long-standing history of dull pain in the tibia and often have bowing of the extremity.[16] This lesion, like classic adamantinoma and OFD, has a strong predilection for the anterior diaphysis of the tibia, and may involve the fibula.[52]

RADIOGRAPHIC FEATURES OF ADAMANTINOMA

Radiographically, classic adamantinoma is an expansile, lytic, intracortical mass. It often causes significant cortical disruption with extension of tumor into the adjacent extraosseous soft tissue and intramedullary canal.[16,46,52,73] The lesion is longitudinally oriented and appears to be multilocular owing to radiolucencies surrounded by ring-shaped sclerotic septations resulting in a "soap bubble" appearance (**Fig. 18**).[52] In addition, multifocality can be observed within the same bone.[72]

Differentiated adamantinoma is a cortically based lesion that does not involve the extraosseous soft tissues or intramedullary canal. The lesion is expansile, lytic, and fairly well marginated, with sclerosis around the periphery.[52]

Bone scans of both classic and differentiated adamantinomas show increased technetium uptake at the site where the lesion is demonstrated on plain radiographs (**Fig. 19**).[72] In cases of classic adamantinoma, CT and MRI scans can

---

Key Features
ADAMANTINOMA

- Two subtypes: Classic and Differentiated

- Intracortically based lesion radiolucent on imaging

  - Classic often extends to extraosseous soft tissue and intramedullary canal

  - Differentiated is limited to the cortex

- Epithelial and osteofibrous components

  - Classic- the epithelial component predominates

  - Differentiated- the fibrous component predominates

- Age distribution

  - Classic >20 years

  - Differentiated <20 years

- Zonal architecture

- c-fos and c-jun proto-oncogenes

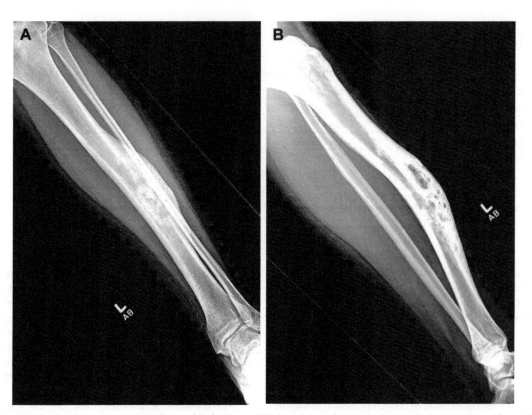

Fig. 18. Classic adamantinoma. Radiographic features. (*A*) This plain radiograph shows a lesion involving the mid tibial diaphysis that appears predominately osteosclerotic on the AP view. (*B*) The lateral radiograph shows a multilocular radiolucent lesion involving the anterior portion of the tibia. It has a "soap bubble" appearance owing to ringlike sclerotic septations.

differentiate between the cortical and extraosseous soft tissue components, and, therefore, provide detail on the extent of the lesion (**Fig. 20**). If present, intramedullary involvement can be determined using MRI scans (**Fig. 21**). These imaging modalities can be useful in staging the patient.

Van der Woude and colleagues[73] studied MRI scans in patients with adamantinoma and distinguished 2 morphologic patterns: a solitary lobulated pattern and a pattern with multiple small nodules separated by normal bone in one or more foci. Although their numbers were small, they noted that multicentricity occurred more frequently in patients with classic adamantinoma.

MRI scans typically show homogeneous low to intermediate signal intensity on T1-weighted images and high signal intensity on T2-weighted images. The degree of homogeneity varies from one patient to the next.

GROSS FEATURES OF ADAMANTINOMA

The gross appearance of both lesions is fleshy, yellow-gray to gray-white with areas of gritty fibrous tissue.[16,72] Resection specimens from classic adamantinomas may reveal cortical disruption with tumor extension beyond the periosteum into the soft tissues and/or involvement of the intramedullary canal (**Fig. 22**A–B). Differentiated adamantinomas are typically confined to the cortex and may be more solid owing to the presence of large bone-forming areas. Occasionally, small cystic spaces are observed.[72]

HISTOLOGIC FEATURES OF ADAMANTINOMA

Classic adamantinoma is a biphasic tumor characterized by cytokeratin-positive epithelial cells and osteofibrous components in various proportions and a variety of patterns (**Fig. 23**).[72] The variants include squamoid, basaloid, spindle, and tubular.

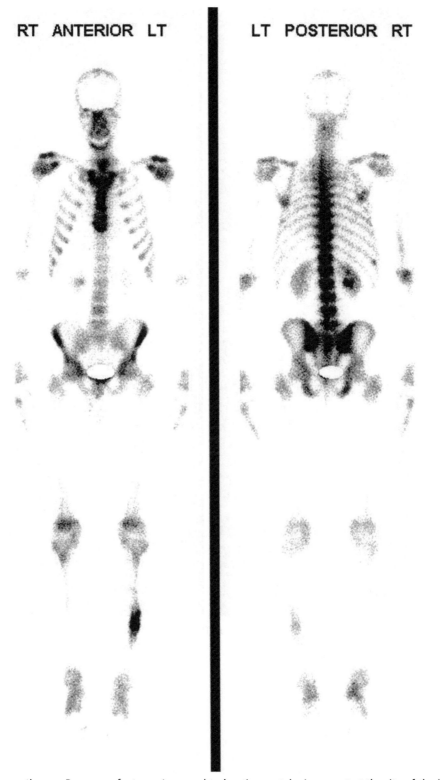

Fig. 19. Adamantinoma. Bone scan features. Increased technetium uptake is present at the site of the lesion.

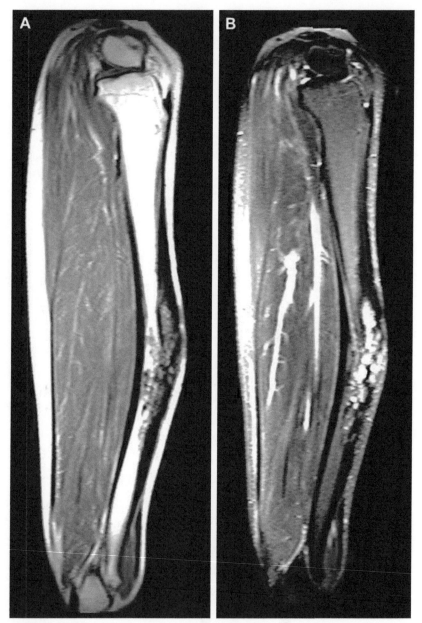

Fig. 20. Classic adamantinoma. MRI features. (*A* and *B*) These coronal imaging studies demonstrate cortical and extraosseous extension of the lesion.

Basaloid and tubular patterns are more common; however, all 4 patterns may be present in one lesion (**Fig. 24**).[46,74] In local recurrences and metastases, the spindle-cell variant tends to be more common.[46] Regardless of the cell pattern, the epithelial component is predominant over the fibrous component.

Histologically, the lesion resembles OFD. Fascicles of loose fibroblastic cells are arranged in a storiform pattern with trabeculae of bone rimmed by prominent osteoblasts. A zonal pattern of architecture is present with the center dominated by epithelial islands and few small immature trabeculae, whereas the periphery has abundant mature

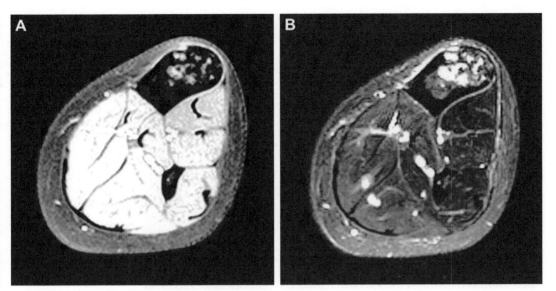

Fig. 21. Classic adamantinoma. MRI features. (*A* and *B*) Axial images reveal intramedullary involvement.

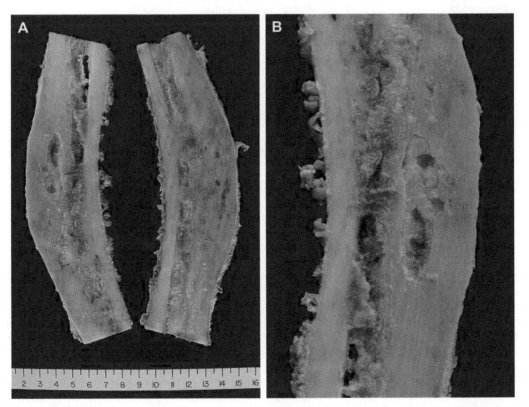

Fig. 22. Classic adamantinoma. Gross features. (*A* and *B*) The resection specimen from the tibia shows a destructive cortically based lesion that involves the intramedullary cavity and has resulted in a bowing deformity.

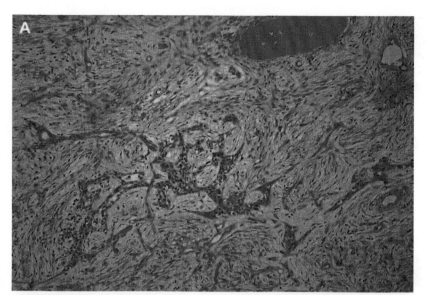

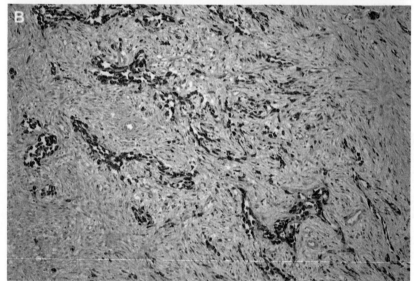

Fig. 23. Classic adamantinoma. Microscopic features. (*A*) The lesion is biphasic with epithelial and osteofibrous components (H&E, original magnification ×10). (*B*) In classic adamantinomas, the keratin-positive epithelial component is predominant over the fibrous component (cytokeratin AE1/AE3, original magnification ×10).

trabeculae and less of the epithelial component.[74] The epithelial tumor cells vary in size and number with individual cells and nests, as well as solid areas scattered throughout the fibrous stroma.[16] The neoplastic cells generally have a bland appearance with fine smooth chromatin. They lack marked atypia, and mitotic activity is low, with 0 to 2 mitoses seen per 10 high power fields.[72]

Differentiated adamantinoma is histologically intermediate between the classic adamantinoma and OFD. In differentiated adamantinomas, the lesion resembles OFD but an epithelial component is present (**Fig. 25**). It has a zonal pattern of architecture, but in contrast to classic adamantinomas, the fibrous component is predominant and the epithelial component is inconspicuous with small nests or individual tumor cells that are often difficult to identify.[74]

There is no consensus on the criteria needed to distinguish among OFD, differentiated adamantinoma, and classic adamantinoma.[61] In the World Health Organization Classification of Tumors of

Fig. 24. Adamantinoma variants. Microscopic features. (*A*) Basaloid variant (H&E, original magnification ×20). (*B*) Spindle cell variant (H&E, original magnification ×20).

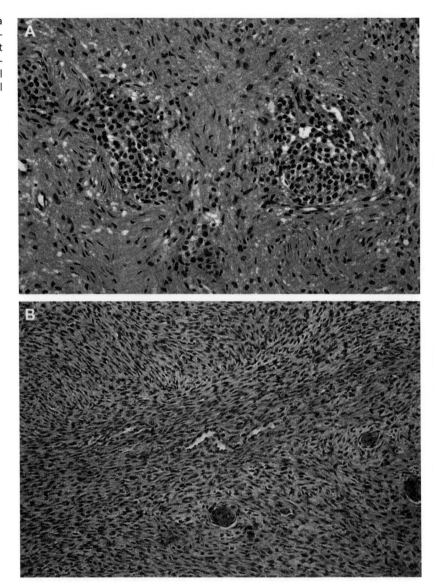

Soft-tissue and Bone, OFD is described as a lesion without epithelial differentiation and defines a tumor as OFD-like (differentiated) adamantinoma if small groups of keratin-positive epithelial cells are present.[46,74,75] Because OFD can have rare individual epithelial cells that are identified only by immunohistochemistry, some feel that a diagnosis of differentiated adamantinoma requires small epithelial nests that are visible by routine H&E staining.[46,61] When it comes to classic versus differentiated adamantinoma, the number of epithelial cells required to make the distinction between the 2 varies from one group to the next. Some groups require a minimal number of

epithelial cells within the nests (<25) for differentiated adamantinoma, and other groups having less specific criteria, requiring "abundant" epithelial cells for classic adamantinoma.[61] It is often difficult to distinguish between these lesions, as the amount and distribution of fibrous and epithelial components can vary widely within the same lesion. Therefore, thorough sampling is critical for establishing the correct diagnosis.[46,53]

Controversy still exists over the histopathogenetic relationship among the 3 neoplasms. Similarities in age distribution, radiographic appearance, histologic features, and strong predilection for the tibia led to the belief that there is

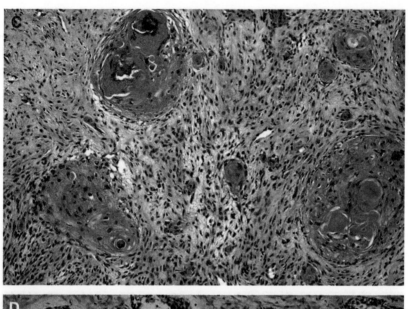

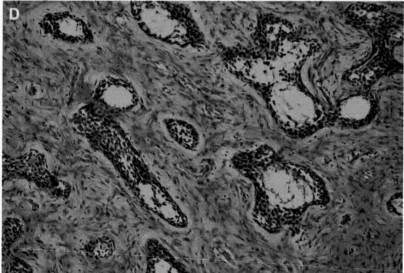

Fig. 24. (*C*) Squamoid variant (H&E, original magnification ×20). (*D*) Tubular variant (H&E, original magnification ×20).

a spectrum of related osteofibrous diseases and raised the question of a process of progression among them.[46,70]

Another variant that should be mentioned is the Ewing-like adamantinoma (or adamantinoma-like Ewing). This rare variant is composed of anastomosing cords of small, uniform, round cells in a myxoid stroma.[72] The tumor cells demonstrate both epithelial and neural antigens by immunohistochemistry including the Ewing sarcoma–related antigen O13. Ultrastructural features of both cell types have also been demonstrated, such as desmosomes (epithelial cells) and dense core granules (neuroendocrine cells).[52] Cytogenetic studies performed by Bridge and colleagues[76] revealed the presence of the 11;22 translocation in nuclei of the cytokeratin-positive cells. Therefore, they considered these tumors to be variants of Ewing sarcoma (adamantinoma-like Ewing) rather than Ewing-like adamantinoma. Hauben and colleagues[77] provided further support for this interpretation using reverse transcription polymerase chain reaction (RT-PCR) and demonstrating t(11;22) and t(21;22) in cases of Ewing sarcoma but not in the cases of adamantinoma that were studied.

Fig. 25. Differentiated adamantinoma. Microscopic features. (*A*) Histology is intermediate between osteofibrous dysplasia and classic adamantinoma. Trabeculae of immature woven bone rimmed by osteoblasts are present in a bland fibrous stroma. Small clusters of epithelial cells are inconspicuous but can be seen on routine H&E-stained slides (original magnification ×10). (*B*) The epithelial cells are more evident with cytokeratin immunohistochemistry (AE1/AE3, original magnification ×10).

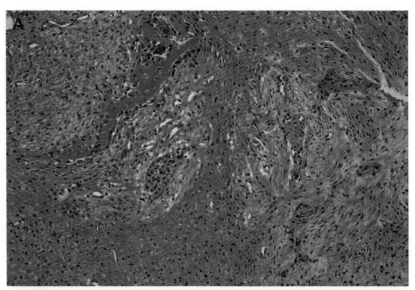

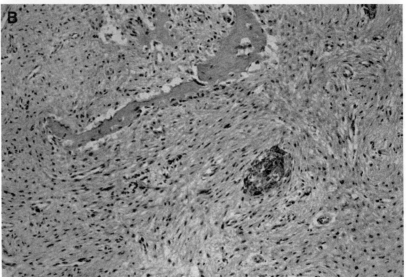

DIFFERENTIAL DIAGNOSIS OF ADAMANTINOMA

The main radiographic and histologic differential for adamantinoma is OFD. Both entities have intracortical lytic lesions that target the tibia. By imaging, OFD and differentiated adamantinoma are nearly indistinguishable.[16] Classic adamantinoma varies in that a soft tissue and/or intramedullary component may be present.

Histologically, the presence of nests of keratin-positive epithelial cells supports the diagnosis of adamantinoma. Cytokeratin-positive cells may be

Differential Diagnosis
ADAMANTINOMA

- Osteofibrous dysplasia
- Metastatic carcinoma
- Brodie abscess
- Osteoid osteoma
- Lymphoma
- Eosinophilic granuloma

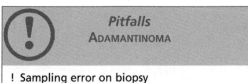

Pitfalls
ADAMANTINOMA

! Sampling error on biopsy

! Inadequate imaging studies

present in OFD; however, they are usually inconspicuous and detected only by performing immunohistochemical studies. Lesions of differentiated adamantinoma are predominately fibrous with small nests of epithelial cells that are visible on routine H&E staining. If the epithelial component predominates, or there is soft tissue and/or intramedullary involvement, a diagnosis of classic adamantinoma should be rendered. In addition, the classic adamantinoma generally affects patients older than 20 years, as compared with differentiated adamantinomas, where the patients are younger than 20 years.

Other entities for consideration are osteoid osteoma, Brodie abscess, eosinophilic granuloma, lymphoma, and metastatic carcinoma. Of these, the only one that may be problematic is metastatic carcinoma, because of its epithelial histology. Metastatic carcinoma, however, usually involves the medullary canal, whereas adamantinomas are cortically based neoplasms. In addition, because adamantinomas have a distinct predilection for the tibia and tend to occur in younger patients, the possibility of a metastatic carcinoma can usually be eliminated.

MOLECULAR PATHOLOGY
OF ADAMANTINOMA

Using immunohistochemistry, Maki and Athanasou[65] identified c-fos and c-jun proto-oncogenes in the nuclei of the fibrous and epithelial components of differentiated and classic adamantinoma. Immunoreactivity has also been observed in the spindle cell nuclei from lesions of OFD[65] and fibrous dysplasia.[63]

c-fos and c-jun are members of a family of genes whose products form the heterodimer complex AP-1 (activator protein 1), which regulates transcription of target genes by binding DNA. c-fos and c-jun control bone cell proliferation and differentiation, and ultimately play a role in the production of bone tumors.[63,65,78]

Cytogenetic analysis has demonstrated the presence of extra copies of chromosomes 7, 8, 12, 19, and 21 in both differentiated and classic adamantinomas. Extra copies of the same chromosomes, except chromosome 19, have been reported in OFD as well, providing further support to a common histopathogenetic relationship between OFD and adamantinomas.[64]

TREATMENT AND PROGNOSIS
OF ADAMANTINOMA

Classic adamantinomas are locally aggressive and extremely slow growing. They have a tendency to recur, with the recurrent tumor behaving much more like a sarcoma. These tumors can also metastasize by both hematogenous and lymphatic routes and most often go to the lungs or nearby lymph nodes.[72] Recurrences have been reported up to 7 years after the initial diagnosis and metastases up to 27 years later.[52]

Over time, treatment strategies for classic and differentiated adamantinomas have varied. With the knowledge that the lesions can recur and that late metastases are possible, treatment now is typically marginal or wide resection of the lesion.

The current treatment protocol for classic adamantinoma is limb salvage with en bloc tumor resection and wide operative margins. Limb salvage with limb reconstruction provides lower rates of local recurrence. Options for reconstruction include vascularized and nonvascularized autografts, allografts, metallic segmental implants, and distraction osteogenesis.[46,72] Radiation therapy and chemotherapy have not been proven to be effective in the treatment of this tumor.[52,53] Because of their tendency to recur and metastasize, long-term follow-up is necessary.

Differentiated adamantinomas behave in a more benign manner, with a lower risk of metastasis and a more favorable prognosis; therefore, treatment strategies tend to be more conservative. It is recommended that surgical intervention be delayed until the patient reaches puberty and used only for extensive or deforming lesions.[52]

REFERENCES

1. Lichtenstein L. Polyostotic fibrous dysplasia. Arch Surg 1938;36:874–98.
2. Garlock JH. The differential diagnosis of hyperparathyroidism: with special reference to polyostotic fibrous dysplasia. Ann Surg 1938;108(3):347–61.
3. Lichtenstein L, Jaffe HL. Fibrous dysplasia of bone: condition affecting one, several, or many bones, graver cases of which may present abnormal pigmentation of skin, premature sexual development, hyperthyroidism or still other extraskeletal abnormalities. Arch Pathol 1942;33:777–816.

4. Coley BL. Neoplasms of bone and related conditions; etiology, pathogenesis, diagnosis, and treatment. 2nd edition. New York: Hoeber; 1960.

5. Campanacci M. Bone and soft tissue tumors: clinical features, imaging, pathology and treatment. 2nd edition. New York: Springer; 1999.

6. Smith SE, Kransdorf MJ. Primary musculoskeletal tumors of fibrous origin. Semin Musculoskelet Radiol 2000;4(1):73–88.

7. Harris WH, Dudley HR Jr, Barry RJ. The natural history of fibrous dysplasia. An orthopaedic, pathological, and roentgenographic study. Am J Orthop 1962;44:207–33.

8. Nakashima Y, Kotoura Y, Nagashima T, et al. Monostotic fibrous dysplasia in the femoral neck. A clinicopathologic study. Clin Orthop Relat Res 1984; 191:242–8.

9. Kaplan FS, Fallon MD, Boden SD, et al. Estrogen receptors in bone in a patient with polyostotic fibrous dysplasia (McCune-Albright syndrome). N Engl J Med 1988;319:421–5.

10. Leet AI, Magur E, Lee JS, et al. Fibrous dysplasia in the spine: prevalence of lesions and associations with scoliosis. J Bone Joint Surg Am 2004; 86:531–7.

11. Frodel JL, Funk G, Boyle J, et al. Management of aggressive midface and orbital fibrous dysplasia. Arch Facial Plast Surg 2000;2:187–95.

12. DiCaprio MR, Enneking WF. Fibrous dysplasia. Pathophysiology, evaluation, and treatment. J Bone Joint Surg Am 2005;87:1848–64.

13. Parekh SG, Donthineni-Rao R, Ricchetti E, et al. Fibrous dysplasia. J Am Acad Orthop Surg 2004; 12(5):305–13.

14. Telford ED. A case of osteitis fibrosa (with formation of hyaline cartilage). Br J Surg 1930;18:409–14.

15. Kyriakos M, McDonald DJ, Sundaram M. Fibrous dysplasia with cartilaginous differentiation ("fibrocartilaginous dysplasia"): a review, with an illustrative case followed for 18 years. Skeletal Radiol 2004; 33(1):51–62.

16. Dorfman HD, Czerniak B. Fibroosseous lesions. Bone tumors. St Louis (MO): Mosby; 1998. p. 441–91.

17. Bell SN, Campbell PE, Cole WG, et al. Tibia vara caused by focal fibrocartilaginous dysplasia: three case reports. J Bone Joint Surg Br 1985;67: 780–4.

18. Dahlin DC, Bertoni F, Beabout JW, et al. Fibrocartilaginous mesenchymoma with low-grade malignancy. Skeletal Radiol 1984;12(4):263–9.

19. Bulychova IV, Unni KK, Bertoni F, et al. Fibrocartilagenous mesenchymoma of bone. Am J Surg Pathol 1993;17(8):830–6.

20. Dorfman HD. New knowledge of fibro-osseous lesions of bone. Int J Surg Pathol 2010;18(Suppl 3): 62S–5S.

21. Weinstein LS, Chen M, Liu J. Gs(alpha) mutations and imprinting defects in human disease. Ann N Y Acad Sci 2002;968:173–97.

22. Weinstein LS. G(s)alpha mutations in fibrous dysplasia and McCune-Albright syndrome. J Bone Miner Res 2006;21(Suppl 2):P120–4.

23. Charpurlat RD, Meunier PJ. Fibrous dysplasia of bone. Bailliere's Clin Rheumatol 2000;14:385–98.

24. Marie PJ, de Pollak C, Chanson P, et al. Increased proliferation of osteoblastic cells expressing the activating Gs alpha mutation in monostotic and polyostotic fibrous dysplasia. Am J Pathol 1997;150: 1059–69.

25. Feller L, Wood NH, Khammissa RA, et al. The nature of fibrous dysplasia. Head Face Med 2009;5:22.

26. Corsi A, Collins MT, Riminucci M, et al. Osteomalacic and hyperparathyroid changes in fibrous dysplasia of bone: biopsy studies and clinical correlations. J Bone Miner Res 2003;18:1235–46.

27. Chapurlat RD, Hugueny P, Delmas PD, et al. Treatment of fibrous dysplasia of bone with intravenous pamidronate: long-term effectiveness and evaluation of predictors of response to treatment. Bone 2004;35:235–42.

28. Yamamoto T, Ozono K, Kasayama S, et al. Increased IL-6 production by cells isolated from the fibrous bone dysplasia tissues in patients with McCune-Albright syndrome. J Clin Invest 1996;98:30–5.

29. Kim IS, Kim ER, Nam HJ, et al. Activating mutation of GS alpha in McCune-Albright syndrome causes skin pigmentation by tyrosinase gene activation on affected melanocytes. Horm Res 1999;52(5): 235–40.

30. Rahman AM, Madge SN, Billing K, et al. Craniofacial fibrous dysplasia: clinical characteristics and long-term outcomes. Eye (Lond) 2009;23(12):2175–81.

31. Ogunsalu CO, Lewis A, Doonquah L. Benign fibro-osseous lesions of the jaw bones in Jamaica: analysis of 32 cases. Oral Dis 2001;7:155–62.

32. Ben hadj Hamida F, Jlaiel R, Ben Rayana N, et al. Craniofacial fibrous dysplasia: a case report. J Fr Ophtalmol 2005;28(8):e6.

33. Lisle DA, Monsour PA, Maskiell CD. Imaging of craniofacial fibrous dysplasia. J Med Imaging Radiat Oncol 2008;52(4):325–32.

34. McCune DJ. Osteitis fibrosa cystica: the case of a nine-year-old girl who also exhibits precocious puberty, multiple pigmentation of the skin and hyperthyroidism. Am J Dis Child 1936;52:743–4.

35. Albright F, Butler A, Hampton A, et al. Syndrome characterized by osteitis fibrosa disseminata, areas of pigmentation and endocrine dysfunction, with precocious puberty in females: report of five cases. N Engl J Med 1937;216:727–46.

36. Dumitrescu CE, Collins MT. McCune-Albright syndrome. Orphanet J Rare Dis 2008;3:12.

37. Mazabraud A, Semat P, Roze R. Apropos of the association of fibromyxomas of the soft tissues with fibrous dysplasia of the bones. Presse Med 1967; 75:2223–8 [in French].

38. Zoccali C, Teori G, Prencipe U, et al. Mazabraud's syndrome: a new case and review of the literature. Int Orthop (SICOT) 2009;33:605–10.

39. Enneking WF, Gearen PF. Fibrous dysplasia of the femoral neck. Treatment by cortical bone-grafting. J Bone Joint Surg Am 1986;68:1415–22.

40. Keijser LC, Van Tienen TG, Schreuder HW, et al. Fibrous dysplasia of bone: management and outcome of 20 cases. J Surg Oncol 2001;76(3):157–66.

41. Liens D, Delmas PD, Meunier PJ. Long-term effects of intravenous pamidronate in fibrous dysplasia of bone. Lancet 1994;343(8903):953–4.

42. Ruggieri P, Sim FH, Bond JR, et al. Malignancies in fibrous dysplasia. Cancer 1994;73:1411–24.

43. Yabut SM Jr, Kenan S, Sissons HA, et al. Malignant transformation of fibrous dysplasia. A case report and review of the literature. Clin Orthop Relat Res 1988;228:281–9.

44. Azouz EM. Magnetic resonance imaging of benign bone lesions: cysts and tumors [review]. Top Magn Reson Imaging 2002;13(4):219–29.

45. Frangenheim P. Angeborne ostitis fibrosa als ursache einer intrauterinen unterschenkelfraktur. Arch Klin Chir 1921;117:22–9.

46. Most MJ, Sim FH, Inwards CY. Osteofibrous dysplasia and adamantinoma. J Am Acad Orthop Surg 2010; 18(6):358–66.

47. Lee RS, Weitzel S, Eastwood DM, et al. Osteofibrous dysplasia of the tibia. Is there a need for a radical surgical approach? J Bone Joint Surg Br 2006; 88(5):658–64.

48. Kempson RL. Ossifying fibroma of the long bones. A light and electron microscopic study. Arch Pathol 1966;82(3):218–33.

49. Campanacci M, Laus M. Osteofibrous dysplasia of the tibia and fibula. J Bone Joint Surg Am 1981; 63(3):367–75.

50. Schajowicz F, Santini-Araujo E. Adamantinoma of the tibia masked by fibrous dysplasia. Report of three cases. Clin Orthop Relat Res 1989;(238): 294–301.

51. Campanacci M. Osteofibrous dysplasia of long bones a new clinical entity. Ital J Orthop Traumatol 1976;2(2):221–37.

52. Kahn LB. Adamantinoma, osteofibrous dysplasia and differentiated adamantinoma. Skeletal Radiol 2003;32(5):245–58.

53. Papagelopoulos PJ, Mavrogenis AF, Galanis EC, et al. Clinicopathological features, diagnosis, and treatment of adamantinoma of the long bones. Orthopedics 2007;30(3):211–5.

54. Sunkara UK, Sponseller PD, Hadley Miller N, et al. Bilateral osteofibrous dysplasia: a report of two cases and review of the literature. Iowa Orthop J 1997;17:47–52.

55. Unni KK, Inwards CY, Bridge JA, et al. AFIP Atlas of Tumor Pathology series 4, tumors of the bones and joints. Washington, DC: American Registry of Pathology; 2005. p. 337–45.

56. Smith NM, Byard RW, Foster B, et al. Congenital ossifying fibroma (osteofibrous dysplasia) of the tibia—a case report. Pediatr Radiol 1991;21(6): 449–51.

57. Anderson MJ, Townsend DR, Johnston JO, et al. Osteofibrous dysplasia in the newborn. Report of a case. J Bone Joint Surg Am 1993;75(2):265–7.

58. Hindman BW, Bell S, Russo T, et al. Neonatal osteofibrous dysplasia: report of two cases. Pediatr Radiol 1996;26(4):303–6.

59. Vigorita VJ, Ghelman B, Hogendoorn PCW. World Health Organization Classification of tumors. Pathology and genetics of soft tissue and bone. Lyon (France): IARC Press; 2002. p. 343–4.

60. Forest M, Tomeno B, Vanel D, et al. Orthopedic surgical pathology. London (England): Churchill Livingstone; 1988. p. 385–93, 595–619.

61. Gleason BC, Liegl-Atzwanger B, Kozakewich HP, et al. Osteofibrous dysplasia and adamantinoma in children and adolescents: a clinicopathologic reappraisal. Am J Surg Pathol 2008;32(3):363–76.

62. Parham DM, Bridge JA, Lukacs JL, et al. Cytogenetic distinction among benign fibro-osseous lesions of bone in children and adolescents: value of karyotypic findings in differential diagnosis. Pediatr Dev Pathol 2004;7:148–58.

63. Sakamoto A, Ode Y, Iwamoto Y, et al. A comparative study of fibrous dysplasia and osteofibrous dysplasia with regard to expressions of c-fos and c-jun products and bone matrix proteins: a clinicopathological review and immunohistochemical study of c-fos, c-jun, type 1 collagen, osteonectin, osteopontin and osteocalcin. Hum Pathol 1999;30: 1418–26.

64. Kanamori M, Antonescu CR, Scott M, et al. Extra copies of chromosomes 7, 8, 12, 19, and 21 are recurrent in adamantinoma. J Mol Diagn 2001;3: 16–21.

65. Maki M, Athanasou N. Osteofibrous dysplasia and adamantinoma: correlation of proto-oncogene product and matrix protein expression. Hum Pathol 2004;35(1):69–74.

66. Bridge JA, Dembinski A, DeBoer J, et al. Clonal chromosomal abnormalities in osteofibrous dysplasia: implications for histopathogenesis and its relationship with adamantinoma. Cancer 1994; 73(6):1746–52.

67. Wagner EF, Eferl R. Fos/AP-1 proteins in bone and the immune system. Immunol Rev 2005;208:126–40.

68. Wagner EF. Functions of AP1(Fos/Jun) in bone development. Ann Rheum 2002;61(Suppl 2):ii40–2.

69. Hahn SB, Kim SH, Cho NH, et al. Treatment of osteo-fibrous dysplasia and associated lesions. Yonsei Med J 2007;48(3):502–10.

70. Czerniak B, Rojas-Corona RR, Dorfman HD. Morphologic diversity of long bone adamantinoma: the concept of differentiated (regressing) adamanti-noma and its relationship to osteofibrous dysplasia. Cancer 1989;64(11):2319–34.

71. Springfield DS, Rosenberg AE, Mankin HJ, et al. Rela-tionship between osteofibrous dysplasia and ada-mantinoma. Clin Orthop Relat Res 1994;309:234–44.

72. Jain D, Jain VK, Vasishta RK, et al. Adamantinoma: a clinicopathological review and update. Diagn Pathol 2008;3:8.

73. Van der Woude HJ, Hazelbag HM, Bloem JL, et al. MRI of adamantinoma of long bones in correlation with histopathology. AJR Am J Roentgenol 2004; 183(6):1737–44.

74. Hogendoor PC, Hashimoto H. World Health Organi-zation classification of tumours: pathology and genetics of tumours of soft tissue and bone. Lyon (France): IARC Press; 2002. p.332–4.

75. Hatori M, Watanabe M, Hosaka M, et al. A classic adamantinoma arising from osteofibrous dysplasia-like adamantinoma in the lower leg: a case report and review of the literature. Tohoku J Exp Med 2006;209(1):53–9.

76. Bridge JA, Fuller ME, Neff JR, et al. Adamantino-ma-like Ewing's sarcoma: genomic confirmation, phenotypic drift. Am J Surg Pathol 2000;24: 322–3.

77. Hauben E, van den Broek LC, Van Marck E, et al. Adamantinoma-like Ewing's sarcoma and Ewing's-like adamantinoma. The T (11;22), T (21;22) status. J Pathol 2001;195:218–21.

78. Gaiddon C, Boutillier AL, Monnier D, et al. Genomic effects of the putative oncogene G alpha s. Chronic transcriptional activation of the c-fos proto-oncogene in endocrine cells. J Biol Chem 1994; 269(36):22663–71.

SMALL ROUND CELL TUMORS OF BONE

Justin L. Seningen, MD[a], Carrie Y. Inwards, MD[b],*

KEYWORDS

- Ewing sarcoma • Bone tumors • Small round cell tumors • Hematopoietic neoplasms
- Primary bone lymphoma • Mesenchymal chondrosarcoma • Small cell osteosarcoma

ABSTRACT

Diagnosing small round cell tumors (SCRTs) can be a difficult task for pathologists due to overlapping clinicopathologic features. This review highlights the clinical, radiographic, histologic, immunohistochemical, and genetic features of the most common SRCTs involving bone with an emphasis on differential diagnosis. SRCTs are a heterogeneous group of neoplasms characterized by poorly differentiated cells with small, blue, round nuclei and scant cytoplasm. They can occur as primary tumors in bone or soft tissue.

Key Points
EWING SARCOMA

- Affected patients are usually in the first or second decade of life. Most tumors are located in the diaphysis or metadiaphysis of the long bones.

- The histologic spectrum includes classic Ewing sarcoma, primitive neuroectodermal tumor (PNET), and atypical Ewing sarcoma. They share the same immunohistochemical and genetic features.

- CD99 is a highly sensitive (99%) immunostain, but it is not specific. Up to 30% of tumors express cytokeratin and 75% are immunoreactive with FLI1. The *EWSR1-FLI1* fusion gene is seen in more than 90% of tumors and ~5% have the *EWSR1-ERG* fusion gene.

- Radiographically, the tumors are typically permeative, lytic, and destructive. CT and MR images are helpful in determining the extent of osseous involvement and whether there is a soft tissue mass.

EWING SARCOMA/PRIMITIVE NEUROECTODERMAL TUMOR (EWING SARCOMA FAMILY OF TUMORS)

OVERVIEW

Terminology for Ewing sarcoma (ES) has evolved over the years as a better understanding of its molecular biology has been gained. In 1918, the first report of ES involving bone was published by James Ewing who used the designation, *diffuse endothelioma.*[1] The concept of a primitive neuroectodermal tumor (PNET) involving bone was introduced in 1984 by Jaffe and coworkers.[2] Currently, ES and PNET are considered manifestations of a single neoplastic entity referred to as the ES family of tumors (ESFT). They share the same molecular features and differ only in the extent of neural differentiation. Although the cell of origin of ESFTs has been debated over the years, mesenchymal stem cells are currently considered the most likely cell of origin.[3,4] A majority of these tumors originate in bone. Approximately 15% to 20% arise primarily in soft tissue and rare examples occurring at visceral sites have also been described.[5–8]

[a] Department of Laboratory Medicine and Pathology, Mayo Clinic, 200 First Street SW, Rochester, MN 55905, USA
[b] Division of Anatomic Pathology, Department of Laboratory Medicine and Pathology, Mayo Clinic, 200 First Street SW, Rochester, MN 55905, USA
* Corresponding author.
E-mail address: inwards.carrie@mayo.edu

Surgical Pathology 5 (2012) 231–256
doi:10.1016/j.path.2011.10.003
1875-9181/12/$ – see front matter © 2012 Elsevier Inc. All rights reserved.

CLINICAL FEATURES

The ESFT is the second most frequent primary malignant bone tumor in children and adolescents, composing 3% of all pediatric malignancies.[9] Approximately 60% of affected patients are in the second decade of life.[10] Only rarely does the tumor occur in patients younger than age 5 years or older than 45 years. It has a predilection for men and is uncommon in African Americans and Asians.[9] Most patients present with pain and swelling around the affected site. Pathologic fractures are an uncommon finding.

Although any bone of the body may be affected by ESFT, most tumors are located in the extremities. The femur is the most commonly affected long bone. Approximately 60% of ESFT in a Mayo Clinic series involved the lower extremities and pelvic girdle, whereas 10% involved the sacrum and spinal column.[10]

RADIOGRAPHIC FEATURES

Radiographically, ESFTs typically present as permeative lytic destructive lesions with poorly defined margins (Fig. 1). A mixed lytic and sclerotic pattern is more commonly seen with tumors involving the flat bones. Most tumors are associated with a large soft tissue mass. It is not uncommon for ES to involve a long segment of the bone, a feature that can be subtle on conventional radiographs but readily apparent in magnetic resonance imaging (MRI) and on CT images. Most tumors are intramedullary, but occasionally they arise in the cortex or between the periosteum and cortex where they are associated with extrinsic erosion (saucerization) of the cortex. Tumors involving the long bones are usually located in the diaphyseal or metadiaphyseal region. As the tumor permeates through the cortex, rapid and repeated periosteal elevation may result in an aggressive multilaminated onion-skin pattern of periosteal new bone formation characteristic of ES. The periosteal reaction is frequently mixed, however, with a combination of multilaminated onionskin, sunburst hair-on-end, and Codman triangles, which may create difficulty in the distinction from osteosarcoma.

GROSS PATHOLOGY

Grossly, ESFT can be solid or have an almost liquid consistency or a combination of both. Solid tumor characteristically has a glistening gray-white or tan cut surface. Less solid areas have more hemorrhage and necrosis, resulting in an appearance that can mimic pus. Because ESFTs are usually responsive to neoadjuvant chemotherapy, resected specimens typically reflect necrotic tumor with a yellow gray-white appearance.

HISTOLOGY

The earliest reports of ESFT primarily included tumors with a homogeneous microscopic appearance. In 1980, a histomorphology-based study by Nascimento and colleagues[11] recognized a subset of ESFT, termed, *atypical ES* or *large cell ES*, characterized by a greater degree of cytologic variability. More recent studies incorporating immunohistochemical, cytogenetic, and molecular data have further expanded the spectrum to include PNET, a tumor with a greater degree of neural differentiation, and a few additional morphologic patterns.[12–18] Currently, histologic classification of ESFT is broken down into 3 major subtypes, including conventional or classic (typical) ES, PNET, and atypical ES.[16,17] All ESFTs are considered high-grade tumors. Conventional ES and PNETs can be diagnosed based on morphologic and immunohistochemical findings. Atypical ES poses a greater diagnostic challenge, however, with a broader differential diagnosis, often requiring molecular testing for a definitive diagnosis.

Conventional or Classic ES

The majority of ESFT falls into the histologic category of conventional ES. These tumors are highly cellular and composed of a monotonous population of undifferentiated small round cells. The nuclei are round to oval-shaped with smooth nuclear contours, finely dispersed chromatin, and inconspicuous nucleoli (Figs. 2 and 3). Moderate to scant amounts of clear to slightly eosinophilic cytoplasm without well-defined boundaries surround the nuclei. Cytologic pleomorphism is minimal and mitotic activity is scarce (approximately 2 to 3 per 40× in 10 consecutive fields). Necrosis varies from slight to extensive and, at times, is associated with viable tumor arranged in a perivascular pattern. The tumor cells are arranged in a diffuse or sheet-like growth pattern, but some show lobulation or a nested pattern created by fibrous septae separating groups of tumor cells. This is seen particularly in areas where the tumor extends beyond the confines of the bone, a feature easier to appreciate with larger biopsies or resected specimens. A filigree pattern can also be seen when the tumor infiltrates dense fibrous tissue. The extent of necrosis and pattern of growth have not been found to influence prognosis.[16]

PNET

Large series of ESFTs arising in bone and soft tissue report the incidence of PNETs at

Fig. 1. Ewing sarcoma involving the ulna of an 18-year-old male. (*A*) Radiograph shows a subtle ill-definded permeative lesion involving a long segment of the diaphysis with marked malignant periosteal new bone formation. (*B*) An MRI more clearly demonstrates a large associated soft tissue mass.

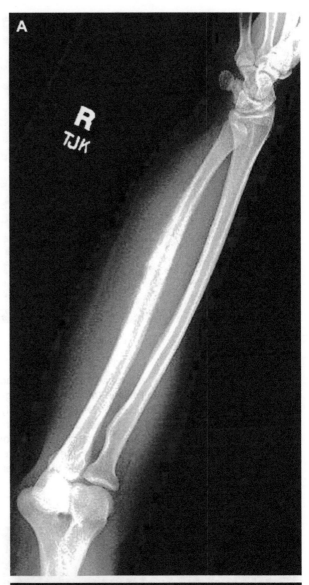

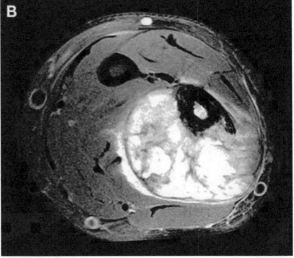

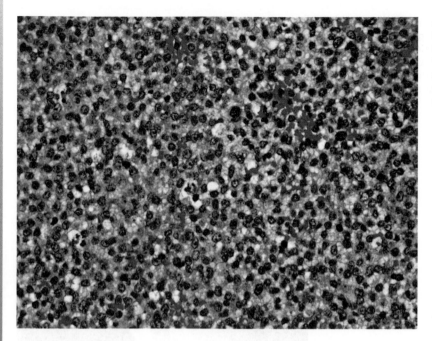

Fig. 2. Conventional ES showing uniform cells with round, regular nuclei containing finely dispersed chromatin and scant clear to slightly eosinophilic cytoplasm.

approximately 15%.[14,16] As a group, they are probably more common in soft tissue than bone. Their neuroectodermal phenotype is reflected in the form of typical Homer Wright rosettes containing a central core of neuropil. The background histologic features most often resemble those of conventional ES. Rosettes are required for the diagnosis of PNET; however, there are no criteria regarding a minimal number. Some tumors contain only a few rosettes whereas in others they are numerous. This variability makes it difficult to know the true incidence of PNET because ES is oftentimes diagnosed on needle biopsy specimens, thus raising the risk of sampling error.

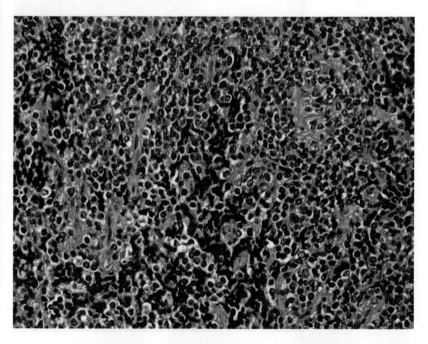

Fig. 3. Conventional ES containing areas with dark cells, a feature that represents degenerative change.

Atypical ES

Atypical ESs account for approximately 15% to 20% of genetically proved ES occurring in bone and soft tissue.[14,16,17] When compared with conventional ES, these tumors have a greater degree of cytologic variability and/or unusual growth patterns. This can lead to misdiagnosis if pathologists are not aware of the histologic heterogeneity and, therefore, overlook atypical ES in the differential diagnosis of a wide variety of primary and metastatic small round cell tumors (SRCTs) involving bone.

Large cell ES refers to tumors within this group characterized by cells that are larger than those of conventional ES and contain nuclei with irregular nuclear membranes and more prominent nucleoli (Fig. 4). The cytoplasm may be abundant and occasionally clear, imparting an epithelioid, rhabdoid, or hypernephroid appearance (Figs. 5 and 6). Most atypical ES grow in a diffuse sheet-like pattern,

Fig. 4. Uniform small round cells of conventional ES (*A*) compared with atypical (large cell) ES composed of larger, irregular cells (*B*).

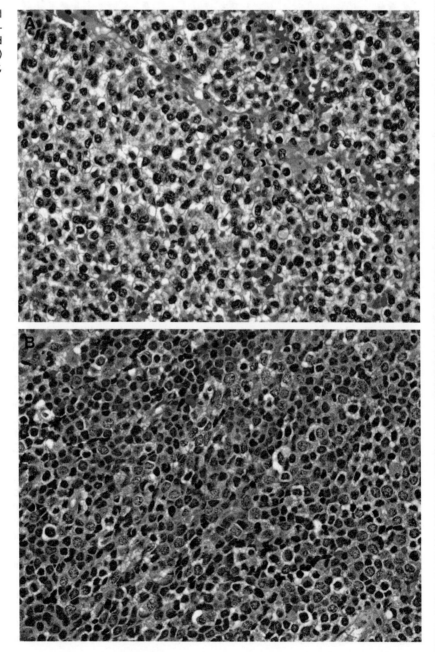

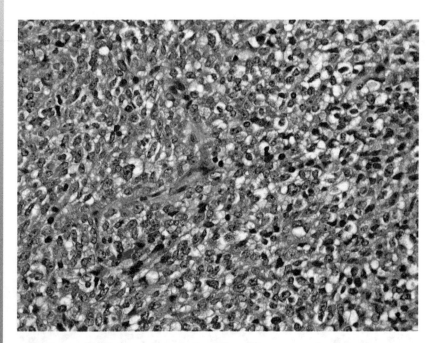

Fig. 5. Atypical ES showing variably shaped large cells. Some of the cells have clear cytoplasm.

similar to conventional ES. Much less common morphologic patterns that have been described include adamantinoma-like pattern, vascular-like pattern, sclerosing pattern, spindle cell sarcoma–like pattern, and synovial sarcoma–like pattern (Fig. 7).[13,14,16,17,19–21] These patterns are usually found in combination with other areas resembling more classic ES. Llombart-Bosch and colleagues[16] group all of the morphologic patterns with large cell ES under the category of atypical ES.[17] The authors agree with this approach because it avoids cumbersome classification schemes.

The adamantinoma-like pattern is one of the more curious variants of atypical ES. It has the same fusion genes as ES but bears little morphologic resemblance. Adamantinoma-like ES contains nests of large, hyperchromatic cells with an epithelioid growth pattern, prominent peripheral pallisading, and stromal desmoplasia (Fig. 8). The tumor cells are positive with CD99, FLI1, pankeratin, and high molecular weight keratin.

The diagnosis of atypical ES requires careful correlation of clinical, histologic, immunohistochemical, and genetic information. Atypical ES can mimic a wide variety of other neoplasms. Therefore, molecular studies are oftentimes an important part of the final diagnosis.

IMMUNOHISTOCHEMISTRY

Immunohistochemical studies are essential in the diagnosis of ESFT. A panel of immunostains, in combination with the histologic features, can lead to a correct diagnosis in many cases. It is important to carefully plan what stains are included in the panel to ensure that enough tissue is available for those cases that require subsequent molecular analysis.

Although immunohistochemistry is a helpful and necessary adjunct in the diagnosis of ESFT, none of the immunohistochemical stains currently available is entirely specific for ESFT. The most useful and sensitive marker is CD99 (MIC2 gene product, O13).[22,23] Up to 99% of ES, including all histologic subtypes, show CD99 expression.[14,16] A diffuse strong membranous staining pattern is most common, but occasional tumors show cytoplasmic or combined membranous and cytoplasmic staining (Fig. 9). Although CD99 is a sensitive marker for ES, it is not specific. Immunoreactivity can also be seen in other SRCTs, such as lymphoblastic lymphoma (LBL)/acute lymphoblastic leukemia, small cell osteosarcoma, poorly differentiated synovial sarcoma, rhabdomyosarcoma, desmoplastic SRCT, and mesenchymal chondrosarcoma, but the staining pattern is generally focal and weak compared with the strong and diffuse pattern characteristic of ES.[15,24–29] Metastatic carcinoma, in particular neurendocrine carcinomas, can also express CD99.[30,31] Rare examples of genetically confirmed, CD99-negative ESFT have been reported in the literature.[16] For practical purposes, it is so uncommon that a diagnosis other than ESFT should be considered for CD99-negative tumors.

Fig. 6. (*A*) Atypical ES composed of large cells with prominent nucleoli and eosinophilic cytoplasm imparting a rhabdoid appearance. (*B*) The tumor cells are diffusely immunoreactive with CD99. (*C*) Some of the tumor cells are also immunoreactive with low molecular weight cytokeratin stain (OSCAR cytokeratin). An RT-PCR study showed that the tumor was positive for the *EWSR1-ERG* fusion transcript.

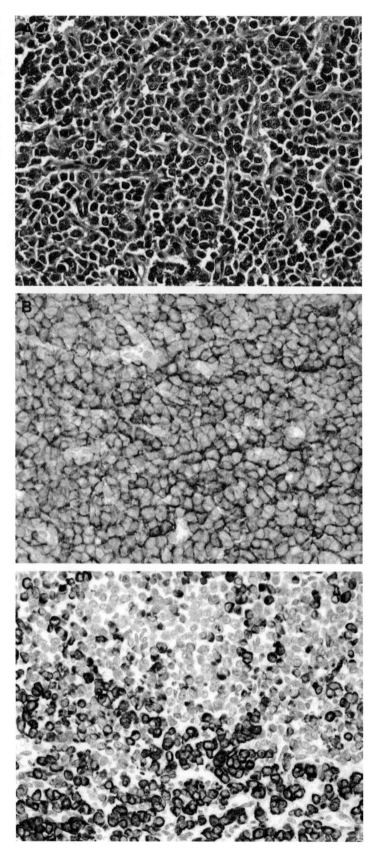

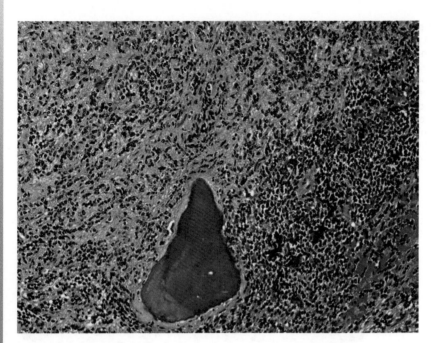

Fig. 7. Atypical ES with sclerosing fibrosis.

FLI1, a polyclonal antibody to the carboxyl terminus of FLI1 protein, is another sensitive marker for ES (**Fig. 10**). Positive immunoreactivity has been observed in approximately 75% of ESs that have been examined.[14,16,32–35] Small round cell sarcomas and carcinoma are negative with FLI1. It is a nuclear stain that is expressed in all ES histologic subtypes. As with CD99, it is not specific marker for ES. It is normally expressed in endothelial cells and T lymphocytes. Most importantly, it is frequently expressed in LBL, one of the important considerations in the differential diagnosis of SRCTs involving bone.[36] Nevertheless, FLI1 can be a helpful marker when used in a panel of immunostains, particularly in difficult cases when molecular studies are not feasible.

Keratin immunoreactivity is seen in approximately 20% to 30% of ES (see **Fig. 9**).[14,16,37,38] The staining is usually focal and more likely to be seen with pancytokeratins and high molecular weight keratins. Desmin expression has been reported in ES, but it is a rare finding.[14,39] Neuroendocrine differentiation in ES is demonstrated by variable immunopositivity for synaptophysin, Leu7, chromogranin, neurofilaments, and S-100 protein. These markers are much less sensitive and specific, however, when compared with CD99 and FLI1, thus significantly reducing their diagnostic usefulness.

MOLECULAR GENETICS

Molecular studies play a critical role in the diagnosis of ES, particularly in the evaluation of tumors

with atypical histologic features and in the setting of limited tissue for ancillary studies.[17,25,40] As for immunohistochemical stains, molecular tests must be interpreted in combination with clinical features, histologic findings, and an immunohistochemical panel. Conventional cytogenetic analysis provides a full karyotype but requires fresh tissue, is expensive, and has a slower turnaround time than fluorescence in situ hybridization (FISH) or reverse transcription–polymerase chain reaction (RT-PCR) (typically 7–15 days). Both RT-PCR and FISH can be performed on formalin-fixed paraffin-embedded tissue to detect the most commonly identified rearrangements in ES/PNET with high sensitivity and specificity (ranging from 93% to 98% or 70% to 98%).[41,42] They also have the advantage of a short turnaround time (1–4 days).

More than 90% of ES/PNETs are characterized by the balanced translocation t(11;22)(q24;q12) producing the *EWSR1-FLI1* fusion transcript.[43–46] Approximately 5% of tumors have the t(21;22) (p22;q12) resulting in *EWSR1-ERG* transcript.[47] Other translocations, including the t(7;22)(p22; q12) (*EWSR1-ETV1*), t(17;22) (q12;q12) (*EWSR1-E1AF*), and t(2;22) (q33;q12) (*EWS-FEV*), are rare and identified in less than 1% of cases. These ES/PNET fusion transcripts can be detected by RT-PCR (see **Fig. 10**). Limitations of RT-PCR include RNA degradation, especially in paraffin-embedded tissues, resulting in inconclusive results. Also, some of the uncommon translocation or splice variants can be missed because the test

Fig. 8. (*A*) Adamantinoma-like variant of ES composed of small blue cells arranged in nests and epithelial-like cords, in association with a hyalinized background. (*B*) Higher-power view showing irregular nuclear contours and prominent nucleoli. The tumor cells expressed high molecular weight cytokeratin and CD99. The tumor was also positive for an *EWSR1-ERG* fusion transcript by RT-PCR.

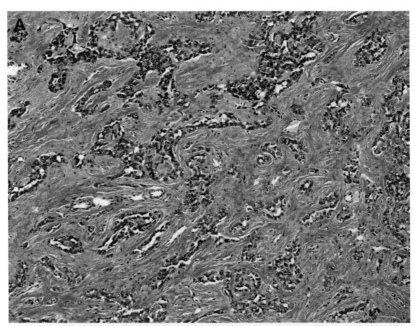

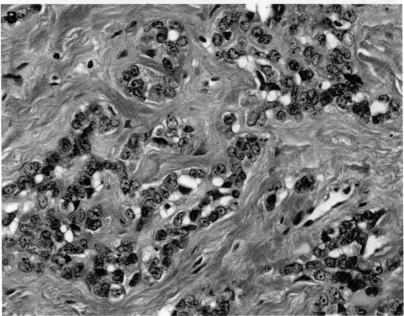

is typically limited to targeting the most common *EWS-FLI1* and *EWS-ERG* transcripts.

FISH analysis for ES involves the use of a dual-color break-apart cocktail of DNA probes that detect translocations involving *EWSR1* (**Fig. 11**).[48] As a result, only one-half of the fusion transcript is targeted. Thus, one of the main advantages of this method is the ability to detect uncommon fusion transcripts because all of the pairs include the *EWSR1* gene. Its specificity, however, is more limited than RT-PCR because other tumors can harbor mutations in the *EWSR1* gene, including desmoplastic SRCT *(EWSR1-WT1)*, clear cell sarcoma (*EWSR1-ATF1*), angiomatoid (malignant) fibrous histiocytoma (*EWSR1-ATF1* and *EWSR1-CREB1*), extraskeletal myxoid chondrosarcoma (*EWSR1-CHN*), myoepithelial tumors (*EWSR1/ZNF444* and *EWSR1/FEV*), and occasional examples of acute myelogenous leukemia.[29,49] Most of these tumors are commonly found in soft tissue,

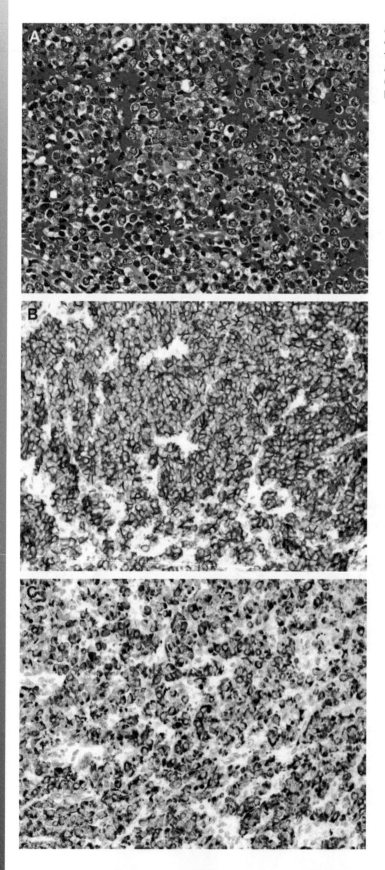

Fig. 9. (*A*) Conventional ES composed of a monotonous population of uniform round blue cells. The tumor cells are immunoreactive with (*B*) CD99, (*C*) high molecular weight cytokeratin.

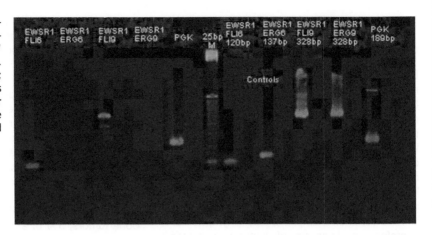

Fig. 10. Agarose gel showing RT-PCR products consistent with *EWSR1-FL1* fusion in a case of ES. Patient sample (*left lanes*); positive control samples (*right lanes*); and marker lane (*center lane*). Observe that tumor was tested negative for *EWSR1-FLI1*.

but rare examples of each have been reported as arising primarily in bone. From a practical standpoint, the histologic overlap of these tumors with conventional ES is minimal and primarily involves only atypical ES.

TREATMENT AND PROGNOSIS

The treatment plan for patients with ES generally consists of 3 stages: neoadjuvant chemotherapy, surgery with or without RT, and consolidation chemotherapy.[50,51] Metastatic disease at the time of presentation is the most important prognostic factor affecting outcome.[52] Patients who present with metastatic tumor have an estimated survival of only 20% to 25%.[53] In contrast, the DFS for patients with localized disease approaches 70%, and OS may exceed 80%.[54–57] Patients with lung metastases have a better survival than those with bone metastases or bone marrow involvement. Histologic assessment of chemotherapy-induced tumor necrosis plays an impo rtant role in the care of patients with ES, because a good histologic response (>90% necrosis) is strongly related to good clinical behavior.[58,59] Pelvic primary tumor and large tumor size (larger than 8 cm) have been associated with a worse prognosis. Some studies have suggested that biologic factors, such as Ki67 expression, atypical ES histologic subtype, overexpression of p53, and mutations in *INK41*, gene are useful prognostic indicators, but additional studies are needed to confirm these results.[16,52,60–64]

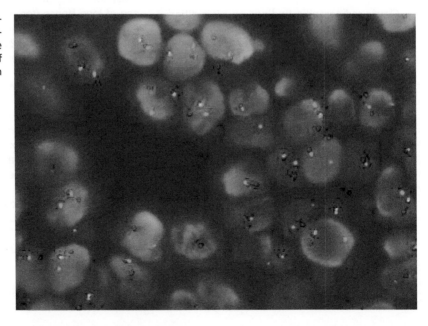

Fig. 11. Molecular cytogenetic analysis (FISH) showing rearrangement of the *EWSR1* locus in a case of ES (separation of green and orange signals).

HEMATOPOIETIC NEOPLASMS OF BONE

OVERVIEW

Lymphomas primarily involve lymph nodes and most present with lymphadenopathy. Ten percent to 35% of non-Hodgkin lymphomas have extranodal disease, most commonly in the gastrointestinal tract, skin testes, kidney, and, rarely, bone.[65] When lymphoma involves the skeleton, it most commonly does so as a component of widespread disease, taking the form of multiple destructive lesions or diffuse marrow infiltrates. Skeletal involvement by a primary extraosseous lymphoma is more common than primary bone lymphoma.[66] Therefore, a diagnosis of lymphoma creating a mass lesion in bone should prompt a clinical work-up and staging with appropriate studies, including chest, abdomen, and pelvis CT and MRI, to determine whether the bone lesion is a manifestation of systemic disease or a primary

Key Points
LYMPHOMA

- Lymphoma involving bone is usually a manifestation of widespread disease. Primary bone lymphoma (PBL) is defined as lymphoma originating in bone with no evidence of extraskeletal disease or disseminated bone marrow involvement.

- PBL most commonly affects middle-aged to elderly patients. It usually involves the metadiaphysis of the long bones.

- Classic radiographic findings on plain films include a radiolucency with permeative margins and minimal periosteal reaction. However, plain films may be normal or show only subtle abnormalities. CT and MR images are useful in assessing extent of marrow and soft tissue involvement.

- The majority of PBLs are B-cell lymphomas, most commonly diffuse large B-cell lymphoma (up to 90%). Less common types include lymphoblastic lymphoma, periperal T-cell lymphoma and anaplastic large cell lymphoma. Crush artifact and fibrosis are frequent problems with bone biopsies of all histologic types.

- Most lymphomas are negative with CD99 and positive with CD45 and either B-cell or T-cell markers. However, lymphoblastic lymphoma can be negative with CD45 and positive with CD99 and FLI1, an immunoprofile that overlaps with Ewing sarcoma.

bone lymphoma (PBL).[67] Because most published series of bone lymphoma conventionally exclude the discussion of secondary bone involvement by extraosseous lymphoma,[68] this discussion focuses on PBL.

PBL is defined as lymphoma originating in bone with no evidence of extraskeletal disease or disseminated bone marrow involvement developing during a minimum of 6 months after diagnosis.[66,69] PBL was first described in 1928 by Oberling, and the first case series (then termed, *reticulum cell sarcoma of bone*) was reported in 1939 by Jackson and Parker.[65] PBL is rare, accounting for 5% to 7% of primary malignant bone tumors, 5% of extranodal lymphomas, and less than 1% of all malignant lymphomas.[67,68] Although some investigators regard the separation of PBL from lymphomatous involvement of bone by systemic disease as purely academic, the current trend is that this is a clinically significant distinction, because studies have suggested that PBL has a more favorable prognosis compared with skeletal involvement by primary extraosseous lymphoma.[65,70] Due to the rarity of PBL and the paucity of large controlled studies, its precise diagnostic criteria, categorization, and treatment remain controversial.[65,66]

CLINICAL FEATURES OF PRIMARY BONE LYMPHOMA

PBL is typically a disease of middle-aged to elderly men; 50% of patients are over 40 years old, and reported male-to-female ratios range from 1.0 to 1.8:1.[65,71] Multiple studies show that the bones most commonly affected include the metadiaphyses of long bones (femur in 20%–32% of cases, humerus in 10%–14%, and tibia in 14%) and axial skeleton (pelvis in 15%–20% and vertebrae in 9%–10%).[67,71] Other locations include the mandible (2% of cases), radius or ulna (1%), scapula (1%), small bones of the hands and feet (rare), and multiple bones (13% to 25%).[67] The most common presenting symptoms are localized pain and swelling; focal neurologic deficits may result from nerve involvement in axial tumors, and 25% of patients present with pathologic fractures when PBL occurs in weight-bearing bones.[67] B symptoms, including fever, weight loss, and night sweats as well as hypercalcemia, are unusual but have also been reported.[65,67,72]

RADIOGRAPHIC FEATURES OF OSSEOUS LYMPHOMA

Overall, imaging studies of osseous lymphoma are variable and nonspecific.[65] Moreover, plain radiographs may appear normal or demonstrate only subtle changes.[69] When present, classic findings on plain films include a radiolucency with moth-eaten or permeative tumor margins, bony sequestra, a minimal onionskin periosteal reaction in 60% of cases, and an associated soft tissue mass in 50% of cases (**Fig. 12**).[69] Less commonly, and in rare cases of primary Hodgkin lymphoma of bone, the lymphoma elicits osteosclerosis and may subsequently appear radiodense, resembling an osteoblastic metastasis or Paget disease.[67,69] CT and T2-weighted MRI have been useful studies as well, particularly when assessing extent of marrow and soft tissue involvement when plain radiographs may appear normal.[65] Positron emission tomography, however, has become the most

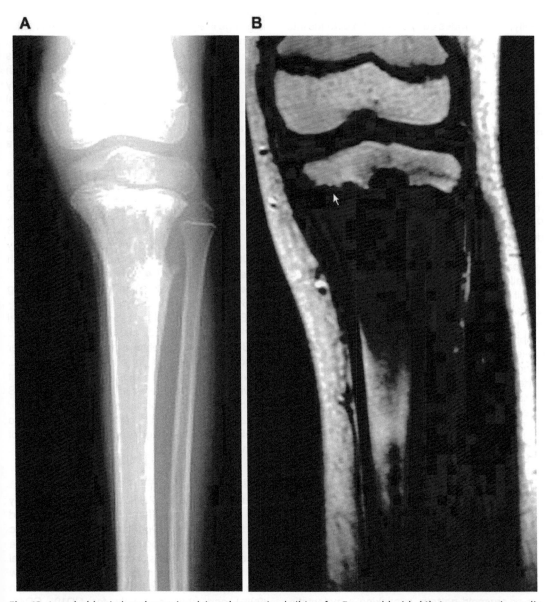

A **B**

Fig. 12. Lymphoblastic lymphoma involving the proximal tibia of a 5-year-old girl. (*A*) Anteroposterior radiograph of the proximal left leg demonstrates a poorly marginated mixed lytic and sclerotic lesion in the proximal tibial metaphysis with cortical destruction and periosteal new bone formation laterally. (*B*) The coronal T1-weighted MRI shows that the lesion is predominantly located in the metaphysis but crosses the growth plate to involve a small portion of the epiphysis and is associated with a soft tissue mass laterally. In addition to lymphoma, the radiographic differential diagnosis includes osteosarcoma and Ewing sarcoma.

important nuclear medicine technique and is routinely used in treatment, staging, and remission assessment of lymphoma.[73]

GROSS PATHOLOGY OF PRIMARY BONE LYMPHOMA

Although not a common surgical specimen, grossly PBL is soft and fleshy and may be necrotic.[67,74] The tumor is usually a large poorly defined osteolytic mass centered in the medullary cavity, which erodes bony cortex and extends into adjacent soft tissue, the proposed result of osteoclast-stimulating factors.[69]

HISTOLOGIC FEATURES OF PRIMARY BONE LYMPHOMA

PBLs demonstrate the same histologic features as their extraosseous counterparts and are classified by the same criteria. There are no reliable histologic or immunohistochemical features that permit distinguishing PBL from secondary bone involvement by extraosseous lymphoma.[69] A majority of PBLs are B-cell lymphomas, most commonly diffuse large B-cell lymphoma (DLBCL). T-cell PBLs are rare in the West but are more common in Japan and China (where T-cell lymphomas are overall more common).[75] Additional non-Hodgkin B-cell lymphomas, including follicular lymphoma (5.7%), marginal zone lymphoma (1.9%), mantle cell lymphoma (1.9%), and small lymphocytic lymphoma (1.9%), have also been reported to present as PBLs.[66] A few examples of primary Hodgkin lymphoma of bone have also been reported in the literature.[76]

Many lymphomas of bone are associated with a dense inflammatory cell infiltrate, many of which are T cells, which may obscure the nature of the underlying lymphoma or lead one to an erroneous diagnosis of chronic osteomyelitis. Crush and distortion artifacts are a frequent problem with biopsy specimens, particularly when dealing with smaller-gauge needle biopsies (Fig. 13). Open biopsy is usually preferred because the technique obtains more tissue and yields better cytologic preservation.[65,71]

Fibrosis elicited by the lymphoma may also lead to several diagnostic difficulties. Fibrous bands may envelop tumor cells, thus simulating an alveolar or organoid pattern, mimicking a metastatic carcinoma. Fibrosis may also be associated with reactive bone and distorted architecture, causing spindling and storiform formations, leading to the morphologic consideration of a sarcoma.[67,77] Cytoplasmic clearing may also exist, imparting a signet ring-like appearance and subsequent confusion with metastatic adenocarcinoma.[77]

Diffuse Large B-Cell Lymphoma

DLBCL is by far the most common PBL, ranging from 75% to 92% of PBLs in published studies.[65,78] On hematoxylin-eosin stain, DLBCL is histologically diverse but common to all tumors is a diffuse round cell marrow infiltrate that leaves bony trabeculae intact. Tumor cells grow in sheets, permeating between trabeculae and medullary fat, and exhibiting large irregular cleaved and multilobated nuclei, prominent nucleoli, clumped chromatin, scant eosinophilic cytoplasm, and abundant mitoses (Figs. 14 and 15). Immunoblastic (large cells with a single prominent nucleolus) and more commonly centroblastic (medium-sized cells with several membrane-bound nucleoli) cells are present, as in extraosseous DLBCLs.[67,79] Background infiltrates of mature T cells and accompanying fibrosis are seen, which may confound the diagnosis.

By immunohistochemistry, primary bone DLBCLs in bone maintain the same staining patterns as extraosseous tumors, being positive for CD45 and pan–B-cell markers (CD19, CD20, CD79a, and PAX5) and negative for T-cell markers (CD3 and CD5). In one study, tumors were also variably positive for BCL2 (81%) and TP53 (52%), with a mean MIB index of 57%.[68] Hans and colleagues[80] have proposed an algorithm for further separating DLBCL into germinal center–like (GCB) and non-GCB immunophenotypes using the additional markers CD10, BCL6, and MUM1. In systemic DLBCLs, the GCB subtype is associated with better clinical outcome.[79,80] In primary bone DLBCL, however, one study to date found no significant survival difference between GCB and non-GCB subtypes or immunohistochemical positivity for BCL2, TP53, or MIB.[68] There are currently no published studies of gene expression profiles of primary bone DLBCL.[67]

Lymphoblastic Lymphoma

LBLs accounted for 2.2% of PBLs in one study and may enter the differential diagnosis of round cell tumors of bone, particularly in the pediatric age group.[70] Histologically mimicking ES, the tumor grows as sheets of cells with rounded nuclei and fine stippled chromatin infiltrating the marrow (Fig. 16). A majority of LBLs are of T-cell origin (90%) and stain positively for CD10, CD43, CD79a, CD99, FLI1,[36] and terminal deoxynucleotidyl transferase (Tdt). CD45 may be weakly positive or negative. When considering the differential diagnosis of ES, LBL may be positive for CD99 and negative for CD45.[81]

Fig. 13. DLBCL involving the femur of a 41-year-old man. (*A*) Cytologic distortion due to crush artifact is a common problem with bone biopsies. (*B*) Better cytologic preservation in other areas of the biopsy tissue allowed for diagnostic histologic and immuno-histochemical evaluation.

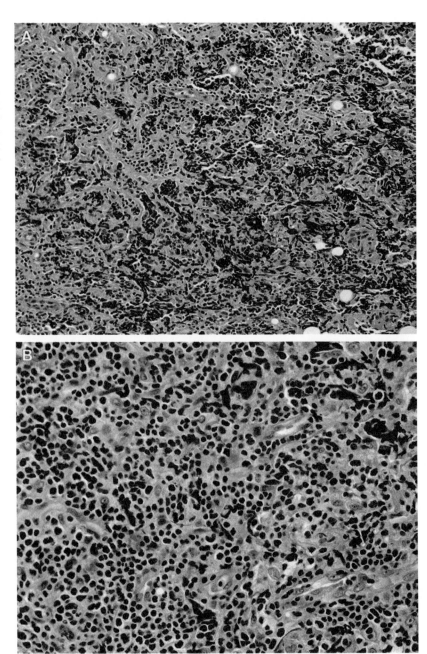

Peripheral T-Cell Lymphomas

Primary bone peripheral T-cell lymphomas are rare in Western countries, reported as 0.2% to 3.8% of PBLs[66,77] but up to 8.8% of PBLs in a Japanese series.[75] This is likely due to the inherently higher prevalence of T-cell lymphomas in Asia. Few case numbers of primary bone peripheral T-cell lymphoma shave prevented reliable immunohisto-chemical characterization, but variable staining for

T-cell markers CD2, CD3, CD4, CD5, CD7, and CD8 and demonstration of T-cell receptor gene rearrangements are useful for confirming T-cell lymphoma.[67,82]

Anaplastic Large Cell Lymphoma

Anaplastic large cell lymphoma (ALCL) is a T-cell lymphoma rarely presenting as PBL and has only been described in a few case reports.[67] The

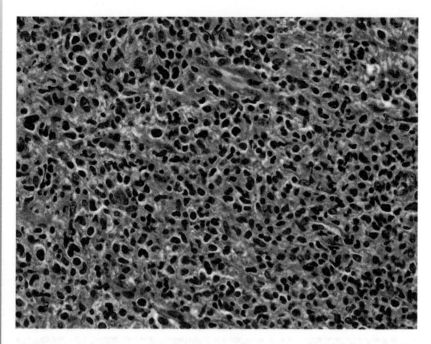

Fig. 14. DLBCL showing a more polymorphous cytologic appearance than what is usually seen in ES.

cytologic features can overlap with atypical ES. ALCL tumor cells are large and contain markedly variable nuclei and horseshoe shapes. They stain positively with CD30; are generally positive with CD3, CD4, and FLI1[83]; and are variable with CD45, EMA, TIA1, perforin, and granzyme B. Most are also reactive for ALK1, which results from the characteristic t(2;5)(p23;q35) translocation between *ALK*

and *NPM*. As in extraosseous ALCL, poorer prognosis is associated with multifocality, ALK1-negativity, tumor necrosis, and advanced age.[67]

Myeloid Sarcoma

Myeloid sarcoma (MS) is also known as granulocytic sarcoma, myeloblastoma, and chloroma (for

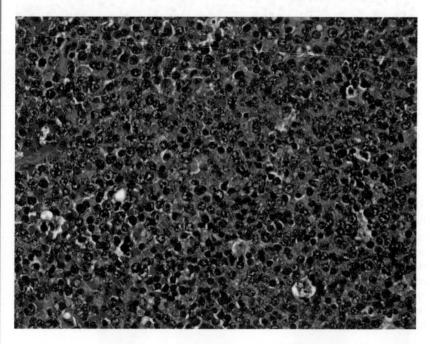

Fig. 15. DLBCL involving the proximal humerus of a 50-year-old man. The features resemble those of atypical ES.

Fig. 16. Biopsy tissue from lymphoblastic lymphoma illustrated in **Fig. 12.** (*A*) The tumor contains a diffuse monotonous population of small round cells. (*B*) Immunohistochemical stain for TdT showing strong nuclear immunoreactivity in tumor cells. The tumor cells were also focally positive with CD99.

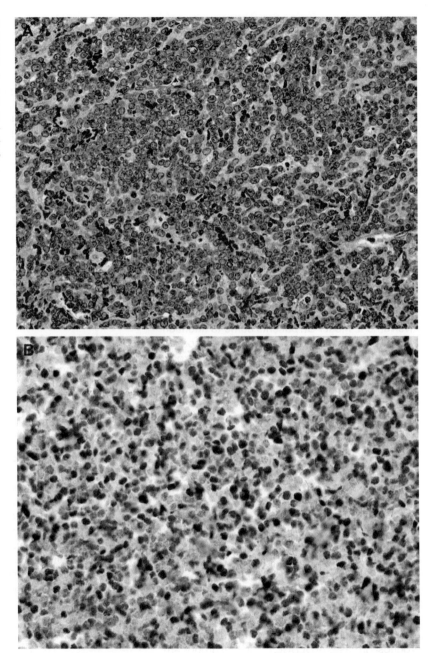

its green color on cut section due to tumor cell myeloperoxidase). MS is rare, occurring in 0.7 per million children and 2 per million adults. Presenting mostly in bone, soft tissues, and lymph nodes, MS is associated with underlying leukemia, occurring in 5% and 13% of adults and children with myeloid leukemia, respectively.[84] Morphologically, it is a tumor composed of eosinophilic myeloblasts without an associated lymphoid component.[67] The tumor cells are positive for myeloperoxidase, lysozyme, and CD43; they stain variably for CD34 and are negative for CD3 and CD20. MS has been shown to express CD99, thus limiting the usefulness of this marker in distinguishing MS from other round cell tumors.

Plasma Cell Neoplasm

Plasma cell myeloma, a malignant proliferation of monoclonal plasma cells, is the most common primary malignant tumor of bone.[85] It can present as a solitary lesion (solitary plasmacytoma) or more commonly as part of widespread disease (multiple myeloma). Histologically, well-differentiated myeloma is easily recognized by plasma cells with eccentric nuclei, clock-face chromatin, and the amphophilic perinuclear golgi apparatus. Poorly differentiated myeloma, however, is more morphologically challenging, with significant pleomorphism and large nucleoli lacking the general nuclear features of plasma cells. Immunohistochemically, myeloma cells are light chain restricted and positive with CD138. Although carcinomas may also stain positively for CD138, malignant plasma cells are positive for both CD138 and MUM-1.[85]

STAGING

By definition, PBL begins with localized bone involvement in the absence of any lymph node involvement. Most PBL patients come to attention in this stage and their disease is thus categorized as stage IE. In one study, 64% of PBL patients presented in stage IE, 18% in stage IIE, and another 18% in stage IVE.[71,86] A more recent study reported 66% of PBL patients presenting in stage IE, 11% in stage IIE, and 23% in stage IVE.[66] PBL tends to spread over time to other osseous sites rather than lymph nodes.[66]

TREATMENT

Surgery has essentially no role in the treatment of PBL, except in enabling an open biopsy or treating pathologic fractures.[65] In the past, PBL was treated with radiation therapy (RT) alone at doses of 40 Gy to 60 Gy[65]; however, recent studies suggest—to varying degrees of statistical significance—that combined modality therapy (CMT) consisting of RT and anthracycline-based chemotherapy decreases the risk of relapse compared with RT alone.[65] The addition of rituximab further improves prognosis in cases of DLBCL.[66,67] Other groups are more skeptical, suggesting that there is no significant difference between CMT versus single-modality therapy.[66,70,71] Nevertheless, one group showed significantly increased disease-free survival (DFS) and overall survival (OS) for CMT versus RT alone,[87] another group found significantly increased DFS but not OS with CMT versus RT alone,[88] whereas yet another group found no significant difference in either DFS or OS with CMT versus RT alone.[70] Despite the need for more data-driven treatment principles for PBL, the consensus in the literature, even from groups whose studies reported no statistically significant change in survival, is that CMT is a reasonable and logical treatment for PBL.[65,66,70,71]

PROGNOSIS

PBL is rare and the number of large reports is small, but a recent study reported a 5-year OS of 88%, DFS of 96%, and freedom from treatment failure of 81%.[78] As described previously, the GCB immunophenotype of DLBCL is associated with improved prognosis by some investigators[67,89] but not others.[68] Ostrowski and colleagues[77] concluded that differences in histologic type and grade had no significant prognostic significance and that disease stage was the single most important prognostic predictor of OS in PBL, reporting 58% 5-year OS for patients with single-bone involvement, 42% for multifocal PBL, and 22% for PBL with subsequent nodal involvement. A more recent study found that age under 60 years and a complete response to initial therapy were the only measured variables associated with a statistically significant difference in survival.[68]

SMALL CELL OSTEOSARCOMA

Small cell osteosarcoma is a rare histologic subtype of osteosarcoma, representing approximately 1% of all osteosarcomas.[10,90–92] As the name implies, it is composed of small cells with cytologic features that resemble those of ESFT and lymphoma. The distinguishing histologic feature of small cell osteosarcoma is the presence of malignant osteoid production. Small cell osteosarcoma has similar age, gender, and skeletal distribution as conventional osteosarcoma. Radiographically it has an aggressive malignant appearance that oftentimes overlaps with lymphoma and ES. The presence of mineralized matrix that differs from the type of reactive new bone occasionally seen in ESFT and

Key Points
SMALL CELL OSTEOSARCOMA AND MESENCHYMAL CHONDROSARCOMA

- The cytologic features of both tumors can resemble Ewing sarcoma, particularly atypical Ewing sarcoma. The amount of matrix production is variable, creating the risk of sampling error.

- Both tumors can be immunoreactive with CD99, but typically negative with FLI1.

- *EWSR1* gene rearrangements are not seen in small cell osteosarcoma or mesenchymal chondrosarcoma.

lymphoma, however, can be an important radiographic clue to the diagnosis of osteosarcoma. There are no differences in the treatment and prognosis of small cell osteosarcoma when compared with conventional osteosarcoma.

Histologically, there is some variation in the cytologic features of the small cells in small cell osteosarcoma.[93] The nuclei can be small, round, and uniform, thus resembling conventional ESFT (Fig. 17). Alternatively, they may be more irregular and even show some spindling, features that more closely mimic atypical ES or lymphoma. Osteoid production also varies from focal to abundant. This creates the problem of sampling error in tumors where the amount of osteoid is minimal.

Ancillary studies play a critical role in cases where osteoid production is questionable or when radiographic studies suggest mineralized matrix but there is no clear-cut histologic evidence of osteoid production. A panel of immunostains can usually distinguish lymphoma from other considerations in the differential diagnosis. CD99 is not useful in separating small cell osteosarcoma from ES because small cell osteosarcomas can be CD99 positive.[28,94,95] FLI1 is a better immunohistochemical marker in this differential because ESFTs are usually positive whereas small cell osteosarcomas are negative.[96] Molecular studies provide the most definitive information because the ESFT t(11;22) translocation has not been described in small cell osteosarcoma.[28]

MESENCHYMAL CHONDROSARCOMA

Mesenchymal chondrosarcoma is another tumor with a small round cell component that can mimic other types of SRCTs. First described in 1959, and later called "primitive multipotential primary sarcoma of bone" and "polyhistiocytoma of bone and soft tissue," mesenchymal chondrosarcoma is rare, accounting for 0.7% of malignant tumors of bone and soft tissue.[10] A majority (70%–75%) are primary tumors in bone, with the remainder extraosseous. The tumor tends to affect patients in their third and fourth decades, with no gender predilection.[10] There is a wide skeletal distribution, with the more common sites, including the mandible, rib, vertebrae, pelvic bones, and femur.[97,98] Like any malignant bone tumor, symptoms are nonspecific and include pain and swelling. Radiographic features demonstrate an intramedullary lytic lesion, with calcification, mineralization, cortical thickening, and poor margination.

Gross pathology reveals a lobulated, necrotic, hemorrhagic mass. Histologically, they are biphasic, exhibiting hypercellular and hypocellular regions. The hypercellular regions contain anaplastic small round cells, which may mimic atypical ES, whereas the hypocellular regions demonstrate chondroid islands of varying size with or without ossification (Fig. 18).[97,98] Spindle cell, hemangiopericytomatous, and alveolar patterns have been described.[10] Mesenchymal chondrosarcoma enters the differential of SRCTs of

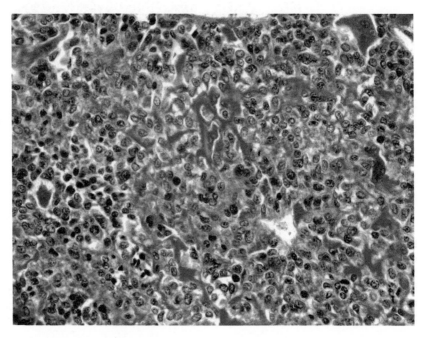

Fig. 17. The neoplastic cells in small cell osteosarcoma are small, round, and only occasionally spindle-shaped. The lace-like pattern of osteoid production differs from reactive bone sometimes seen in other types of SRCTs of bone.

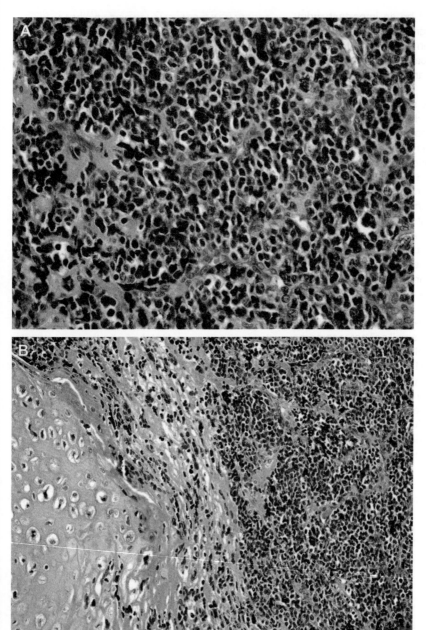

Fig. 18. (*A*) The small blue cell portion of mesenchymal chondrosarcoma resembling other types of SRCTs, in particular atypical ES. (*B*) A diagnosis of mesenchymal chondrosarcoma can be made in another microscopic field containing the low-grade chondrosarcoma component.

bone when the cartilaginous component is not evident, most often due to limited tissue samples. Mesenchymal chondrosarcomas can show some immunoreactivity with CD99. They are negative, however, for FLI1 whereas ESFTs typically are FLI1 positive.[96]

METASTATIC DISEASE AND OTHER RARE TUMORS

Metastatic tumors to bone with small round cell features, such as neuroblastoma, small cell carcinoma, and rhabdomyosarcoma, usually do not pose a diagnostic problem in surgical pathology because these patients usually have disseminated disease or an obvious primary tumor. A chest and abdominal CT scan usually detects the primary site in cases where the initial diagnosis is made or suggested via a bone biopsy. Patients with metastatic neuroblastoma are almost always younger than age 5 years, whereas all of the other tumors in the differential diagnosis typically occur in patients older than 5 years. Rare cases of rhabdomyosarcoma, desmoplastic SRCT, and synovial sarcoma occurring as primary bone tumors have been reported.[99–101] Immunohistochemical (Table 1) and molecular studies are necessary in diagnosing these tumors. Myoepithelial tumors and chordoid sarcoma (extraskeletal myxoid chondrosarcoma) can also occur primary in bone and mimic SRCTs, particularly with small biopsy specimens.[49,102–104]

DIAGNOSTIC APPROACH TO THE DIFFERENTIAL DIAGNOSIS

SRCTs of bone typically have an aggressive radiographic appearance that leads clinicians to a needle biopsy or, at times, open biopsy in an attempt to obtain diagnostic tissue. As a result, pathologists often deal with a small amount of tissue in the face of a differential diagnosis that requires ancillary studies. A limited amount of tissue also increases the risk of sampling error in the assessment of matrix production. Nevertheless, a thoughtful approach that takes all of the clinical and radiographic information into account leads to a definitive diagnosis in the vast majority of cases.

The first step is obtaining a hematoxylin-eosin stain and several unstained slides. Tissue should be sent for cytogenetic karyotyping only if ample amounts are available. Review of the histologic features is followed by a careful plan for ancillary studies that aid in sorting through the differential diagnosis. The most common SRCTs that present as a mass lesion involving bone are ESFTs and hematopoietic malignancies followed by other rare types of sarcoma and metastatic tumors with small round cell features.

Most osseous lymphomas are DLBCLs, characterized by a polymorphous histologic appearance. The histologic features overlap with those of atypical ES but usually differ from the diffuse sheets of uniform round blue cells typically seen in conventional ES. LBL is less common in bone but more problematic because of its more monomorphic histologic appearance and immunohistochemical features that overlap with conventional ES. A suggested initial panel of immunstains includes CD99, CD45, CD20, and CD3. ESFT is positive with CD99 and negative with the B-cell (CD20) and T-cell (CD3) markers. A majority of lymphomas, with the exception of LBLs, are negative with CD99 and positive with CD45 and either B-cell or T-cell markers. FLI1 is not helpful in the differential diagnosis, because LBL and ESFT are both positive with this marker. If the initial panel points toward a B-cell lymphoma, histologic assessment is the next step in determining whether the subsequent panel focuses on subclassification into DLBCL or a small B-cell lymphoma. Because the vast majority is DLBCL, further subclassification can be accomplished with additional immunostains, including CD10, CD21, bcl-2, bcl-6, MIB-1, and MUM-1. The differential diagnosis for hematopoietic tumors that are negative or weakly positive for CD45 includes LBL, ALCL, MS, and myeloma. Table 1 summarizes immunohistochemical features that are helpful in separating these tumors.

Table 1
Immunohistochemical profile of ESFT and hematopoietic malignancies

Tumor	CD45	CD20	CD3	CD43	CD99	FLI1	Tdt	ALK-1	CD30	MPO	CD138 and MUM1	PAX5
ESFT	−	−	−	−	+	+	−	−	−	−	−	−
DLBCL	+	+	−	±	−	−	−	−	±	−	−	+
T-LBL	±	−	+	+	+	+	+	−	−	−	−	+
B-LBL	±	+	−	+	+	+	+	−	−	−	−	+
ALCL	±	−	±	+	−	+	−	+	+	−	−	−
Myeloid sarcoma	+	−	−	+	−	−	−	−	−	+	−	−
Myeloma	±	−	−	±	−	−	−	−	−	−	+	−

Abbreviations: ALCL, anaplastic large cell lymphoma; B-LBL, B-cell lymphoblastic lymphoma; DLBCL, diffuse large B cell lymphoma; ESFT, Ewing sarcoma family tumors; T-LBL, T-cell lymphoblastic lymphoma.

Table 2
Immunohistochemical profile of ESFT and non-hematopoietic round cell tumors

Tumor	CD99	FLI1	CK	TLE-1	Desmin	Myogenin
ESFT	+	+	±	−	−	−
Mesenchymal chondrosarcoma	+	−	−	−	−	−
Small cell osteosarcoma	±	−	±	−	−	−
Rhabdomyosarcoma	±	−	−	−	+	+
Desmoplastic SRCT	−	−	+	−	+	−
Poorly differentiated synovial sarcoma	+	−	±	+	−	−
Carcinoma	±	−	+	−	−	−

In cases where immunohistochemical stains have ruled out hematopoietic malignancies, the differential diagnosis is narrowed down to ESFT, other rare small cell sarcomas (small cell osteosarcoma, mesenchymal chondrosarcoma, rhabdomyosarcoma, poorly differentiated synovial sarcoma, and desmoplastic SRCT), and metastatic disease (carcinoma and neuroblastoma). A negative CD99 essentially rules out ESFT. Particularly with tumors showing cytologic variability, however, it is important to remember that a positive CD99 does not separate ESFT from the other types of sarcoma or metastatic neuroendocrine carcinoma. At this point, molecular analysis (FISH, RT-PCR, or cytogenetics) is the most sensitive and specific means of determining whether a tumor is EFT. RT-PCR for *EWS-FLI1* and *EWS-ERG* identifies approximately 95% of ESFTs. FISH using an *EWSR1* probe is a more sensitive test because it also targets the remaining (<5%) of ESFT. Because *EWSR1* rearrangements are also present in DSRCT and a subset of myoepithelial tumors, correlation with the histologic features and immunohistochemical profile or additional molecular studies may be necessary in distinguishing these tumors.

If molecular studies are not available, additional immunostains can be helpful in sorting through the differential diagnosis (Table 2). Most synovial sarcomas are immunoreactive with TLE-1 and lack FLI1 expression. Ideally, however, molecular analysis for the t(X:18) translocation confirms the diagnosis of synovial sarcoma. Desmin and myogenin or myo-D1 aid in identifying rhabdomyosarcoma. A positive FLI1 lends support to a diagnosis of ESFT and helps exclude mesenchymal chondrosarcoma and small cell osteosarcoma. Metastatic carcinomas, in particular neuroendocrine carcinomas, may show some expression of CD99 but stronger cytokeratin and synaptophysin expression than ESFT. Metastatic neuroblastoma is negative for CD99 and positive for synaptophysin and chromogranin.

SUMMARY

SRCTs comprise a heterogeneous group of neoplasms with overlapping features.[95,105] Histologically, they are all characterized by poorly differentiated cells with small, blue, round nuclei and scant cytoplasm. The most common primary SRCTs involving bone include ESFT and non-Hodgkin lymphoma followed by small cell osteosarcoma and mesenchymal chondrosarcoma. Rarely, metastatic carcinoma and neuroblastoma present as a mimic of primary SRCT of bone. Clinical symptoms and imaging studies are usually not immediately useful in differentiating these tumors, because these lesions may all present with nonspecific pain and demonstrate permeative lytic growth radiographically. Careful histologic review, however, in combination with strategic use of immunohistochemical stains and molecular studies lead pathologists to a correct diagnosis.

REFERENCES

1. Ewing J. Diffuse endothelioma of bone. Proc NY Path Soc 1921;12:17–24.
2. Jaffe R, Santamaria M, Yunis EJ, et al. The neuroectodermal tumor of bone. Am J Surg Pathol 1984; 8(12):885–98.
3. Riggi N, Cironi L, Provero P, et al. Development of Ewing's sarcoma from primary bone marrow-derived mesenchymal progenitor cells. Cancer Res 2005;65(24):11459–68.
4. Tirode F, Laud-Duval K, Prieur A, et al. Mesenchymal stem cell features of Ewing tumors. Cancer Cell 2007;11(5):421–9.
5. Dedeurwaerdere F, Giannini C, Sciot R, et al. Primary peripheral PNET/Ewing's sarcoma of the

dura: a clinicopathologic entity distinct from central PNET. Mod Pathol 2002;15(6):673–8.

6. Jimenez RE, Folpe AL, Lapham RL, et al. Primary Ewing's sarcoma/primitive neuroectodermal tumor of the kidney: a clinicopathologic and immunohistochemical analysis of 11 cases. Am J Surg Pathol 2002;26(3):320–7.

7. Parham DM, Roloson GJ, Feely M, et al. Primary malignant neuroepithelial tumors of the kidney: a clinicopathologic analysis of 146 adult and pediatric cases from the National Wilms' Tumor Study Group Pathology Center. Am J Surg Pathol 2001; 25(2):133–46.

8. Welsch T, Mechtersheimer G, Aulmann S, et al. Huge primitive neuroectodermal tumor of the pancreas: report of a case and review of the literature. World J Gastroenterol 2006;12(37):6070–3.

9. Esiashvili N, Goodman M, Marcus RB Jr. Changes in incidence and survival of Ewing sarcoma patients over the past 3 decades: surveillance epidemiology and end results data. J Pediatr Hematol Oncol 2008;30(6):425–30.

10. Unni KK, Inwards CY. Mesenchymal chondrosarcoma. Dahlin's bone tumors: general aspects and data on 10,165 cases. Philadelphia: Lippincott Williams & Wilkins; 2010. p. 92–7.

11. Nascimento AG, Unii KK, Pritchard DJ, et al. A clinicopathologic study of 20 cases of large-cell (atypical) Ewing's sarcoma of bone. Am J Surg Pathol 1980;4(1):29–36.

12. Askin FB, Rosai J, Sibley RK, et al. Malignant small cell tumor of the thoracopulmonary region in childhood: a distinctive clinicopathologic entity of uncertain histogenesis. Cancer 1979;43(6):2438–51.

13. Bridge JA, Fidler ME, Neff JR, et al. Adamantinoma-like Ewing's sarcoma: genomic confirmation, phenotypic drift. Am J Surg Pathol 1999;23(2): 159–65.

14. Folpe AL, Goldblum JR, Rubin BP, et al. Morphologic and immunophenotypic diversity in Ewing family tumors: a study of 66 genetically confirmed cases. Am J Surg Pathol 2005;29(8):1025–33.

15. Llombart-Bosch A, Contesso G, Peydro-Olaya A. Histology, immunohistochemistry, and electron microscopy of small round cell tumors of bone. Semin Diagn Pathol 1996;13(3):153–70.

16. Llombart-Bosch A, Machado I, Navarro S, et al. Histological heterogeneity of Ewing's sarcoma/ PNET: an immunohistochemical analysis of 415 genetically confirmed cases with clinical support. Virchows Arch 2009;455(5):397–411.

17. Machado I, Noguera R, Mateos EA, et al. The many faces of atypical Ewing's sarcoma. A true entity mimicking sarcomas, carcinomas and lymphomas. Virchows Arch 2011;458(3):281–90.

18. Shanfeld RL, Edelman J, Willis JE. Immunohistochemical analysis of neural markers in peripheral

primitive neuroectodermal tumors (pPNET) without light microscopic evidence of neural differentiation. Appl Immunohistochem 1997;5:78–86.

19. Fukunaga M, Ushigome S. Periosteal Ewing-like adamantinoma. Virchows Arch 1998;433(4):385–9.

20. Hauben E, van den Broek LC, Van Marck E, et al. Adamantinoma-like Ewing's sarcoma and Ewing's-like adamantinoma. The t(11; 22), t(21; 22) status. J Pathol 2001;195(2):218–21.

21. Ishida T, Kikuchi F, Oka T, et al. Case report 727. Juxtacortical adamantinoma of humerus (simulating Ewing tumor). Skeletal Radiol 1992;21(3):205–9.

22. Stevenson AJ, Chatten J, Bertoni F. CD99 (p30/ 32MIC2) neuroectodermal/Ewing's sarcoma antigen as an immunohistochemical marker: review of more than 600 tumors and the literature experience. Appl Immunohistochem 1994;2(2):231–40.

23. Weidner N, Tjoe J. Immunohistochemical profile of monoclonal antibody O13: antibody that recognizes glycoprotein p30/32MIC2 and is useful in diagnosing Ewing's sarcoma and peripheral neuroepithelioma. Am J Surg Pathol 1994;18(5): 486–94.

24. Buxton D, Bacchi CE, Gualco G, et al. Frequent expression of CD99 in anaplastic large cell lymphoma: a clinicopathologic and immunohistochemical study of 160 cases. Am J Clin Pathol 2009;131(4):574–9.

25. Bovee JV, Hogendoorn PC. Molecular pathology of sarcomas: concepts and clinical implications. Virchows Arch 2010;456(2):193–9.

26. Granter SR, Renshaw AA, Fletcher CD, et al. CD99 reactivity in mesenchymal chondrosarcoma. Hum Pathol 1996;27(12):1273–6.

27. Lae ME, Roche PC, Jin L, et al. Desmoplastic small round cell tumor: a clinicopathologic, immunohistochemical, and molecular study of 32 tumors. Am J Surg Pathol 2002;26(7):823–35.

28. Machado I, Alberghini M, Giner F, et al. Histopathological characterization of small cell osteosarcoma with immunohistochemistry and molecular genetic support. A study of 10 cases. Histopathology 2010;57(1):162–7.

29. Romeo S, Dei Tos AP. Soft tissue tumors associated with EWSR1 translocation. Virchows Arch 2010; 456(2):219–34.

30. Malone VS, Dobin SM, Jones KA, et al. CD99-positive large cell neuroendocrine carcinoma with rearranged EWSR1 gene in an infant: a case of prognostically favorable tumor. Virchows Arch 2010;457(3):389–95.

31. Pelosi G, Fraggetta F, Sonzogni A, et al. CD99 immunoreactivity in gastrointestinal and pulmonary neuroendocrine tumours. Virchows Arch 2000; 437(3):270–4.

32. Llombart-Bosch A, Navarro S. Immunohistochemical detection of EWS and FLI-1 proteins in Ewing

sarcoma and primitive neuroectodermal tumors: comparative analysis with CD99 (MIC-2) expression. Appl Immunohistochem Mol Morphol 2001; 9(3):255–60.

33. Folpe AL, Hill CE, Parham DM, et al. Immunohistochemical detection of FLI-1 protein expression: a study of 132 round cell tumors with emphasis on CD99-positive mimics of Ewing's sarcoma/primitive neuroectodermal tumor. Am J Surg Pathol 2000;24(12):1657–62.

34. Mhawech-Fauceglia P, Herrmann F, Penetrante R, et al. Diagnostic utility of FLI-1 monoclonal antibody and dual-colour, break-apart probe fluorescence in situ (FISH) analysis in Ewing's sarcoma/primitive neuroectodermal tumour (EWS/PNET). A comparative study with CD99 and FLI-1 polyclonal antibodies. Histopathology 2006;49(6):569–75.

35. Rossi S, Orvieto E, Furlanetto A, et al. Utility of the immunohistochemical detection of FLI-1 expression in round cell and vascular neoplasm using a monoclonal antibody. Mod Pathol 2004;17(5):547–52.

36. Lin O, Filippa DA, Teruya-Feldstein J. Immunohistochemical evaluation of FLI-1 in acute lymphoblastic lymphoma (ALL): a potential diagnostic pitfall. Appl Immunohistochem Mol Morphol 2009;17(5): 409–12.

37. Collini P, Sampietro G, Bertulli R, et al. Cytokeratin immunoreactivity in 41 cases of ES/PNET confirmed by molecular diagnostic studies. Am J Surg Pathol 2001;25(2):273–4.

38. Gu M, Antonescu CR, Guiter G, et al. Cytokeratin immunoreactivity in Ewing's sarcoma: prevalence in 50 cases confirmed by molecular diagnostic studies. Am J Surg Pathol 2000;24(3):410–6.

39. Parham DM, Dias P, Kelly DR, et al. Desmin positivity in primitive neuroectodermal tumors of childhood. Am J Surg Pathol 1992;16(5):483–92.

40. Jambhekar NA, Bagwan IN, Ghule P, et al. Comparative analysis of routine histology, immunohistochemistry, reverse transcriptase polymerase chain reaction, and fluorescence in situ hybridization in diagnosis of Ewing family of tumors. Arch Pathol Lab Med 2006;130(12):1813–8.

41. Bridge RS, Rajaram V, Dehner LP, et al. Molecular diagnosis of Ewing sarcoma/primitive neuroectodermal tumor in routinely processed tissue: a comparison of two FISH strategies and RT-PCR in malignant round cell tumors. Mod Pathol 2006;19(1):1–8.

42. Qian X, Jin L, Shearer BM, et al. Molecular diagnosis of Ewing's sarcoma/primitive neuroectodermal tumor in formalin-fixed paraffin-embedded tissues by RT-PCR and fluorescence in situ hybridization. Diagn Mol Pathol 2005;14(1):23–8.

43. Aurias A, Rimbaut C. Chromosomal translocations in Ewing's sarcoma. N Engl J Med 1983;309:496–7.

44. Delattre O, Zucman J, Melot T, et al. The Ewing family of tumors–a subgroup of small-round-cell tumors defined by specific chimeric transcripts. N Engl J Med 1994;331(5):294–9.

45. Delattre O, Zucman J, Plougastel B, et al. Gene fusion with an ETS DNA-binding domain caused by chromosome translocation in human tumours. Nature 1992;359(6391):162–5.

46. Toomey EC, Schiffman JD, Lessnick SL. Recent advances in the molecular pathogenesis of Ewing's sarcoma. Oncogene 2010;29(32):4504–16.

47. Sorensen PH, Lessnick SL, Lopez-Terrada D, et al. A second Ewing's sarcoma translocation, t(21;22), fuses the EWS gene to another ETS-family transcription factor, ERG. Nat Genet 1994;6(2):146–51.

48. Yamaguchi U, Hasegawa T, Morimoto Y, et al. A practical approach to the clinical diagnosis of Ewing's sarcoma/primitive neuroectodermal tumour and other small round cell tumours sharing EWS rearrangement using new fluorescence in situ hybridisation probes for EWSR1 on formalin fixed, paraffin wax embedded tissue. J Clin Pathol 2005;58(10):1051–6.

49. Antonescu CR, Zhang L, Chang NE, et al. EWSR1-POU5F1 fusion in soft tissue myoepithelial tumors. A molecular analysis of sixty-six cases, including soft tissue, bone, and visceral lesions, showing common involvement of the EWSR1 gene. Genes Chromosomes Cancer 2010;49(12):1114–24.

50. Bacci G, Ferrari S, Longhi A, et al. Local and systemic control in Ewing's sarcoma of the femur treated with chemotherapy, and locally by radiotherapy and/or surgery. J Bone Joint Surg Br 2003;85(1):107–14.

51. Granowetter L, Womer R, Devidas M, et al. Dose-intensified compared with standard chemotherapy for nonmetastatic Ewing sarcoma family of tumors: a Children's Oncology Group Study. J Clin Oncol 2009;27(15):2536–41.

52. Pinto A, Dickman P, Parham D. Pathobiologic markers of the ewing sarcoma family of tumors: state of the art and prediction of behaviour. Sarcoma 2011;2011:856190.

53. Tageja N. Prognostic indicators for Ewing's sarcoma. Lancet 2010;376(9737):232.

54. Bacci G, Longhi A, Ferrari S, et al. Prognostic factors in non-metastatic Ewing's sarcoma tumor of bone: an analysis of 579 patients treated at a single institution with adjuvant or neoadjuvant chemotherapy between 1972 and 1998. Acta Oncol 2006;45(4):469–75.

55. Paulussen M, Ahrens S, Dunst J, et al. Localized Ewing tumor of bone: final results of the cooperative Ewing's Sarcoma Study CESS 86. J Clin Oncol 2001;19(6):1818–29.

56. Rodriguez-Galindo C, Navid F, Liu T, et al. Prognostic factors for local and distant control in Ewing sarcoma family of tumors. Ann Oncol 2008;19(4): 814–20.

57. Rodriguez-Galindo C, Spunt SL, Pappo AS. Treatment of Ewing sarcoma family of tumors: current status and outlook for the future. Med Pediatr Oncol 2003;40(5):276–87.

58. Picci P, Rougraff BT, Bacci G, et al. Prognostic significance of histopathologic response to chemotherapy in nonmetastatic Ewing's sarcoma of the extremities. J Clin Oncol 1993;11(9):1763–9.

59. Schoedel K, Dickman PS, Krailo M, et al. Histologic response to chemotherapy and prognosis in Ewing's sarcoma/primitive neuroectodermal tumor (ES/PNET). Int Surg Pathol 1995;2:443.

60. de Alava E, Antonescu CR, Panizo A, et al. Prognostic impact of P53 status in Ewing sarcoma. Cancer 2000;89(4):783–92.

61. van Doorninck JA, Ji L, Schaub B, et al. Current treatment protocols have eliminated the prognostic advantage of type 1 fusions in Ewing sarcoma: a report from the Children's Oncology Group. J Clin Oncol 2010;28(12):1989–94.

62. Le Deley MC, Delattre O, Schaefer KL, et al. Impact of EWS-ETS fusion type on disease progression in Ewing's sarcoma/peripheral primitive neuroectodermal tumor: prospective results from the cooperative Euro-E.W.I.N.G. 99 trial. J Clin Oncol 2010; 28(12):1982–8.

63. Lee J, Hoang BH, Ziogas A, et al. Analysis of prognostic factors in Ewing sarcoma using a population-based cancer registry. Cancer 2010;116(8): 1964–73.

64. Lopez-Guerrero JA, Machado I, Scotlandi K, et al. Clinicopathological significance of cell cycle regulation markers in a large series of genetically confirmed Ewing's sarcoma family of tumors. Int J Cancer 2011;128(5):1139–50.

65. Gill P, Wenger DE, Inwards DJ. Primary lymphomas of bone. Clin Lymphoma Myeloma 2005;6(2): 140–2.

66. Alencar A, Pitcher D, Byrne G, et al. Primary bone lymphoma—the University of Miami experience. Leuk Lymphoma 2010;51(1):39–49.

67. Bhagavathi S, Fu K. Primary bone lymphoma. Arch Pathol Lab Med 2009;133(11):1868–71.

68. Bhagavathi S, Micale MA, Les K, et al. Primary bone diffuse large B-cell lymphoma: clinicopathologic study of 21 cases and review of literature. Am J Surg Pathol 2009;33(10):1463–9.

69. Krishnan A, Shirkhoda A, Tehranzadeh J, et al. Primary bone lymphoma: radiographic-MR imaging correlation. Radiographics 2003;23(6):1371–83 [discussion: 1384–7].

70. Dubey P, Ha CS, Besa PC, et al. Localized primary malignant lymphoma of bone. Int J Radiat Oncol Biol Phys 1997;37(5):1087–93.

71. Baar J, Burkes RL, Gospodarowicz M. Primary non-Hodgkin's lymphoma of bone. Semin Oncol 1999; 26(3):270–5.

72. Moses AM, Spencer H. Hypercalcemia in patients with malignant lymphoma. Ann Intern Med 1963; 59:531–6.

73. Jerusalem G, Hustinx R, Beguin Y, et al. Positron emission tomography imaging for lymphoma. Curr Opin Oncol 2005;17(5):441–5.

74. Unni KK, Hogendoorn PC. Malignant lymphoma. In: Fletcher CD, Unni KK, Mertens F, editors. WHO classification of tumours: pathology and genetics of tumours of soft tissue and bone. Lyon (France): IARC; 2002. p. 306–8.

75. Ueda T, Aozasa K, Ohsawa M, et al. Malignant lymphomas of bone in Japan. Cancer 1989;64(11): 2387–92.

76. Ozdemirli M, Mankin HJ, Aisenberg AC, et al. Hodgkin's disease presenting as a solitary bone tumor. A report of four cases and review of the literature. Cancer 1996;77(1):79–88.

77. Ostrowski ML, Unni KK, Banks PM, et al. Malignant lymphoma of bone. Cancer 1986;58(12):2646–55.

78. Beal K, Allen L, Yahalom J. Primary bone lymphoma: treatment results and prognostic factors with long-term follow-up of 82 patients. Cancer 2006;106(12):2652–6.

79. Stein H, Warnke RA, Chan WC, et al. Diffuse large B-cell lymphoma, not otherwise specified. In: Swerdlow SH, Campo E, Harris NL, et al, editors. WHO Classification of tumours of haematopoietic and lymphoid tissues. Lyon (France): IARC; 2008. p. 233–7.

80. Hans CP, Weisenburger DD, Greiner TC, et al. Confirmation of the molecular classification of diffuse large B-cell lymphoma by immunohistochemistry using a tissue microarray. Blood 2004; 103(1):275–82.

81. Ozdemirli M, Fanburg-Smith JC, Hartmann DP, et al. Precursor B-Lymphoblastic lymphoma presenting as a solitary bone tumor and mimicking Ewing's sarcoma: a report of four cases and review of the literature. Am J Surg Pathol 1998;22(7):795–804.

82. Gudgin E, Rashbass J, Pulford KJ, et al. Primary and isolated anaplastic large cell lymphoma of the bone marrow. Leuk Lymphoma 2005;46(3):461–3.

83. Gustafson S, Medeiros LJ, Kalhor N, et al. Anaplastic large cell lymphoma: another entity in the differential diagnosis of small round blue cell tumors. Ann Diagn Pathol 2009;13(6):413–27.

84. Haresh KP, Joshi N, Gupta C, et al. Granulocytic sarcoma masquerading as Ewing's sarcoma: a diagnostic dilemma. J Cancer Res Ther 2008; 4(3):137–9.

85. Martinez-Tello FJ, Calvo–Asensio M, Lorenzo-Roldan JC. Plasma cell myeloma. In: Fletcher CD, Unni KK, Mertens F, editors. WHO classification of tumours: pathology and genetics of tumours of soft tissue and bone. Lyon (France): IARC; 2002. p. 302–5.

86. Edge SB, Fritz AG, Byrd DR, et al. Lymphoid neoplasm. 7th edition. New York: American Joint Committee on Cancer (AJCC) Cancer Staging Manual; 2010.

87. Fidias P, Spiro I, Sobczak ML, et al. Long-term results of combined modality therapy in primary bone lymphomas. Int J Radiat Oncol Biol Phys 1999;45(5):1213–8.

88. Fairbanks RK, Bonner JA, Inwards CY, et al. Treatment of stage IE primary lymphoma of bone. Int J Radiat Oncol Biol Phys 1994;28(2):363–72.

89. Fu K, Weisenburger DD, Choi WW, et al. Addition of rituximab to standard chemotherapy improves the survival of both the germinal center B-cell-like and non-germinal center B-cell-like subtypes of diffuse large B-cell lymphoma. J Clin Oncol 2008; 26(28):4587–94.

90. Ayala AG, Ro JY, Raymond AK, et al. Small cell osteosarcoma. A clinicopathologic study of 27 cases. Cancer 1989;64(10):2162–73.

91. Sim FH, Unni KK, Beabout JW, et al. Osteosarcoma with small cells simulating Ewing's tumor. J Bone Joint Surg Am 1979;61(2):207–15.

92. Bertoni F, Present D, Bacchini P, et al. The Istituto Rizzoli experience with small cell osteosarcoma. Cancer 1989;64(12):2591–9.

93. Nakajima H, Sim FH, Bond JR, et al. Small cell osteosarcoma of bone. Review of 72 cases. Cancer 1997;79(11):2095–106.

94. Devoe K, Weidner N. Immunohistochemistry of small round-cell tumors. Semin Diagn Pathol 2000;17(3):216–24.

95. Hameed M. Small round cell tumors of bone. Arch Pathol Lab Med 2007;131(2):192–204.

96. Lee AF, Hayes MM, Lebrun D, et al. FLI-1 distinguishes Ewing sarcoma from small cell osteosarcoma and mesenchymal chondrosarcoma.

Appl Immunohistochem Mol Morphol 2011;19(3): 233–8.

97. Nakashima Y, Unni KK, Shives TC, et al. Mesenchymal chondrosarcoma of bone and soft tissue. A review of 111 cases. Cancer 1986;57(12): 2444–53.

98. Vencio EF, Reeve CM, Unni KK, et al. Mesenchymal chondrosarcoma of the jaw bones: clinicopathologic study of 19 cases. Cancer 1998;82(12): 2350–5.

99. Lucas DR, Ryan JR, Zalupski MM, et al. Primary embryonal rhabdomyosarcoma of long bone. Case report and review of the literature. Am J Surg Pathol 1996;20(2):239–44.

100. Murphy A, Stallings RL, Howard J, et al. Primary desmoplastic small round cell tumor of bone: report of a case with cytogenetic confirmation. Cancer Genet Cytogenet 2005;156(2):167–71.

101. Thomas F, Lipton JF, Barbera C, et al. Primary rhabdomyosarcoma of the humerus: a case report and review of the literature. J Bone Joint Surg Am 2002; 84(5):813–7.

102. Jung SC, Choi JA, Chung JH, et al. Synovial sarcoma of primary bone origin: a rare case in a rare site with atypical features. Skeletal Radiol 2007;36(1):67–71.

103. Kilpatrick SE, Inwards CY, Fletcher CD, et al. Myxoid chondrosarcoma (chordoid sarcoma) of bone: a report of two cases and review of the literature. Cancer 1997;79(10):1903–10.

104. O'Donnell P, Diss TC, Whelan J, et al. Synovial sarcoma with radiological appearances of primitive neuroectodermal tumour/Ewing sarcoma: differentiation by molecular genetic studies. Skeletal Radiol 2006;35(4):233–9.

105. Li S, Siegal GP. Small cell tumors of bone. Adv Anat Pathol 2010;17(1):1–11.

PSEUDOTUMORS AND REACTIVE LESIONS

Edward F. McCarthy, MD

KEYWORDS

- Heterotopic ossification • Tumoral calcinosis • Giant cell reparative granuloma • Florid osteolysis

ABSTRACT

This article discusses reactive or degenerative processes in bone or periosteal soft tissue that occasionally masquerade as neoplasms. Presentation of the clinical, radiologic, and pathologic features of these processes is provided with an emphasis on the avoidance of overdiagnosis. Clinical, radiologic, and pathologic features of pseudotumors are presented in detail. This article approaches these tumor-like lesions in 2 categories: (1) those in the soft tissue next to bone and (2) those inside bones from the aspect of mineralization and calcification.

OVERVIEW

Pseudotumors fall into 2 major categories—periosteal radiodensities or intraosseous radiolytic processes. The periosteal densities are due to either bone formation or soft tissue calcifications. These lesions may masquerade as bone-forming neoplasms. Intraosseous radiolytic processes may be aggressive on radiograph and these may be confused radiologically with malignant neoplasms. Awareness of the clinical and radiologic features of these lesions is critical for the correct pathologic diagnosis.

HETEROTOPIC BONE

Heterotopic ossification is the formation of the bone outside the skeletal system. This pathologic process may occur in sites, such as the skin, subcutaneous tissue, skeletal muscle, and fibrous tissue adjacent to joints. Bone may also form in the walls of blood vessels as well as in ligaments.[1] Occasionally, it may form in intraabdominal sites, such as the mesentery.[2] The spectrum of this disorder is wide. Lesions range from small clinically

Key Features
PSEUDOTUMORS AND REACTIVE LESIONS

- Awareness of the clinical and radiologic features of pseudotumors is critical for the correct pathologic diagnosis.

- Fibrodysplasia ossificans progressive (FOP), the most severe genetic bone-forming disease, is extremely rare—only approximately 400 cases in the United States.

- Histologic features of myositis ossificans evolve parallel to the radiologic features.

- In contrast to radiodensity produced by some tumor-like lesions of the soft tissues, many intraosseous reactive lesions are radiolucent.

- An important intraosseous reactive process is giant cell reactive granuloma, a lesion that may be mistaken for a giant cell tumor of bone.

- Other radiolytic processes, such as idiopathic pubic osteolysis, are destructive and may mimic infection or a malignant neoplasm.

- In contrast to radiolytic processes, stress fractures or avulsion injuries may produce radiodensities, which may be misdiagnosed as osteosarcoma.

insignificant foci of ossification to massive deposits of bone, which are deposited throughout the body.

Four factors are necessary in the pathogenesis of heterotopic bone[3]:

1. There must be an inciting event. This is usually an episode of trauma, which may result in a hematoma. Often the trauma may be minimal and consist of only a few torn muscle or collagen fibers.

Department of Pathology, Johns Hopkins Hospital, 401 North Broadway, Weinberg 2261, Baltimore, MD 21231, USA
E-mail address: mccarthy@jhmi.edu

Surgical Pathology 5 (2012) 257–286
doi:10.1016/j.path.2011.07.014
1875-9181/12/$ – see front matter © 2012 Elsevier Inc. All rights reserved.

2. There is a signal from the site of injury. This signal is most probably a protein secreted from cells of the injured tissue or from inflammatory cells arriving in response to the tissue injury.
3. There must be a supply of mesenchymal cells whose genetic machinery is not fully committed. Given the appropriate signal, genes that synthesize osteoid and chondroid are activated and cause these mesenchymal cells to differentiate into osteoblasts or chondroblasts. Heterotopic bone formation may occur anywhere where these uncommitted mesenchymal cells reside. These sits include skeletal muscle, perivascular tissue, and fibrous tissue.
4. There must exist an appropriate environment conducive to the continued production of the heterotopic bone.

Of these 4 factors, signaling agents seem to play the most important role in the formation of heterotopic bone, and recent progress has been made in understanding of these agents. These signaling agents are known as bone morphogenic proteins (BMPs) and there are at least 15 proteins in this family.

Important BMPs include types 1 through 12 and growth differentiation factors types 5 through 7.[4] Most of these molecules are members of the transforming growth factor β superfamily of molecules.

Heterotopic bone occurs in 5 broad clinical settings:

1. Genetic
2. Posttraumatic
3. Neurogenic
4. Postsurgical
5. As distinctive reactive lesions most often seen in the hands and feet.

In the genetic setting, the most important disorder is fibrodysplasia ossificans progressiva (FOP). This disorder is characterized by massive deposits of heterotopic bone, which progressively accumulate around multiple joints. This process eventually causes severe disability and early death.

In the second setting, known as myositis ossificans circumscripta, a localized self-limited proliferation of fibroblasts and heterotopic bone form in skeletal muscle after trauma. Sometimes patients with this localized presentation recall no injury.

Neurogenic ossification, the third setting, occurs in muscle and periarticular fibrous tissue at multiple sites in patients who have sustained head trauma or spinal cord injury. Patients who have been in long comas may also develop this form of heterotopic bone.

The fourth clinical setting is heterotopic formation in periarticular soft tissue, which occasionally follows total joint arthroplasties. Finally, heterotopic bone may occur in the hands and feet. In these locations, the clinical, radiographic, and histologic presentations are distinct.

FIBRODYSPLASIA OSSIFICANS PROGRESSIVA

FOP is the most severe genetic bone-forming disease. In this disorder, extensive heterotopic ossification progressively develops at multiple periarticular sites and eventually causes complete immobilization. Fortunately, this disease is rare; only approximately 400 patients are known in the United States. FOP almost always arises by a spontaneous mutation, and no sexual, racial, or ethnic prevalence has been observed. Because the reproductive capacity of most patients is limited, familial transmission is rare; however, a few familial cases suggest an autosomal dominant mode of transmission.[5]

The heterotopic ossification of FOP begins in the first decade of life, usually at approximately age 3. The first lesions usually occurs in the back when a soft mass becomes palpable adjacent to the upper spine and shoulder girdle.[6] As the patient ages, other masses appear. The manner of progression is consistent. Lesions develop from cranial to caudal and from the axial to the appendicular skeleton (Fig. 1). Many patients develop a severe scoliosis. Although the disease progresses at different rates in different patients, by the third decade most patients are usually severely crippled with widespread periarticular ossification. Although a few patients survive into middle adulthood (one patient survived to age 70),[7] most die in the third or fourth decade from pneumonia. Patients uniformly have characteristic congenital skeletal abnormalities. For example, almost all patients have short great toes due to synostoses or deformities of the phalanx, and some have short thumbs (Fig. 2). These phalangeal features are essential to the diagnoses of this disorder.[8]

The development of lesions in FOP follows an orderly progression:

• First, it induces an inflammatory reaction in the injured soft tissue. The earliest lesions show muscular degeneration and lymphoid infiltrate.
• This is followed by proliferation of a highly muscular fibrous tissue in which BMPs 2 and 4 have been demonstrated.[9]
• Then, osteoid forms in this fibroblastic stroma. The zonal pattern typical of other forms of

Fig. 1. Heterotopic bone formation in the shoulder girdle of a patient with FOP. This is usually the first site of ossification in this disorder.

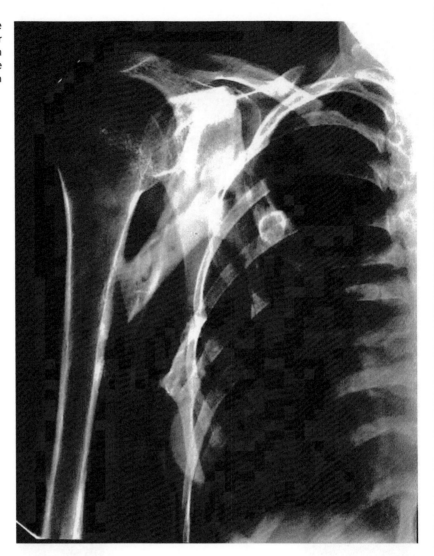

heterotopic ossification is not usually present in FOP.

- In addition, hyaline cartilage, which is undergoing endochondral ossification, is abundant in FOP. Endochondral ossification seems to be the principal mechanism of bone formation in this disorder.[10]

MYOSITIS OSSIFICANS CIRCUMSCRIPTA

The second clinical setting of heterotopic ossification, myositis ossificans circumscripta, is the most common form of heterotopic bone formation. This process is characterized by the intramuscular proliferation of fibroblasts, new bone, and, occasionally, cartilage. In this common, self-limited disorder, an osseous mass develops next to bones and joints. Although myositis ossificans may develop spontaneously, the process is initiated by trauma in 60% to 75% of cases. A distinctive feature of myositis ossificans is lesional maturation, which is apparent clinically, radiologically, and histologically.

One or 2 days after trauma to a muscle, a painful mass appears. Sometimes there is no history of a single episode of severe trauma. Instead, multiple episodes of minor injury may initiate the process. The lump may even appear spontaneously. The mass grows steadily for a month or 2 and reaches a size of from 4 to 10 cm. Thereafter, the mass becomes hard and ceases to grow. Often, after a year or so, the firm mass becomes smaller and, rarely, it may disappear completely.

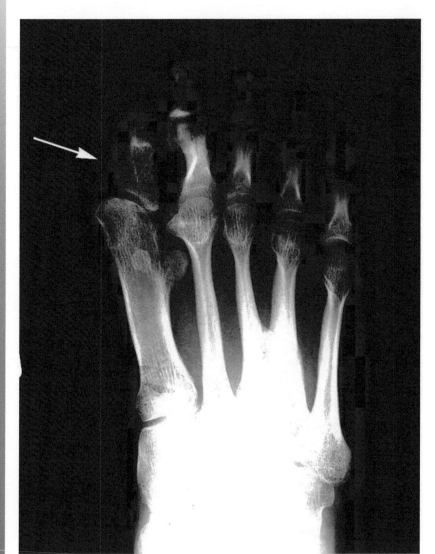

Fig. 2. Characteristic shortening of the proximal phalanx of the great toe seen in patients with FOP (*arrow*).

Patients with myositis ossificans are usually in their teens and 20s, although patients as old as age 84 and as young as age 5 months have been reported.[11] The most common locations are the muscles of the thigh, buttock, or upper arm. These sites correspond to muscles most easily traumatized in young athletic adults, the most common patients to be affected.

The radiologic features of myositis ossificans evolve as the lesion matures. For the first few weeks after clinical presentation, a soft tissue mass, best seen on MRI, shows no mineralization. On routine MRI, the soft tissue mass is nonspecific.[12] After gadolinium administration, however, the lesion may show rim enhancement, a feature rarely seen in other soft tissue masses.[13] After 3 to 5 weeks, fluffy radiodensities appear in the mass, and a periosteal reaction is often present in the adjacent bone (**Fig. 3**). After approximately 6 weeks, the mineralization shows a characteristic zonal pattern; mineralization is denser at the periphery of the lesion. This zonal pattern is best visualized with a CT scan (**Fig. 4**). As the lesion ages, orderly lines of mature trabecular bone become distinct (**Fig. 5**).

The histologic features of myositis ossificans evolve parallel to the radiologic features. The early lesion shows cellular sheets of plump fibroblasts, and mitotic figures are numerous. These early lesions have the appearance of a tissue culture of fibroblasts (**Fig. 6**). The cells are spindle-shaped or stellate and seem to float in a myxoid

Fig. 3. Myositis ossificans. This earlier lesion shows only faint radiodensity in the soft tissues adjacent to the greater trochanter (*arrow*).

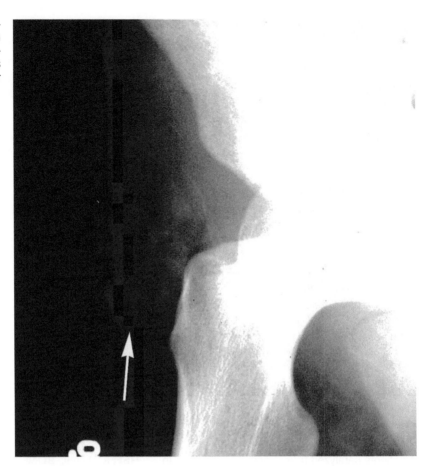

extracellular matrix. As early as 1 week after the mass becomes clinically palpable, seams of osteoid appear in the peripheral portions (Fig. 7). Because of the dense cellularity and osteoid production, lesions at this early stage of evolution have been called "pseudomalignant osseous tumors of soft tissue."[14,15] Despite the high degree of cellularity and frequent mitotic figures, however, cytologic atypia and abnormal mitoses are absent. In some lesions of myositis ossificans, cartilage is present; as the lesion matures, the cartilage undergoes endochondral ossification. A characteristic feature of myositis ossificans is the entrapment of skeletal muscle in the peripheral portions of the mass.

After approximately 6 weeks, the zonal pattern seen on plain radiographs is also apparent on low-power microscopic study. The outer portion of the mass shows dense lamellar bone arranged as a pseudocortex. Spicules of bone are progressively thinner toward the center of the lesion (Fig. 8). After 6 months to a year, lesions of myositis ossificans develop an orderly arrangement of thick,

mature trabecular bone. In these older lesions, the zonal pattern is no longer apparent, and bone marrow may be present.

Differential diagnostic problems arise in both early and late lesions of myositis ossificans. An early lesion may be misdiagnosed as a soft tissue osteosarcoma. Pleomorphic atypical cells with atypical mitotic figures, features characteristic of soft tissue osteosarcoma, however, are absent in myositis ossificans. A late lesion of myositis ossificans may be confused with a parosteal osteosarcoma. Parosteal osteosarcoma, however, does not show a zonal pattern of ossification and lacks orderly lines of mature trabecular bone. Also, in parosteal osteosarcoma, cellular atypia, although mild, is always present.

NEUROGENIC OSSIFICATION

In the third clinical setting, heterotopic bone occasionally develops around joints in patients immobilized after traumatic neurologic lesions.[16] For example, heterotopic bone forms in 20% to 25%

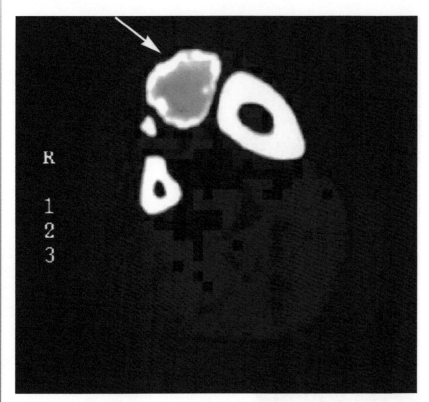

Fig. 4. Heterotopic ossification in the distal extremity. Between the fibula and tibia there is a radiodense lesion with a characteristic zonal pattern of radiodensity. The lesion is most radiodense around the periphery (*arrow*).

of patients paralyzed from a spinal cord injury. In 18% to 35% of these patients, the process is severe enough to cause limitation of joint motion (**Fig. 9**). Patients with low cervical or high thoracic lesions are the most likely to develop this complication. In addition to patients with spinal cord injury, 10% to 20% of patients immobilized due to closed head trauma form heterotopic bone. Approximately 10% of these patients develop severe limitation of joint motion.[17]

Patients with neurogenic heterotopic ossification develop lesions around larger joints. The hip is the most common location, followed by the knees and elbows. A single joint is affected in 40% of patients; in another third, two joints are affected. The heterotopic bone formation begins within 2 months after neurologic injury and is usually fully developed by 2 years. Sometimes the heterotopic bone may be massive and cause complete ankylosis of the affected joint.

The cause of the heterotopic bone formation in these patients is unknown. Vascular stasis, edema, and prolonged swelling are likely contributing factors. In addition, passive manipulation of joints to preserve range of motion may traumatize soft tissue and initiate heterotopic bone formation.[18]

HETEROTOPIC BONE POST–TOTAL JOINT ARTHROPLASTY

The fourth clinical setting is the development of heterotopic bone in periarticular tissues after total hip surgery. From 25% to 7% of patients develop this complication.[19] In many of these patients, resulting limitation in motion necessitates a revision arthroplasty. Although the incidence of clinically significant heterotopic ossification is small, asymptomatic heterotopic bone formation occurs frequently; radiographic evidence is present in as many as 56% of patients.[20,21] Patients with ankylosing spondylitis, Paget disease, and hypertrophic osteoarthritis are at risk of developing this complication.[22] In high-risk patients as well as those requiring revision arthroplasty for this complication, the incidence of heterotopic bone is reduced by prophylactic low-dose irradiation. Beginning 5 days after surgery, 1000 rad is administered in 5 divided doses. Postoperative nonsteroidal antiinflammatory drug therapy also reduces the incidence of heterotopic bone.

Myositis ossificans is rare in the muscles of the hands and feet.[23,24] Other manifestations of heterotopic, however, bone occur in these locations. These reactive lesions in the hands and

Fig. 5. Mature lesion of myositis ossificans adjacent to the humerus. Lines of mature trabecular bone are present within this radiodense mass.

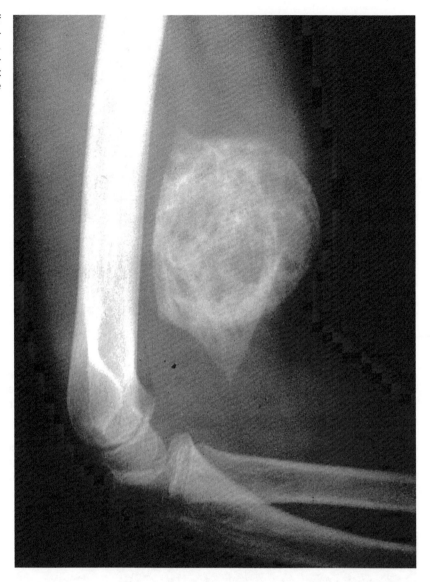

feet occur in 3 important clinicoradiologic settings. The first setting, bizarre parosteal osteochondromatous proliferation (BPOP), also known as Nora's lesion, is a lobular proliferation of reactive bone and cartilage, which forms an exophytic mass adjacent to the bone. Formerly, this process was often regarded as an osteochondroma. The second setting, florid reactive periostitis, is a fusiform proliferation of reactive tissue confined beneath the tight periosteum. These first 2 settings are probably manifestations of the same reactive process in different locations, one subperiosteal and the other involving the loose alveolar tissues outside the periosteum.[25] When these lesions are mature and firmly attached to the bone surface,

they have been referred to as turret exostoses.[26] The third reactive lesion of the hands and feet, subungual exostosis, is a bony projection from the distal phalanx and is probably a response to trauma.

Like lesions of heterotopic bone in other locations, reactive lesions of the hands and feet may be misdiagnosed as osteosarcoma. Therefore, awareness of their distinctive clinicoradiologic features is necessary to prevent this misdiagnosis.

BPOP presents as a painless swelling in the soft tissues of the hand or feet. The most common site is adjacent to a proximal phalanx, a metacarpal, or a metatarsal. Similar lesions have been reported in sites other than the hands and feet, such as

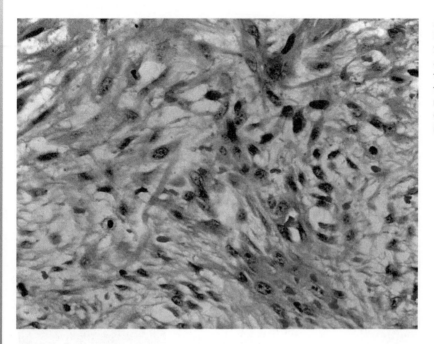

Fig. 6. Myositis ossificans in the earlier phase. Spindle and cellate cells are present in an exomatous matrix. At this stage, the lesion is similar to nodular fasciitis pattern (hematoxylin-eosin, original magnification ×400).

adjacent to the ulna, femur, and radius. Patients range in age from 8 to 73 years, although most patients are between ages 20 and 40. Approximately 12% of patients have a history of trauma.[27]

On plain radiographs, BPOP is a well-circumscribed radiodense mass, which arises from the cortical surface (Fig. 10). An additional unmineralized soft tissue mass is absent. The underlying cortex is always intact but occasionally shows slight surface irregularity. The radiodense mass, which shows a trabecular pattern in later stages of development, ranges in size from 0.4 cm to 3 cm.

Histologically, BPOP consists of irregular aggregates of hyaline cartilage, spindle cells, and new bone (Fig. 11). The cartilage, probably formed by

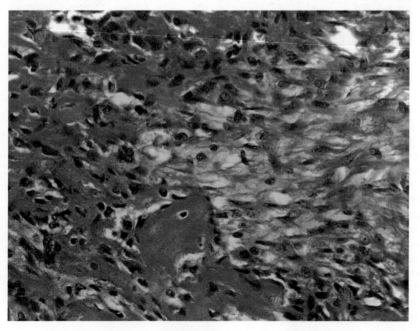

Fig. 7. Photomicrograph of an earlier lesion of myositis ossificans showing osteoid production in a cellular fibrous tissue background pattern (hematoxylin-eosin, original magnification ×100).

Fig. 8. A mature lesion of myositis ossificans showing dense bone at the periphery of the lesion and abundant fibrous tissue in the central portion of the lesion. This is the characteristic zonal pattern as seen on microscopic study.

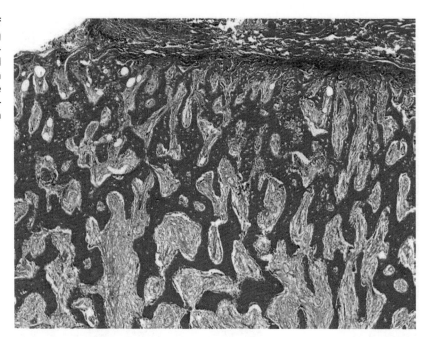

chondroid metaplasia of fibrous tissue, often forms a cap at the periphery of the lesion. The cartilage is usually hypercellular with large chondrocytes, some of which are binucleated and show mild atypia. The cartilage lobules are separated by a florid spindle cell proliferation. The spindle cells show mild to moderate mitotic activity, but atypical mitotic figures are not present. Cellular atypia is also absent. In addition, myxoid change is occasionally present. Irregular new bone or osteoid is abundant and is formed in the cartilage lobules by endochondral ossification or by metaplastic ossification in the spindle cell areas. A characteristic histologic feature of BPOP is deep basophilia of the new bone (**Fig. 12**). Older lesions contain mature lamellar bone.

BPOP should be treated by surgical excision. However, 50% of lesions recur from 2 months to 2 years after the first excision; 20% of patients have more than one recurrence. Recurrent lesions should be excised.

Florid reactive periostitis, like BPOP, affects patients of any age. Also, like BPOP, most patients are between ages 20 and 40. Unlike most patients with BPOP, however, who have painless swelling, almost all patients with florid reactive periostitis present with pain and a fusiform swelling. A history of trauma is present in 40% of patients. Like BPOP, the proximal phalanges, metacarpals, and metatarsals are the most common sites.[28]

Early lesions of florid reactive periostitis show only soft tissue swelling. Later, a smoothly contoured mass of fluffy subperiosteal new bone develops (**Fig. 13**). In the late stages, the new bone matures and becomes incorporated in the cortex. Like BPOP, the underlying bone is unaffected.

Histologically, florid reactive periostitis shows new bone in a fibroblastic proliferation. Although cartilage is occasionally present, it is less conspicuous than in BPOP. In addition, unlike the disorganization of tissue elements in BPOP, florid reactive periostitis tends to have a zonal pattern with more mature bone in the center of the lesion (**Fig. 14**). The fibroblastic component is usually very cellular, the cells having plump nuclei with a large nucleolus. In addition, there is mild pleomorphism, and numerous typical mitotic figures are present. The osteoid is usually lace-like in early stages and is rimmed by plump uniform osteoblasts. Trabecular bone is present in more mature lesions.

Florid reactive periostitis should also be treated by surgical excision. Unlike BPOP, florid reactive periostitis rarely recurs.

Subungual exostosis arises on the dorsal surface of the distal phalanx. Lesions range from a few millimeters to 2 cm. Larger lesions elevate the nail and ulcerate the nail bed. Patients ranging in age from 8 to 55 years (mean 23.5 years) present with pain. Approximately 75% of subungual exostoses arise in the great toe. The remaining 25% of

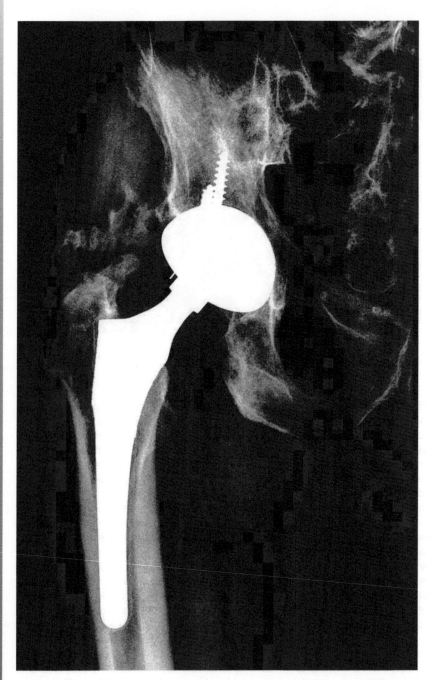

Fig. 9. Heterotopic bone formation in the periarticular tissues of the hip after total hip replacement.

cases affect the other digits of the hands and feet with equal frequency.[29]

Radiologically, a bony projection from the dorsal portion of the distal phalanx is best seen on a lateral plain radiograph (**Fig. 15**). The underlying bone is unremarkable.

Histologically, a cartilage cap, which arises from chondroid metaplasia of spindle cells beneath the nail, covers the projection of trabecular bone. A zonal arrangement of tissues is apparent (**Fig. 16**). Superficially, spindle cells with chondroid metaplasia are present under the nail, and beneath this tissue, mature cartilage changes to endochondral bone. The deepest portion of the lesion consists of mature trabecular bone, which connects with the cortex of the phalanx.

Fig. 10. BPOP of the finger. The lesion is a well-circumscribed radiodensity.

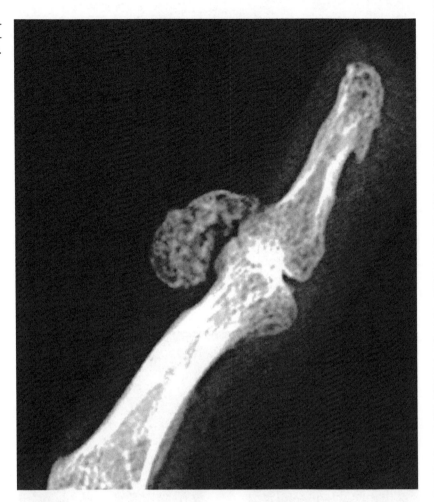

Fig. 11. Photomicrograph of bizarre parosteal chondromatous proliferation. This proliferation shows a haphazard admixture of cartilage, bone, and fibrous tissue pattern (hematoxylin-eosin, original magnification ×100).

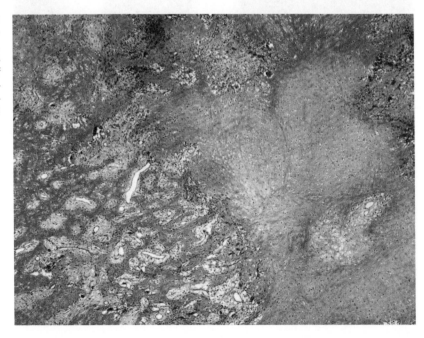

268

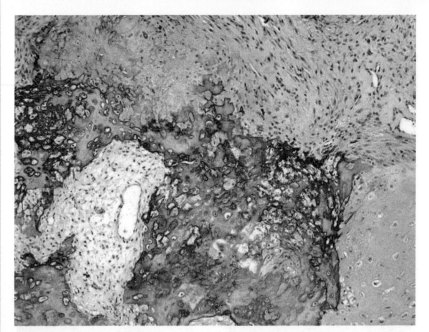

Fig. 12. Bizarre parosteal chondromatous proliferation showing deep basophilia of the new bone. This feature is commonly seen in BPOP pattern (hematoxylin-eosin, original magnification ×100).

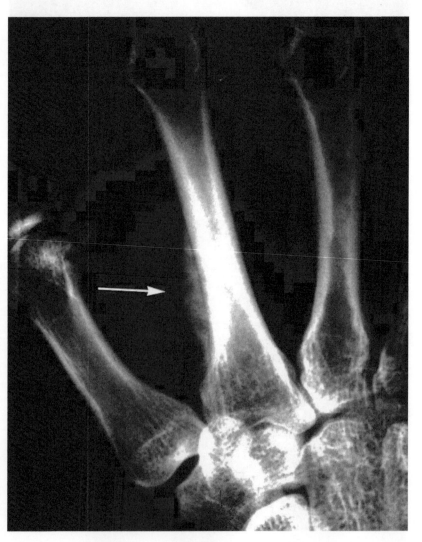

Fig. 13. Florid reactive periostitis of the second metacarpal (*arrow*).

Fig. 14. Photomicrograph of florid reactive periostitis. Broad bands of woven bone are present in a regulating regular pattern perpendicular to the shaft of the bone pattern (hematoxylin-eosin, original magnification ×100).

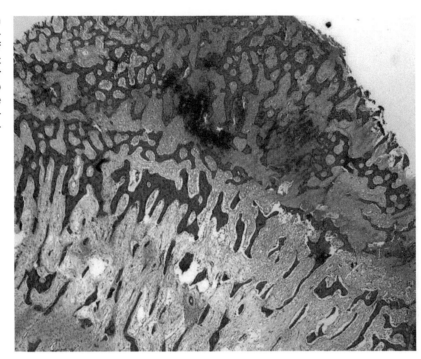

Fig. 15. A subungual exostosis. There is a bony projection from the distal phalanx.

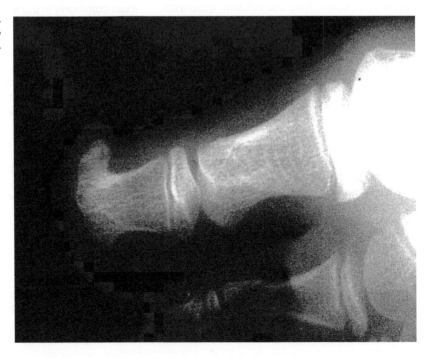

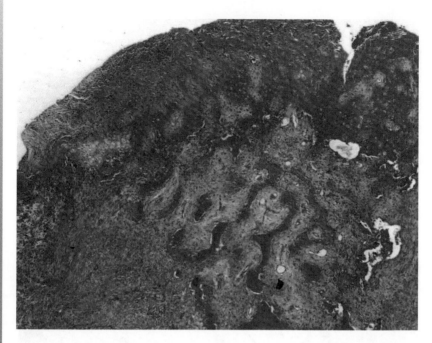

Fig. 16. The histologic features of a subungual exostosis show a zonal arrangement of reactive bone formation beneath the nail bed pattern (hematoxylin-eosin, original magnification ×100).

Subungual exostoses can be cured by simple excision with preservation of the distal phalanx and nail.

TUMORAL CALCINOSIS

CLINICAL PRESENTATION

Tumoral calcinosis is the massive deposition of amorphous calcium salts and calcium hydroxyapatite crystals in periarticular soft tissues. This disease occurs in 3 clinical settings.

1. The first is a sporadic presentation, affecting adult patients and usually only involving one joint. In this setting, the calcification is probably initiated by local tissue damage. A small nodule of this process in tendons is known as calcific tendonitis.
2. The second setting, accounting for one-third of patients with this disease, suggests a familial metabolic abnormality. Several members of a family may be affected in a pattern of autosomal dominant inheritance. These families are usually African American, and affected members first present in childhood, usually with multiple sites of involvement. Hyperphosphatemia and elevated serum levels of 1,25 (OH)$_2$ vitamin D in many of these patients suggests a metabolic abnormality.[30]
3. In the third and last setting, tumoral calcinosis may occur in patients on chronic renal dialysis. Multiple joints are usually involved.[31]

RADIOGRAPHIC FEATURES

Plain radiographic images of tumoral calcinosis show multiple, amorphous periarticular radiodensities (**Fig. 17**). The densities are round or oval and are grouped in a mass, sometimes 20 cm or more in diameter. Favorite sites of involvement are the hips, elbows, and shoulders. The limited form of this disease, calcific tendonitis, occurs most commonly in the shoulder.[32] A small oval radiodensity is present, usually in the supraspinatus tendon.

Tumoral calcinosis may be mistaken radiographically for a bone or cartilage producing neoplasm. Tumoral calcinosis lacks the stippled and ring-like calcification of cartilage, however, and it lacks the trabecular pattern of bone. Furthermore, 2 features of tumoral calcinosis are not present in bone or cartilage lesions. First, the radiodensities of tumoral calcinosis are separated by bands of lucency imparting a cobblestone appearance. Second, fluid-calcium levels within the radiodensities are often present on CT scans or plain radiographs.[33]

HISTOLOGIC FEATURES

Tumoral calcinosis is probably initiated by a soft tissue, periarticular hematoma followed by an infiltrate of histiocytes.[30] Motion of the nearby joint stimulates neobursa formation in the area of hemorrhage. Then, due to systemic problems of

Fig. 17. Tumoral calcinosis of the soft tissues adjacent to the proximal tibia.

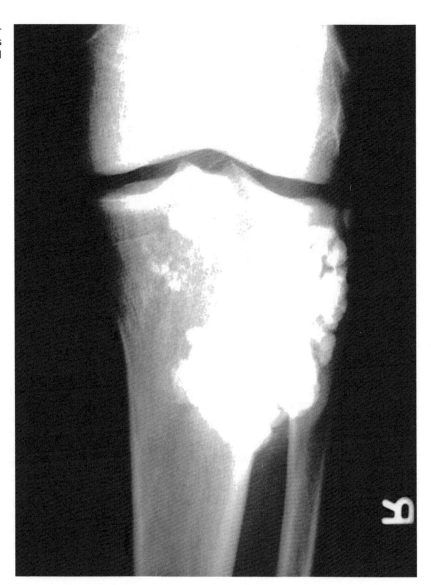

calcium metabolism, local calcification begins. Fully developed lesions of tumoral calcinosis are characterized histologically by locules of amorphous, calcified debris surrounded by a histiocytic and multinucleated giant cell infiltrate (**Fig. 18**). The histiocytes and giant cells show focal degeneration with occasional intracellular calcifications. Extracellular calcification is more prominent, occurring as plates or laminated spherules (psammoma bodies) admixed with amorphous debris (**Fig. 19**). The calcifications are deeply basophilic and are not birefringent in polarized light. Calcification may be absent in early lesions, which show only a histiocytic infiltrate. Occasionally, metaplastic bone develops at the periphery of the lesions.

TREATMENT

Massive lesions of tumoral calcinosis are difficult to eradicate. Large deposits have, in some patients, been reduced by oral administration of phosphate binders, such as aluminum hydroxide.[34] Symptomatic deposits may also be surgically debulked or excised. Smaller lesions may be aspirated or treated symptomatically.

In contrast to the calcium hydroxyapatite deposition characteristic of tumoral calcinosis, calcium pyrophosphate may also be deposited as large soft tissue masses. This condition, known as tumoral calcium pyrophosphate deposition disease (also known as tophaceous pseudogout), is a rare manifestation of calcium pyrophosphate deposition

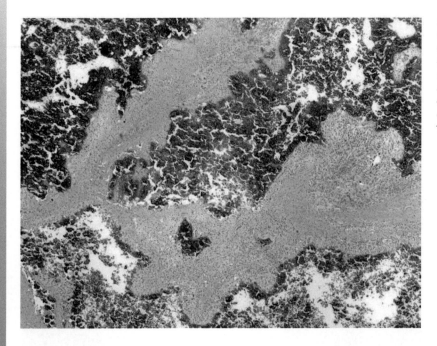

Fig. 18. Low-power photomicrograph of tumoral calcinosis showing locules of calcific debris surrounded by histiocytes and foreign body giant cells pattern (hematoxylin-eosin, original magnification ×40).

disease.[35,36] Although radiographically indistinguishable from tumoral calcinosis, certain microscopic features help distinguish these lesions:

- First, high-power microscopic study of tumoral calcium pyrophosphate deposition disease demonstrates small, uniform, rhomboid calcium pyrophosphate crystals. This contrasts with the plates of calcium hydroxyapatite characteristic of tumoral calcinosis.
- Second, chondroid metaplasia, not seen in tumoral calcinosis, is common in tissues surrounding

deposits of calcium pyrophosphate (**Fig. 20**). This feature, present in most cases, frequently leads to a histologic misdiagnosis of a cartilage neoplasm. The demonstration of polarizable pyrophosphate crystals, not present in cartilage lesions, properly identifies tumoral calcium pyrophosphate deposition disease.

Tumoral calcium pyrophosphate deposition disease most commonly occurs around the temporomandibular joint or in the fingers (**Fig. 21**). Patients present with pain and swelling

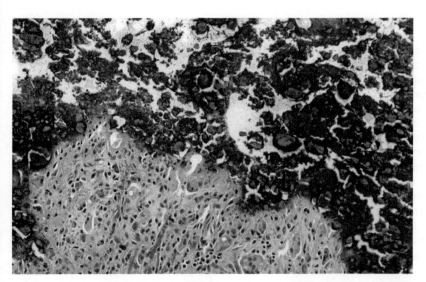

Fig. 19. The calcification occurs as plates or laminated spirules mixed with amorphous debris pattern (hematoxylin-eosin, original magnification ×200).

Fig. 20. Photomicrograph of tumoral calcium pyrophosphate deposition disease. There is chondroid metaplasia associated with the calcium crystals pattern (hematoxylin-eosin, ×200).

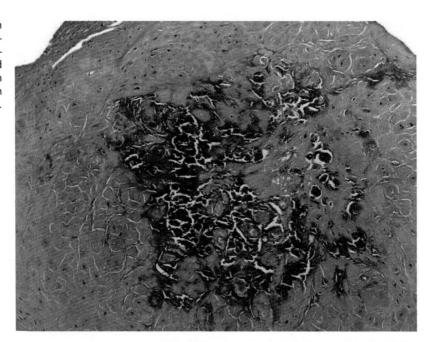

Fig. 21. Calcium pyrophosphate disease of the hand. There are multiple nodules of calcific radiodensities in the periosteal soft tissues.

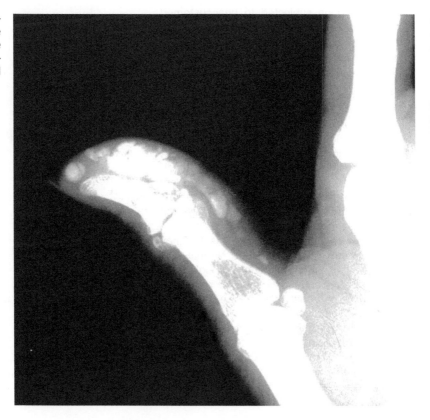

and range in age from 31 to 86 years; most are over age 50. Surgical excision is the treatment of choice, although approximately 20% of patients develop recurrence after this therapy.

DIRECT BONE INJURY MIMICKING NEOPLASMS

Although an occasional occult fracture may be missed on radiographic examination, typical fractures rarely present diagnostic problems. Certain special types of fractures, however, are frequently confused with other bone lesions. Most problematic are stress fractures or avulsion fractures.

STRESS FRACTURES

Unlike a typical fracture, which is a complete break in a bone due to a single trauma, a stress fracture is a partial break secondary to repeated episodes of lesser trauma. The partial break is often accompanied by endosteal and periosteal new bone formation. If the repetitive stress continues, the lesion increases in size and may progress to a complete fracture. Diagnostic problems arise because the stress fracture may not be apparent on plain radiography or because the reactive bone changes mimic a more aggressive lesion.

Stress fractures occur in 2 settings:

1. In normal bone subjected to unaccustomed stress (fatigue fractures)
2. In bone weakened by preexisting disease and subjected to normal stresses (insufficiency fractures).

Fatigue fractures are associated with a new, strenuous activity, which is repeated regularly. Fatigue fractures may occur in any bone. There are at least 25 documented activities that produce lesions at specific sites. For example, fatigue fractures commonly occur in the metatarsals of military recruits who must march all day. Also, runners may develop fatigue fractures in almost any bone in the lower extremities, although the tibia and fibula are the most common sites.[37]

In contrast to fatigue fractures, insufficiency fractures develop in abnormal bone. Normal daily activities cause gradual fracturing through bone that is weak. Most commonly, this occurs in osteoporosis, and the bones affected are the pelvis, sacrum, and femur.

The first stage in the development of a stress fracture is increased bone turnover, which is concentrated in the zone of maximum bone deformation.[38–42] This increased turnover, which is probably mediated by electric streaming potentials, is imbalanced—osteoblastic activity is less than osteoclastic activity. As a result, a thin zone of osteopenia develops. The trabeculae in this zone are thinner and the cortex is porous. Next, a tiny crack develops in the porous cortex, and a periosteal and endosteal reactive bone proliferates. If the activity continues, the crack lengthens to include trabecular bone, and reactive bone formation increases.

Radiologic Features

Early stress fractures may be completely unapparent on plain radiographs. As the lesion develops, however, a small amount of reactive periosteal new bone appears. At this stage, a bone scan is diagnostic—a linear zone of tracer accumulation is present (**Fig. 22**). As this process continues, plain radiographs show a linear zone of osteopenia or mixed osteopenia and sclerosis

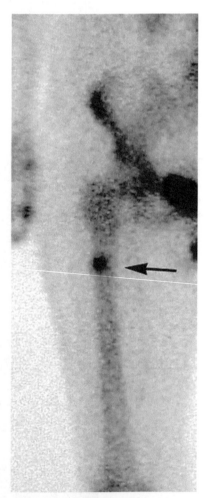

Fig. 22. Bone scan of a patient with a stress fracture. There is a band like zone of increased tracer uptake in the proximal femur (*arrow*).

(Fig. 23). An MRI is useful to delimit the osseous change. The periosteal reaction is sometimes florid and can mimic a neoplasm. In late stress fractures and in healing lesions, the periosteal reaction consolidates into a smoothly contoured surface density.

Pathologic Features

Although the clinical history of pain associated with repeated activity should be a clue to the correct diagnosis, some stress fractures are misdiagnosed as infections or neoplasms and are biopsied. Histologically, a biopsy from a stress fracture shows fracture callus. Irregular seams of osteoid or woven bone are present in granulation tissue or a loose fibrovascular stroma. Islands of cartilage undergoing endochondral ossification are also present (Fig. 24). Sometimes, marked cellularity and abundant osteoid may mimic a bone-forming neoplasm. Unlike a neoplasm, however, acute stress fractures show a zonal pattern—bone is denser and more mature at the periphery of the

lesion. Also, pleomorphic cells are not present in a stress fracture. Chronic or healed stress fractures contain dense trabecular or cortical bone with an intervening fibrous stroma. The zonal pattern may no longer be present, and the bone is lamellar with mature haversian systems.

AVULSION INJURY

An avulsion injury is another special type of fracture. Because tendon and the tendon insertion into bone often has stronger tensile strength than the bone itself, a violent muscle contraction or repetitive muscle contraction may pull off a portion of bone. This avulsion injury, which is occasionally seen in active young patients, causes cortical irregularity and periosteal reactive tissue proliferation. Sometimes a large fragment of bone is detached. Common sites of avulsion include the ischeal tuberosity, the greater or lesser trochanter, the iliac spines, and the humerus at the insertion of the pectoralis major. The 2 most common sites of avulsion, however, are the tibial tuberosity,

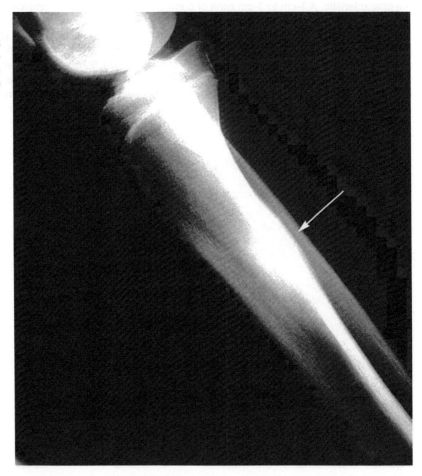

Fig. 23. Plain radiograph of a stress fracture showing a zone of radiodensity. This radio density may sometimes be confused with a bone-forming neoplasm (*arrow*).

a disorder known as Osgood-Schlatter disease, and the medial distal femoral metaphysis.

An avulsion injury of the distal femoral metaphysis is known as the distal femoral cortical irregularity syndrome. Because fibrous tissue proliferation occurs in this lesion, it was formerly called "periosteal desmoid." This process characteristically occurs on the medial surface of the distal femoral metaphysis. Initiated by the pull of the adductor magnus tendon, periosteal reactive bone forms adjacent to a scalloped cortex.[43–51] This lesion occurs exclusively in children and adolescents, the reported age range 3 to 22 years. Small cortical irregularities in this region are present in 11.5% (male) and 3.5% (female), and as many as one-third of patients have bilateral lesions. Although most patients are asymptomatic, some present with pain after strenuous physical activity, a symptom, which prompts radiographic examination.

Radiographic Features

The plain radiographic features of most cases of the distal femoral cortical irregularity syndrome are characteristic. A 1-cm to 3-cm zone of cortical erosion is present on the posterior medial aspect of the distal femoral metaphysis (Fig. 25). Some lesions may cause a poorly defined lytic area, and, in many cases, periosteal new bone is present. Occasionally, the reactive periosteal bone is extensive and has a sunburst appearance, a pattern simulating a malignant neoplasm. The

MRI is useful in florid cases to outline specific intramedullary reactive changes. This imaging modality shows a well-demarcated medullary lesion, which is hypointense on T_1-weighted images and hyperintense on T_2-weighted images. In both images, the lesion is surrounded by a dark rim.

Histologic Features

Like stress fractures, avulsion injuries are often accompanied by extensive reactive bone proliferation and, therefore, mistaken for malignant neoplasms. The distal femoral cortical erosion syndrome may be particularly problematic because it occurs in the same age group and most common location of osteosarcoma. Although awareness of the distal femoral cortical erosion syndrome usually prevents overdiagnosis, these lesions are occasionally biopsied.

Histologically, the distal femoral cortical irregularity syndrome shows a wide range of reactive tissues. Some lesions are densely fibrous with bland fibroblasts in a highly collagenized matrix. Other lesions contain very cellular fibrous tissue (Fig. 26), and abundant osteoid. The osteoid seams are lined by typical osteoblasts. In addition, cartilage is occasionally present.

Although normal mitotic figures may be present in the fibrous tissue, cellular pleomorphism and atypical mitoses, necessary for the diagnosis of osteosarcoma, are not present in the distal femoral cortical irregularity syndrome.

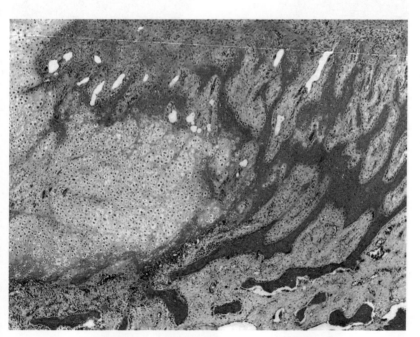

Fig. 24. Photomicrograph of a stress fracture. There is an irregular admixture of bone cartilage and fibrous tissue. This is fracture callous. This may be misdiagnosed, however, as a bone-forming neoplasm pattern (hematoxylin-eosin, original magnification ×100).

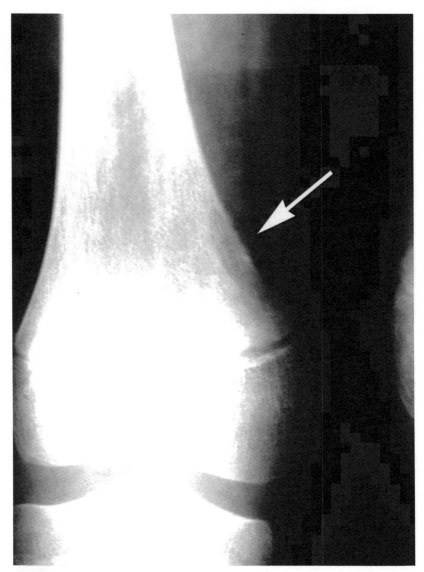

Fig. 25. The distal femoral cortical irregularity syndrome involving the medial aspect of the distal femur. There is a zone of irregular radiolucency in the metaphysis (*arrow*).

FLORID REACTIVE BONE RESORPTION

Rapidly destructive hip arthrosis[52] and idiopathic pubic osteolysis[53] are two reactive bone diseases characterized by rapid dissolution of bone. This process may mimic a neoplasm or infection. Both lesions have similar clinical, radiologic, and pathologic features.

Both rapidly destructive hip arthrosis and pubic osteolysis tend to occur in older patients, usually women. Patients frequently have osteoporosis. Often, the process begins with an insufficiency fracture, although this early change frequently goes unnoticed. In the hip, this insufficiency fracture appears on plain radiographs as a subchondral radiolucency beneath the articular surface of the femoral head. This change mimics the subchondral crescent seen in primary osteonecrosis of the hip, and this has led to the misinterpretation that rapidly destructive hip arthrosis is a primary bone infarction.

Clinically the insufficiency fracture leads to a self-propagating cascade of bone resorption, which can rapidly destroy the entire femoral head (**Fig. 27**) or, in the pubis, broad segments of the pubic or ischial ramus (**Fig. 28**). This process

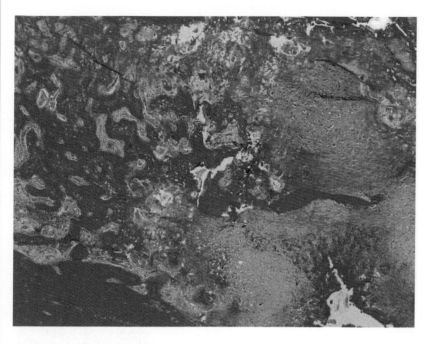

Fig. 26. Photomicrograph of the distal femoral cortical irregularity syndrome showing an admixture of bone, fibrous tissue and cartilage. Like a stress fracture, this histologic pattern may be misdiagnosed as a bone-forming tumor pattern (hematoxylin-eosin, original magnification ×100).

may occur so rapidly that a normal looking femoral head or pubic ramus may be completely destroyed.

RADIOGRAPHIC APPEARANCE

Both lesions show extensive osteolysis. The osteolysis is associated with extensive bone fragments in the adjacent soft tissues. Frequently this appears as a periosteal mass that is filled with fragments of both cartilage and bone.

PATHOLOGIC FEATURES

Pathologically there is extensive detritic bone in the periosteal soft tissues in the joint space

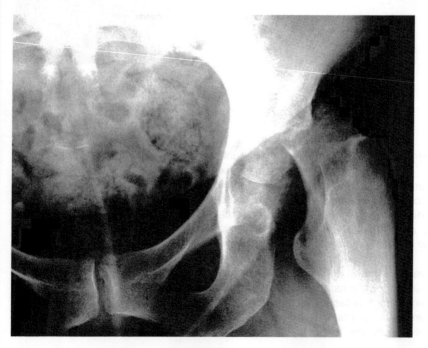

Fig. 27. The plain radiograph of rapidly progressive hip arthrosis. The entire femoral head has been dissolved.

Fig. 28. A plain radiograph of idiopathic pubic osteolysis. The pubic ramus has been completely destroyed. This irregular bone destruction, like that in the femoral head, may be radiographically misdiagnosed as a malignant tumor or an infection.

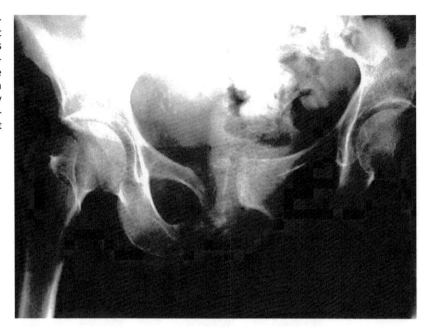

(**Fig. 29**). The detritic bone fragments are necrotic. This is secondary necrosis and does not reflect a primary osteonecrotic lesion. In the hip, there is fragmentation of the subchondral bone and fragments of detritic cartilage are extensively implanted in the joint capsule (**Fig. 30**). There is abundant fibrin and granulation tissue.

DIFFERENTIAL DIAGNOSIS

Rapidly destructive hip arthrosis is often misdiagnosed initially as an infection. All cultures, however, are negative and a purulent exudate is not present. Lesions in the hip are occasionally felt to be a manifestation of Charcot arthropathy. Patients, however, are not the typical patients

Fig. 29. Photomicrograph of the soft tissues adjacent to the femoral in rapidly progressive hip arthrosis. There is extensive detritic bone and cartilage in the periarticular soft tissues pattern (hematoxylin-eosin, original magnification ×200).

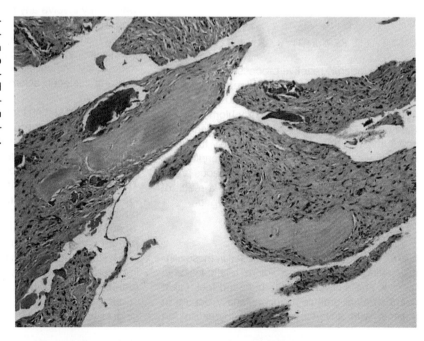

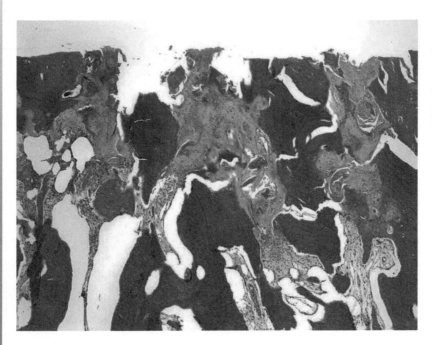

Fig. 30. Photomicrograph of the superficial area of the femoral head. There is extensive fragmentation of the bone. This bone will be shed into the joint space pattern (hematoxylin-eosin, original magnification ×100).

who have Charcot joints, and there is no evidence of somatic denervation. Both lesions may be felt clinically and radiographically to be neoplasms. Even malignant neoplasms, however, rarely grow at such as a rate as the bone destruction seen in these processes.

Awareness of rapidly destructive hip arthrosis and idiopathic pubic osteolysis may prevent the clinical and radiographic misdiagnosis of infection or neoplasm, and unnecessary biopsy procedures may be avoided.

GIANT CELL REPARATIVE GRANULOMA

Unlike radiodense reactive processes on the bone surface or in soft tissue, giant cell reparative granuloma, an intraosseous lesion, causes radiolucency. Giant cell reparative granuloma shares many histologic features with conventional giant cell tumor of bone. Unlike giant cell tumor of bone, however, giant cell reparative granuloma is not a neoplasm. It is a reactive intraosseous proliferation of connective tissue, probably a result of prior incidents of excessive bone resorption.

CLINICAL FEATURES

Giant cell reparative granuloma arises in these clinical settings: hyperparathyroidism, a lytic lesion in the jaw, and a lesion in the hands and feet. Giant cell reparative granuloma occasionally occurs in patients with advanced hyperparathyroidism. In

this setting, the giant cell reparative granuloma is known as a brown tumor due to lesional hemosiderin deposition. Multiple lesions are typical, and the femur and tibia are the most common sites. Because advanced primary hyperparathyroidism is rare nowadays, brown tumors are usually only seen in secondary hyperparathyroidism due to chronic renal failure.

Giant cell reparative granuloma associated with hyperparathyroidism is a well-defined lytic lesion, which may involve any portion of the bone. In the long bones, usually the metaphysis or diaphysis is involved. Multiple lesions are often present. Initially, lesions lack a sclerotic rim. After parathyroidectomy, however, lesions show perilesional and intralesional sclerosis, a manifestation of healing.

The second setting for giant cell reparative granulomas is a lytic lesion in jaw or face in the absence of hyperparathyroidism. Giant cell reparative granuloma in this setting most commonly (two-thirds of cases) affects the anterior portion of the mandible. The maxilla, maxillary sinus, and sphenoid sinus are other sites of involvement.[54] Although patients range in age from 7 to 67 years, most are between 10 and 20 years.[55] The characteristic radiographic pattern is a lytic expansile (Fig. 31). The cause of this lesion is unknown, although trauma has been implicated in some cases. Giant cell reparative granuloma of the jaw is usually cured by simple curettage. Occasionally, this lesion occurs in the gingiva without involving the underlying bone. A

Fig. 31. A CT scan of a giant cell reparative granuloma of the mandible. The lesion is a well-circumscribed radiolytic process.

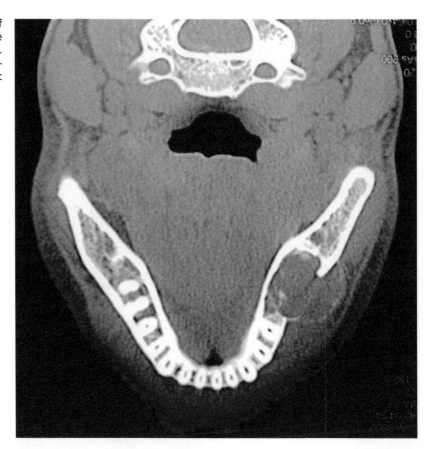

lesion in this setting is called a peripheral giant cell epulis.

A curious syndrome of multiple giant cell reparative granulomas affecting the mandible in children is known as cherubism. In this autosomal dominant disorder, the multiple jaw lesions cause a puffy swelling of the lower face, a feature characteristic of the faces of cherubs in Renaissance paintings. The lesions are symmetric and begin to appear at approximately age 2. They grow until the patients are in their early teens and then begin to regress.[56]

The third setting for giant cell reparative granuloma is in the bones of the hands and feet, also in the absence of hyperparathyroidism. In this setting, there is occasionally a history of trauma, but patients usually have no prior medical problems.[57–59]

Giant cell reparative granuloma of the hands and feet is a lytic lesion, which usually affects the metaphysis or diaphysis (**Fig. 32**). The tubular bones of the hands and feet are more commonly involved than the carpal or tarsal bones. These lesions may appear aggressive and occasionally destroy one cortex.

PATHOLOGIC FEATURES

The histologic features of giant cell reparative granuloma are identical in all clinical settings. Stromal cells are admixed with osteoclast-like giant cells. The most important histologic feature of the lesion is a zonal pattern. The clusters of giant cells aggregate around red blood cells (**Fig. 33**). The giant cells are surrounded by a zone of reactive fibrosis, which, in turn, is bounded by reactive bone (**Fig. 34**). This pattern repeats itself numerous times in any low-power field. Giant cell reparative granuloma may also undergo focal aneurysmal bone cyst change. Lesions with focal aneurysmal bone cyst have been called the *solid variant of aneurysmal bone cyst*.

DIFFERENTIAL DIAGNOSIS

Giant cell reparative granuloma presents an important problem of differential diagnosis—it is

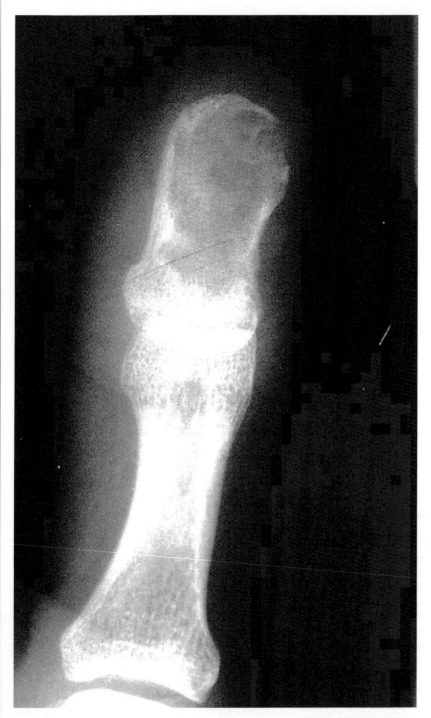

Fig. 32. A giant cell reparative granuloma of the distal phalanx. There is extensive lysis in the central portion of the phalanx.

often confused with giant cell tumor of bone. It is imperative to distinguish these lesions because giant cell tumor of bone is an aggressive neoplasm whereas giant cell reparative granuloma is an indolent process, often cured by simple curettage.

These 2 lesions may be distinguished by clinicoradiographic and histologic means. Although giant cell tumor may rarely be multicentric, multiple giant cell lesions are more likely to be brown tumors of hyperparathyroidism. Serum calcium and parathormone levels should be checked.

Fig. 33. Photomicrograph of a giant cell reparative granuloma. Giant cells tend to cluster around extravasated red blood cells pattern (hematoxylin-eosin, original magnification ×200).

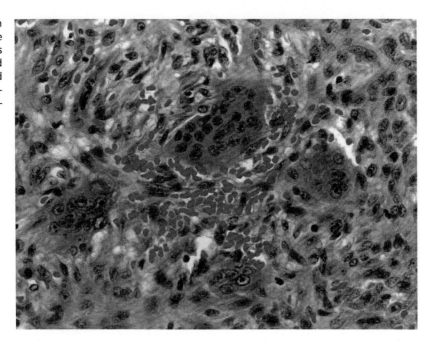

Differences in location also aid in distinguishing these lesions. For example, giant cell tumor rarely occurs in the jaw; lesions in this location are probably reparative granulomas. In the long bones, giant cell tumor is centered in the epiphysis and extends into the metaphysis; patients are skeletally mature. By contrast, giant cell reparative granuloma is usually metaphyseal or diaphyseal; patients may be skeletally immature.

Fig. 34. Low-power photomicrograph of a giant cell reparative granuloma showing the zonal pattern of giant cells and fibroblasts of reactive bone in a repeating pattern (hematoxylin-eosin, original magnification ×60).

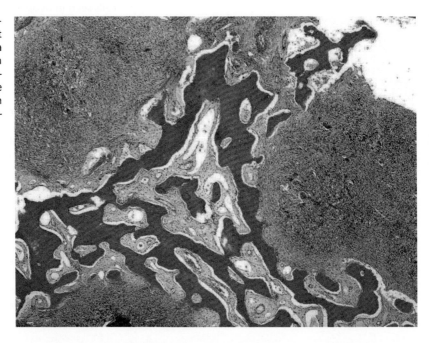

Differential Diagnosis
PSEUDOTUMORS AND REACTIVE LESIONS

Disease	Common Misdiagnosis	Characteristic Features
Myositis ossificans—early	Soft tissue osteosarcoma	Pleomorphic atypical cells with atypical mitotic figures absent in myositis ossificans
Myositis ossificans—late	Parosteal osteosarcoma	Cellular atypia not present in myositis ossificans; zonal pattern of ossification and mature trabecular bone present in myositis ossificans
Tumoral calcinosis	Bone or cartilage producing neoplasms	*Tumoral calcinosis lacks* • Cartilage's stippled and ring-like calcification • Bone's trabecular pattern *Tumoral calcinosis radiodensities* • Separated by bands of lucency imparting a cobblestone appearance. • Fluid-calcium levels within the radiodensities often present on CT scans or plain radiographs
Giant cell reparative granuloma (GCRG)	Giant cell tumor (GCT)	A zonal GCRG distinguish it from GCT
Bone injury	Infections or neoplasms	Bone injury diagnosed by clinical history of pain associated with activity *Stress fracture biopsy shows* • Fracture callus • Irregular seams of osteoid or woven bone in granulation tissue or loose fibrovascular stroma • Islands of cartilage undergoing endochondral ossification • Marked cellularity and abundant osteoid Stress fracture does not reveal pleomorphic cells seen in neoplasm

Pitfalls
PSEUDOTUMORS AND REACTIVE LESIONS

! Pseudotumors may masquerade as bone-forming neoplasms.

! Intraosseous radiolytic processes may be confused radiologically with malignant neoplasms.

! Some stress fractures are misdiagnosed as infections or neoplasms and are biopsied unnecessarily.

! Rapidly destructive hip arthrosis is often misdiagnosed initially as an infection.

Histologic differences are also present. Although both lesions contain giant cells and stromal cells, giant cell tumor lacks the zonal pattern characteristic of giant cell reparative granuloma.

REFERENCES

1. Bostrom K, Watson KE, Horn S, et al. Bone morphogenetic protein expression in human atherosclerotic lesions. J Clin Invest 1993;91(4):1800–9.
2. Wilson J, Montague CJ, Salcuni P, et al. Heterotopic mesenteric ossification ('intraabdominal myositis ossificans'): report of five cases. Am J Surg Pathol 1993;23(12):1464–70.

3. Kaplan FS, Glaser DL, Hebela N, et al. Heterotopic ossification. J Am Acad Orthop Surg 2004;12(2):116–25.

4. Kaplan FS. Skin and bones. Arch Dermatol 1996; 132(7):815–8.

5. Shore EM, Glaser DL, Gannon FH. Osteogenic induction in hereditary disorders of heterotopic ossification. Clin Orthop 2000;(374):303–16.

6. Cohen RB, Hahn GV, Tabas JA, et al. The natural history of heterotopic ossification in patients who have fibrodysplasia ossificans progressiva. A study of forty-four patients. J Bone Joint Surg Am 1993; 75(2):215–9.

7. Campbell RK. Myositis ossificans progressiva. Radiol Rev 1933;55:153.

8. Smith R, Russell RG, Woods CG. Myositis ossificans progressiva. Clinical features of eight patients and their response to treatment. J Bone Joint Surg Br 1976;58(1):48–57.

9. Gannon FH, Kaplan FS, Olmsted E, et al. Bone morphogenetic protein 2/4 in early fibromatous lesions of fibrodysplasia ossificans progressiva. Hum Pathol 1997;28:339–43.

10. Kaplan FS, Tabas JA, Gannon FH, et al. The histopathology of fibrodysplasia ossificans progressiva. An endochondral process. J Bone Joint Surg Am 1993; 75(2):220–30.

11. Heifetz SA, Galliani CA, DeRosa GP. Myositis (fasciitis) ossificans in an infant. Pediatr Pathol 1992;12: 223–9.

12. DeSmet AA, Norris MA, Fisher DR. Magnetic resonance imaging of myositis ossificans: analysis of seven cases. Skeletal Radiol 1992;21:503–7.

13. Cvitanic O, Sedlak J. Acute myositis ossificans. Skeletal Radiol 1995;24:139–41.

14. Ogilvie-Harris DJ, Fornasier VL. Pseudomalignant myositis ossificans: heterotopic new-bone formation without a history of trauma. J Bone Joint Surg Am 1980;62(8):1274–83.

15. Lagier R, Cox JN. Pseudomalignant myositis ossificans. A pathological study of eight cases. Hum Pathol 1975;6(6):653–65.

16. Damanski M. Heterotopic ossification in paraplegia. J Bone Joint Surg Br 1961;43(2):286–99.

17. Garland DE. A clinical perspective on common forms of acquired heterotopic ossification. Clin Orthop 1991;263:13–29.

18. Milgram J. In: Gruhn J, editor. Radiologic and histologic pathology of nontumorous diseases of bones and joints. 1st edition. Northbrook (IL): Northbrook Publishing Co; 1990. p. 454. Chapter. 23.

19. Riegler HF, Harris CM. Heterotopic bone formation after total hip arthroplasty. Clin Orthop 1976;117:209–16.

20. Thomas BJ. Heterotopic bone formation after total hip arthroplasty. Orthop Clin North Am 1992;23: 347–58.

21. Brooker AF, Bowerman JW, Robinson RA, et al. Ectopic ossification following total hip replacement. Incidence and method of classification. J Bone Joint Surg Am 1973;55:1629–32.

22. Kjaersgaard-Andersen P, Ritter MA. Prevention of formation of heterotopic bone after total hip arthroplasty. J Bone Joint Surg Am 1991;73:942–7.

23. Nuovo MA, Norman A, Chumas J, et al. Myositis ossificans with atypical clinical, radiographic, or pathologic findings: a review of 23 cases. Skeletal Radiol 1992;21:87–101.

24. Johnson MK, Lawrence JF. Metaplastic bone formation (myositis ossificans) in the soft tissues of the hand. J Bone Joint Surg Am 1975;57(7):999–1000.

25. Yuen M, Friedman L, Orr W, et al. Proliferative periosteal processes of phalanges: a unitary hypothesis. Skeletal Radiol 1992;21:301–3.

26. Wissinger HA, McClain EJ, Boyes JH. Turret exostosis. Ossifying hematoma of the phalanges. J Bone Joint Surg Am 1966;48(1):105–10.

27. Meneses MF, Unni KK, Swee RG. Bizarre parosteal osteochondromatous proliferation of bone (Nora's lesion). Am J Surg Pathol 1993;17(7):691–7.

28. Spjut HJ, Dorfman HD. Florid reactive periostitis of the tubular bones of the hands and feet. A benign lesion which may simulate osteosarcoma. Am J Surg Pathol 1981;5(5):423–33.

29. Landon GC, Johnson KA, Dahlin DC. Subungual exostoses. J Bone Joint Surg Am 1979;61(2):256–9.

30. Slavin RE, Wen J, Kumar D, et al. Familial tumoral calcinosis. A clinical, histopathologic, and ultrastructural study with an analysis of its calcifying process and pathogenesis. Am J Surg Pathol 1993;17(8):788–802.

31. McGregor DH, Mowry M, Cherian R, et al. Nonfamilial tumoral calcinosis associated with chronic renal failure and secondary hyperparathyroidism: report of two cases with clinicopathological, immunohistochemical, and electron microscopic findings. Hum Pathol 1995;26(6):607–13.

32. Holt PD, Keats TE. Calcific tendinitis: a review of the usual and unusual. Skeletal Radiol 1993;22:1–9.

33. Steinbach LS, Johnston JO, Tepper EF, et al. Tumoral calcinosis: radiologic - pathologic correlation. Skeletal Radiol 1995;24:573–8.

34. Gregosiewicz A, Warda E. Tumoral calcinosis: successful medical treatment. A case report. J Bone Joint Surg Am 1989;71:1244,–1249.

35. Ishida T, Dorfman HD, Bullough PG. Tophaceous pseudogout (tumoral calcium pyrophosphate dihydrate crystal deposition disease). Hum Pathol 1995;6:587–93.

36. Sissons HA, Steiner GC, Bonar F, et al. Tumoral calcium pyrophosphate deposition disease. Skeletal Radiol 1989;18:79–87.

37. McBryde AM Jr. Stress fractures in athletes. J Sports Med 1975;3(5):212–7.

38. Resnick D, Goergen TG, Niwayama G. Physical injury: concepts and terminology. diagnosis of

bone and joint disorders. 3rd edition. Philadelphia: W.B. Saunders Co; 1995. p. 2561–692.

39. Sweet DE, Allman RM. RPC of the month from the AFIP. Radiology 1971;99(3):687–93.

40. Johnson LC. Morphologic analysis in pathology. In: Frost HH, editor. Bone biodynamics. henry ford hospital international symposium. Boston: Little, Brown and Co; 1964. p. 607.

41. Burr DB, Milgrom C, Boyd RD, et al. Experimental stress fractures of the tibia. Biological and mechanical aetiology in rabbits. J Bone Joint Surg Br 1990; 72(3):370–5.

42. Mori S, Burr DB. Increased intracortical remodeling following fatigue damage. Bone 1993;14(2):103–9.

43. Barnes GR, Gwinn JL. Distal irregularities of the femur simulating malignancy. Am J Roentgenol Radium Ther Nucl Med 1974;122(1):180–5.

44. Brower AC, Culver JE, Keats TE. Histological nature of the cortical irregularity of the medial posterior distal femoral metaphysis in children. Radiology 1971;99(2):389–92.

45. Bufkin WJ. The avulsive cortical irregularity. Am J Roentgenol Radium Ther Nucl Med 1971;112(3):487–92.

46. Dunham WK, Marcus NW, Enneking WF, et al. Developmental defects of the distal femoral metaphysis. J Bone Joint Surg Am 1980;62(5):801–6.

47. Johnson LC, Genner BA, Engh CA, et al. Cortical desmoids. J Bone Joint Surg Am 1968;50(4): 828–9.

48. Kimmelstiel P, Rapp I. Cortical defect due to periosteal desmoids. Bull Hosp Joint Dis 1951;12(2):286–97.

49. Kreis WR, Hensinger RN. Irregularity of the distal femoral metaphysis simulating malignancy: case report. J Bone Joint Surg Am 1977;59(6):38.

50. Sontag LW, Pyle SI. The appearance and nature of cyst-like areas in the distal femoral metaphyses of children. Am J Roentgenol 1941;46(2):185–8.

51. Resnick D, Greenway G. Distal femoral cortical defects, irregularities, and excavations. Radiology 1982;143(2):345–54.

52. Batra S, Batra M, McMurtie A, et al. Rapidly destructive osteoarthritis of the hip joint: a case series. J Orthop Surg Res 2008;3:3.

53. McCarthy B, Dorfman HD. Pubic osteolysis. A benign lesion of the pelvis closely mimicking a malignant neoplasm. Clin Orthop Relat Res 1990;(251): 300–7.

54. Rogers LF, Mikhael M, Christ M, et al. Case report 276. Giant cell (reparative) granuloma of the sphenoid bone. Skeletal Radiol 1984;12:48–53.

55. Waldron CA, Shafer WG. The central giant cell reparative granuloma of the jaws. An analysis of 38 cases. Am J Clin Pathol 1966;45(4):437–47.

56. Jones WA. Cherubism. A thumbnail sketch of its diagnosis and a conservative method of treatment. Oral Surg Oral Med Oral Pathol 1965;20: 648–53.

57. Lorenzo JC, Dorfman HD. Giant-cell reparative granuloma of short tubular bones of the hands and feet. Am J Surg Pathol 1980;4(6):551–63.

58. Picci P, Baldini N, Sudanese A, et al. Giant cell reparative granuloma and other giant cell lesions of the bones of the hands and feet. Skeletal Radiol 1986;15:415–21.

59. Wold LE, Dobyns JH, Swee RG, et al. Giant cell reaction (giant cell reparative granuloma) of the small bones of the hands and feet. Am J Surg Pathol 1996;10(7):491–6.

SKELETAL METASTASIS

Andrea T. Deyrup, MD, PhD[a],[b],*

KEYWORDS

• Skeletal metastasis • Bone metastasis • Metastatic carcinoma • Bone tumor

ABSTRACT

The most commonly diagnosed tumor in the skeleton represents metastatic disease. Metastatic carcinoma should be the first consideration in older patients with atypical radiologic findings or clinical features suggestive of a bone lesion. The primary goal in the setting of skeletal metastasis is usually palliation.

OVERVIEW OF BONE METASTASIS

In view of the rarity of primary bone tumors and the much higher incidence of primary malignancies arising outside the skeleton (ie, carcinomas, melanomas, and soft tissue sarcomas), it is not surprising that the most commonly diagnosed tumor in the skeleton represents metastatic disease. Outside the pediatric population, metastatic carcinoma and melanoma are more frequently encountered than metastatic sarcomas. In children, in whom sarcomas are more common, metastatic soft tissue sarcomas as well as metastatic foci of osteosarcoma must be considered.

Bone may be secondarily involved by malignancy by direct extension, in which case the primary disease can be easily identified, or by vascular spread usually via Batson vertebral vein plexus. This valveless venous plexus is intimately involved with vertebral bodies, skull, pelvis, and proximal limb girdles and extends from the sacrum to the calvarium.[1] Active hematopoietic marrow (ie, red marrow) with its sinusoidal vascular architecture predominates in these flat bones and in the epiphyses of the long bones of the pelvic and shoulder girdle. These 2 factors, Batson vascular plexus and the distribution of red marrow, may account for the typical skeletal pattern of metastatic disease.

METASTATIC CARCINOMA

OVERVIEW

Metastatic carcinoma is the most common "bone tumor" and should be the first consideration in older patients with atypical radiologic findings or clinical features suggestive of a bone lesion, such as pathologic fracture. Among carcinomas, those of the breast, lung, prostate, thyroid, and kidney most frequently metastasize to bone.[2] The most common primary carcinomas in cases of metastatic carcinoma of unknown primary are those of the lung and kidney.[3] In the pediatric population, skeletal metastases of carcinoma are reported in the literature primarily as case reports.[4–7]

GROSS FEATURES OF METASTATIC CARCINOMA

Grossly, metastatic carcinoma may mimic a primary bone neoplasm and the gross appearance is rarely of diagnostic usefulness in this instance.

Key Points
METASTATIC CARCINOMA

1. For clinical management, it is critical to differentiate primary sarcoma of bone from metastatic carcinoma.

2. Kidney, lung, breast, thyroid, and prostate are the most common sites of primary disease in this clinical setting.

3. Imaging modalities have strengths and weaknesses and should be used in combination.

---

[a] Department of Orthopaedic Surgery, University of South Carolina School of Medicine - Greenville, Health Sciences Administration Buliding, 701 Grove Road, Greenville, SC 29605, USA
[b] Pathology Consultants of Greenville, 8 Memorial Medical Court, Greenville, SC 29605-4449, USA
* Pathology Consultants of Greenville, 8 Memorial Medical Court, Greenville, SC 29605-4449.
E-mail address: atdeyrup@yahoo.com

Surgical Pathology 5 (2012) 287–300
doi:10.1016/j.path.2012.01.001
1875-9181/12/$ – see front matter

RADIOLOGIC FEATURES OF METASTATIC CARCINOMA

Features that suggest metastatic disease include multifocality and the absence of a periosteal reaction. Solitary bone metastases, however, are not uncommon and multifocality is a characteristic feature of multiple myeloma.

Metastatic carcinoma shows the full spectrum of radiologic appearances: osteolytic, osteoblastic, and mixed osteolytic/osteoblastic. Although exceptions occur, carcinomas of the lung, kidney, thyroid, adrenal, gastrointestinal tract and uterus are usually osteolytic (**Fig. 1**) in contrast to those of prostate and bladder, which are typically osteoblastic (**Fig. 2**). A mixed pattern can be seen in carcinomas of breast, lung, ovary, testis and cervix.[8,9]

The particular bone involved and the site within the bone offer important information. Metastases to the distal extremities most often represent lung or breast carcinoma. The small tubular bones of the hands and feet are rarely involved by metastatic carcinoma and are even less commonly the first manifestation of malignancy.[10,11] Metastasis to the hands is significantly more common than to the feet[11] and there is a predilection for the dominant hand.[10] Carcinomas of the lung, kidney, and gastrointestinal tract are the most frequently described acrometastases.[10] Libson and colleagues[11] noted an increased proportion of subdiaphragmatic

malignancies (eg, colorectal, renal, and uterine) to the feet and have suggested that this may be secondary to venous tumor emboli.

IMAGING MODALITIES FOR PATHOLOGIC FRACTURE

Evaluation of plain radiographs is a useful starting point and is usually the first study done in the setting of a pathologic fracture. This modality lacks sensitivity in recognizing metastatic disease, however, because a significant amount of bone loss can occur before there is a roentgenographic manifestation. In contrast, CT scans can detect metastatic disease within the bone marrow before bony destruction has occurred. Although this modality is not well suited for whole-body screening, evaluation of the skeleton in staging studies may reveal clinically occult metastatic disease.

Radioisotope bone scan with technetium Tc 99 m is more sensitive than plain radiographs in identifying metastatic disease but is limited by decreased specificity (**Fig. 3**). Tracer accumulates in areas with brisk turnover of bone and requires adequate vascular perfusion for uptake; imaging may be limited due to the absence of reactive bone (purely lytic lesions) or lesions confined to marrow or in aggressive tumors with compromised blood flow. Moreover, falsely negative

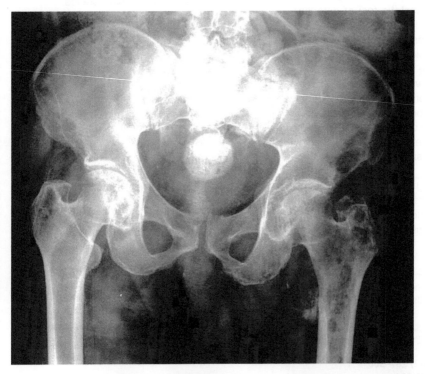

Fig. 1. Plain radiograph of the pelvis showing numerous purely radiolucent metastases in the proximal femur as well as an avulsion of the lesser trochanter.

Fig. 2. Plain radiograph of the pelvis showing numerous osteoblastic metastases (from a breast primary) throughout both femurs and the pelvis.

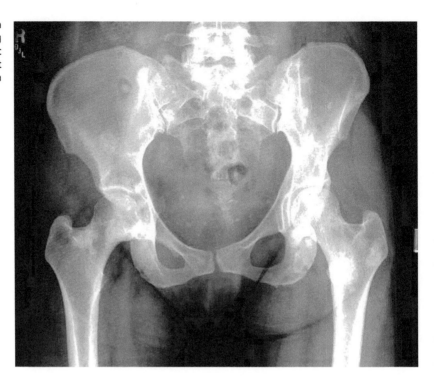

bone scans in a variety of metastatic carcinomas, including thyroid, prostate, lung, and breast, have been documented.[12–14] Furthermore, areas of previous or recent trauma and infection can yield a false-positive result. An additional limitation of this modality is that radionuclide bone scan does not help characterize the lesion as blastic, lytic, or mixed.

Fludeoxyglucose F 18–positron emission tomography (FDG-PET) is another modality related to tumor activity because it measures glucolysis and is, therefore, best suited for evaluation of highly metabolic malignancies. Like scintigraphy, FDG-PET evaluates the entire skeleton but also can assess soft tissue and organs. In addition, FDG-PET provides greater spatial resolution and anatomic localization. An important caveat is that FDG-PET is less sensitive in osteoblastic lesions and is most useful in identifying osteolytic metastases, such as thyroid carcinoma.[13]

Fig. 3. A bone scan demonstrating marked uptake of radioisotope in widely metastatic carcinoma lesions involving the lower extremities.

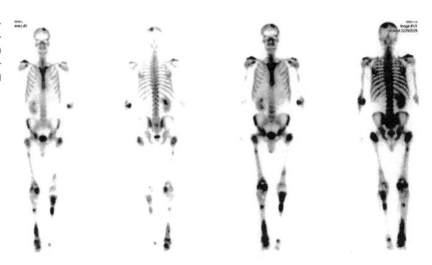

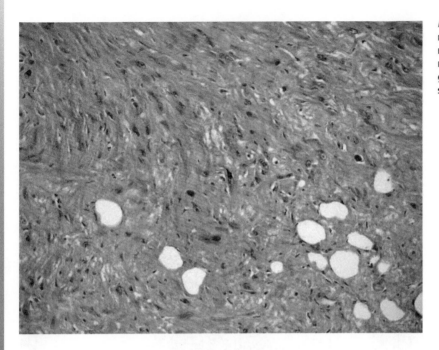

Fig. 4. Metastatic sarcomatoid carcinoma of thyroid origin. Such lesions may be difficult to distinguish from primary bone sarcomas.

MRI is an extremely sensitive modality for evaluating metastatic disease and, like CT, can detect metastasis to bone marrow before bony destruction occurs. T1-weighted images show areas of low signal that can be distinguished from background red bone marrow by the more diffuse signal of the latter. Although MRI offers the possibility of more accurately characterizing a soft tissue component, its sensitivity is also its greatest drawback because previous surgical site changes, areas of antecedent trauma, and treatment effect cannot always be readily distinguished from neoplasia. Moreover, it is impractical to use MRI as a modality for whole-body

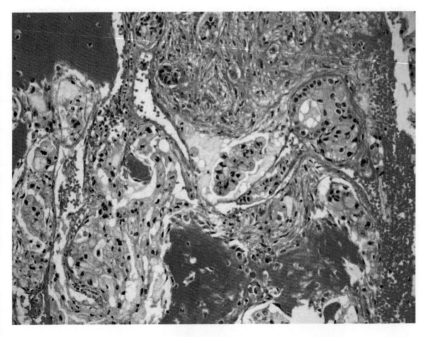

Fig. 5. A typical metastatic adenocarcinoma involving bone.

screening. A retrospective study comparing more limited MRI "marrow" screens and scintigraphic analysis suggested that, although MRI was more sensitive, no significant changes in patient management would have resulted.[15]

MICROSCOPIC FEATURES OF METASTATIC CARCINOMA

Metastatic carcinomas show a wide range of morphologic features, including spindled cells more suggestive of a sarcoma (**Fig. 4**) and lesions with distinct glandular formation (**Fig. 5**), which is essentially pathognomonic for metastatic carcinoma (although adamantinoma may enter the differential diagnosis). Patterns of bone involvement may be diffuse and extensive (eg, carcinomas of breast and prostate) or focal with a nested growth pattern (eg, lung).[2] When malignant cells are not obvious, marrow fibrosis is a clue to metastatic disease.

A panel of immunohistochemical stains should be used, even in the setting of a known primary malignancy. A recent study has shown that antigenicity is maintained in bone marrow biopsies of skeletal metastases.[2] An initial immunohistochemical panel should include cytokeratins 7 and 20; thyroid transcription factor 1; prostate-specific antigen and prostate-specific acid phosphatase (in men); and mammaglobin, estrogen receptor, and gross cystic disease fluid protein (in women).[16] Synaptophysin expression is more prominent in metastatic carcinoma of breast and prostate than in the primary lesions.[2]

With current decalcification solutions and immunohistochemical protocols, only minimal artifact is seen in most bone biopsies.[17,18] Extensive decalcification of cortical bone, however, may have a slight impact on tissue morphology and antigen reactivity; therefore, if possible, a portion of tissue with a minimal bone component should be submitted separately to reduce the risk of false-negative results.

DIAGNOSIS AND DIFFERENTIAL DIAGNOSIS OF METASTATIC CARCINOMA

For clinical management, the most important entity to exclude is a primary sarcoma of bone. Osteosarcoma is readily diagnosed when osteoid formation is prominent; however, reactive bone in the setting of metastatic carcinoma may confound interpretation. Other factors may impede diagnosis in older patients:

1. Osteoid formation may be focal.
2. Like carcinomas, osteosarcomas may range from spindled to epithelioid in appearance.
3. Pancytokeratin may be focally positive in osteosarcoma.

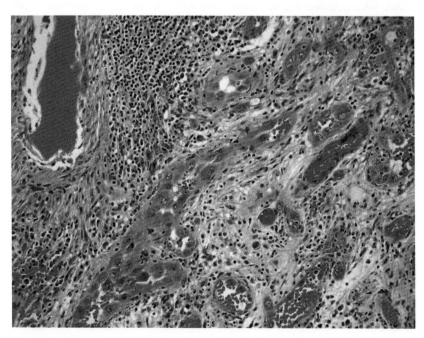

Fig. 6. An epithelioid hemangioma of bone, characterized by well-formed vessels lined by large, tombstone-like endothelial cells accompanied by a background inflammatory infiltrate rich in eosinophils.

Because metastatic carcinoma is exceptional in the pediatric and young adult population, osteosarcoma should be meticulously excluded.[2]

Malignant fibrous histiocytoma of bone is typically a diagnosis of exclusion and, like osteosarcoma, can show a wide range of morphologic appearances. These tumors may show focal staining with epithelial markers but strong, diffuse expression is more indicative of a metastatic carcinoma.

The epithelioid vascular neoplasms (epithelioid hemangioma, epithelioid hemangioendothelioma, and epithelioid angiosarcoma) share with metastatic carcinoma the histologic feature of abundant cytoplasm and can show expression of epithelial antigens, suggesting the possibility of metastatic carcinoma (Fig. 6).[19–22] Furthermore, vascular neoplasms may be multifocal, simulating metastatic disease.[23] Immunohistochemical assessment is essential for cases where the

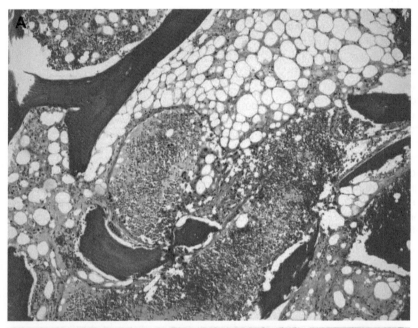
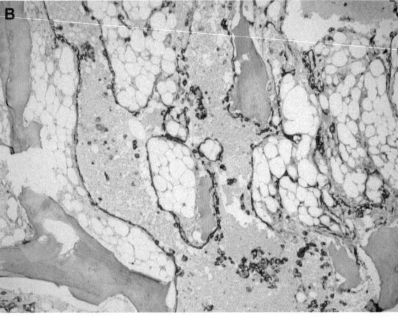

Fig. 7. (A) Well-differentiated angiosarcoma of bone. Well-formed vascular channels are lined by plump endothelial cells. (B) The vascular nature of the tumor is confirmed by the strong immunoreactivity for CD31.

vasoformative nature of neoplasm is not evident. Vascular markers, such as CD34, CD31, and Fli-1, should be used as a panel (Fig. 7). Factor VIII is also used in some laboratories.

Classic adamantinoma is characterized by a biphasic appearance with glands admixed with spindle cells. The presence of glands raises the possibility of metastatic carcinoma. Unlike metastatic carcinoma, however, which is typically centered in the medullary canal, adamantinoma is primarily a cortical lesion (Fig. 8). Furthermore, the clinical setting of adamantinoma, including tibial (rarely fibular) location and younger patients, helps exclude this possibility.

Although plasmacytomas usually present no significant diagnostic challenge, multifocality and anaplastic variants may raise the possibility of metastatic carcinoma (Fig. 9). Furthermore, some plasmacytomas (as well as a variety of other hematological neoplasms) are positive for cytokeratin and EMA.[24] A diagnosis of plasmacytoma can be confirmed by immunohistochemical stains for CD138 and by laboratory studies. Imaging studies that show multifocal lesions with negative radionuclide bone scan are suggestive of multiple myeloma, which is often falsely negative by bone scan.

Melanoma displays a wide range of morphologic appearances and skeletal involvement may be the first manifestation of clinically occult disease. Metastatic melanoma is discussed later in greater detail.

PROGNOSIS OF METASTATIC CARCINOMA

Metastatic disease to the skeleton is high stage by definition. In cases of isolated bone metastases, surgical resection may be warranted; however, the primary goal in the setting of skeletal metastasis is usually palliation.

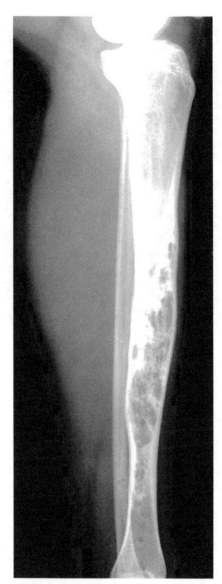

Fig. 8. Plain radiograph of an adamantinoma of the tibia. Adamantinomas typically arise in the anterior cortex of the tibia or fibula.

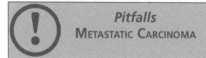

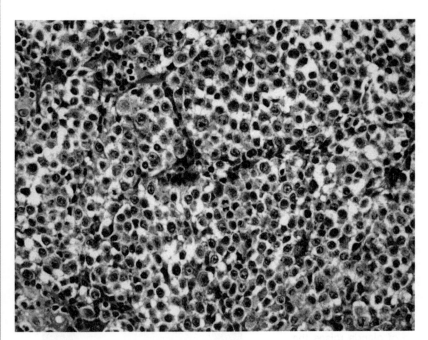

Fig. 9. Anaplastic, or plasmablastic, plasmacytoma, characterized by sheets of large cells containing minimal cytoplasm and a prominent nucleolus.

METASTATIC MELANOMA

OVERVIEW

Melanoma is a rare malignancy (approximately 1%–3% of cancers). As imaging technology has advanced, the ability to recognize melanoma metastatic to bone has increased: although a study from 1978 identified skeletal metastases in 7% of cases using roentgenogram and/or bone scan,[25] a study of known melanoma patients using CT scans limited to the abdomen, pelvis, chest, and neck found skeletal metastases in 17% of cases.[26] Whole-body MRI demonstrated the greatest incidence in patients who had not died of disease: 32%.[27] In a subset of patients who died of their disease and were subsequently autopsied, the incidence ranged from 23% to 49%.[28,29]

> ### *Key Points*
> #### METASTATIC MELANOMA
>
> 1. Metastatic melanoma typically metastasizes to the axial skeleton, especially the ribs and vertebral bodies.
>
> 2. Even in the absence of known melanoma, this entity should be excluded due to the possibility of occult/unknown primary melanoma.

RADIOLOGIC FEATURES OF METASTATIC MELANOMA

Metastatic melanoma typically involves the axial skeleton (incidence 70%–80%) as opposed to the appendicular skeleton and is most common in the ribs and vertebral column.[25,30] The radiologic appearance is usually of an ostelytic lesion that is eccentric and that has a minimal periosteal reaction.[25,30] Pathologic fracture is often the clinical presentation. Metastatic disease commonly affects the diaphysis or metaphysis.[30]

Bone scan may be negative, despite radiologic evidence of metastatic disease.[30] On MRI, melanoma shows increased T1 signal intensity, which may be attributed to melanin pigment.[31] A soft tissue component may be present, a potential pitfall in excluding primary sarcomas of bone.[29]

A comparison of whole-body MRI and whole-body CT showed the former modality to be more sensitive in identifying skeletal metastases and showed the greatest incidence of skeletal metastases except for autopsy studies.[27]

GROSS PATHOLOGY OF METASTATIC MELANOMA

Heavily pigmented metastatic melanoma is perhaps the best example of a correlation between gross appearance and diagnosis. In cases of amelanosis, however, metastatic melanoma has no specific distinguishing features.

MICROSCOPIC FEATURES OF METASTATIC MELANOMA

Melanoma is known as "the great imitator" and this holds true in skeletal metastases. Even in the absence of a history of melanoma or evidence of melanin pigment on microscopic examination, an immunohistochemical panel that includes S-100 protein, HMB-45 and Melan-A should be performed, because there are reports of skeletal metastases from unknown/occult primary (**Fig. 10**).[32,33]

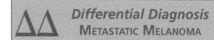

Differential Diagnosis
METASTATIC MELANOMA

- Both epithelial and mesenchymal neoplasms should be considered.

- An immunohistochemical panel should be performed.

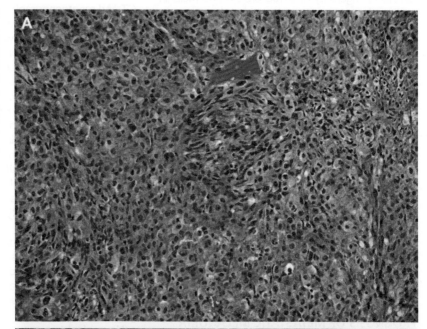
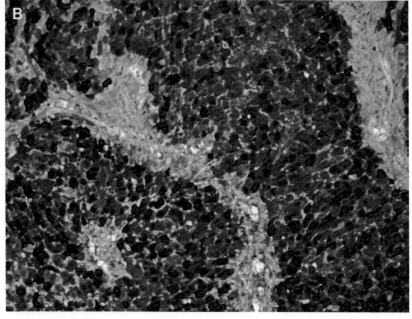

Fig. 10. (*A*) Metastatic melanoma in the scapula, characterized by vague nests of spindled and epithelioid cells, many of which contain prominent nucleoli. (*B*) The diagnosis of metastatic melanoma can be confirmed with immunostains for S-100 protein (shown here), HMB-45, and Melan-A.

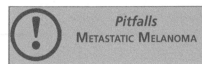

Decalcifying agents seem not to significantly diminish antigenicity of S-100 protein and melanin markers.[17,34] Although metastatic melanoma may express pancytokeratin, expression of CAM 5.2 is usually not seen.[35,36]

DIAGNOSIS AND DIFFERENTIAL DIAGNOSIS OF METASTATIC MELANOMA

Metastatic melanoma can show morphologic and immunhistochemical overlap with metastatic carcinoma. Metastatic carcinomas do not express melanocytic markers or S-100 protein; however, cytokeratin expression in metstatic melanoma is well characterized.[37]

Primary perivascular epithelioid cell tumor of bone is a rare entity that shares expression of melanocytic markers with metastatic melanoma.[34,38] Cytologic atypia, however, is minimal in these tumors. Expression of smooth muscle actin antigens is also helpful in excluding metastatic melanoma.

PROGNOSIS OF METASTATIC MELANOMA

Prognosis is poor in melanoma patients with skeletal metastases. Mean survival time after diagnosis of skeletal metastasis ranges from 3.5 to 8 months with appendicular metastases typically showing the longest survival.[30,39,40]

METASTATIC SARCOMA

OVERVIEW

The most common site of soft tissue sarcoma metastasis is the lung; secondary skeletal involvement, usually to regional bones, occurs only rarely and usually after a longer interval than lung metastases.[41–43] The most commonly encountered entities include myxoid liposarcoma, rhabdomyosarcoma, alveolar soft part sarcoma, dedifferentiated liposarcoma, angiosarcoma, and rhabdomyosarcoma.[41,42,44,45] Cases of chondrosarcoma, cardiac sarcoma, synovial sarcoma, and osteosarcoma have also been reported.[43,46,47]

The most common metastases to bone in children are neuroblastoma, rhabdomyosarcoma, and Ewing sarcoma.[2,48] In addition, clear cell sarcoma of kidney (formerly known as bone metastasizing renal tumor of childhood), has a tendency to metastasize to bone.[49] Rare cases of acrometastases of osteosarcoma have been described and should be considered in younger patients with acral malignancies.[10]

RADIOLOGIC FEATURES OF METASTATIC SARCOMA

CT and roentgenographic evaluation of metastatic sarcoma usually shows osteolysis, with the exception of osteosarcoma, which may be blastic. As with metastatic carcinoma, a periosteal reaction is usually absent. These tumors frequently present with pathologic fracture.

MRI and scintigraphic evaluation of children is complicated by the high cellularity of their hematopoietic marrow, which may obscure marrow metastases and osteoblastic activity of the epiphyseal plates.[50] Although FDG-PET demonstrates great sensitivity in identifying bone metastases in children and young adults, this modality is limited by a higher percentage of false-positive results. Moreover, a small study of FDG-PET in skeletal metastases of primary bone sarcomas showed metastatic osteosarcoma to be frequently falsely negative.[51] FDG-PET is clearly superior to bone scintigraphy, however, perhaps due to late osteoblastic reactivity to marrow metastatic disease and the brisk metabolic activity of these high-grade tumors.[51,52]

Neuroblastoma may metastasize to the skull, pelvis, ribs, and metaphysis of long bones. The lesions are lytic or appear as irregular areas of lucency. Sclerosis may be seen in instances of tumor infarction and there is often a periosteal

Key Points
METASTATIC SARCOMA

1. For clinical management, it is critical to differentiate primary sarcoma of bone from metastatic sarcoma.

2. Myxoid liposarcoma, alveolar rhabdomyosarcoma, and dedifferentiated liposarcoma are the sarcomas that metastasize most frequently to bone.

3. Imaging modalities have strengths and weaknesses and should be used in combination.

reaction. Identification of skeletal metastases in these patients should be based on MRI and/or scintigraphy because CT scan is less sensitive.[53]

In the case of liposarcomas, in particular myxoid liposarcoma, bone scans and PET scan are often negative, despite the presence of metastatic disease.[44,45] Whole-spine MRI scanning has been suggested, at least in as an initial staging modality, in this cohort of patients.[54]

GROSS FEATURES OF METASTATIC SARCOMA

Gross appearance is not particularly useful in predicting if the lesion is primary or secondary. The hemorrhagic appearance of angiosarcoma and the cartilaginous nodules of metastatic chondrosarcoma can be seen in telangiectatic osteosarcoma and chondroblastic osteosarcoma/primary chondrosarcoma, respectively.

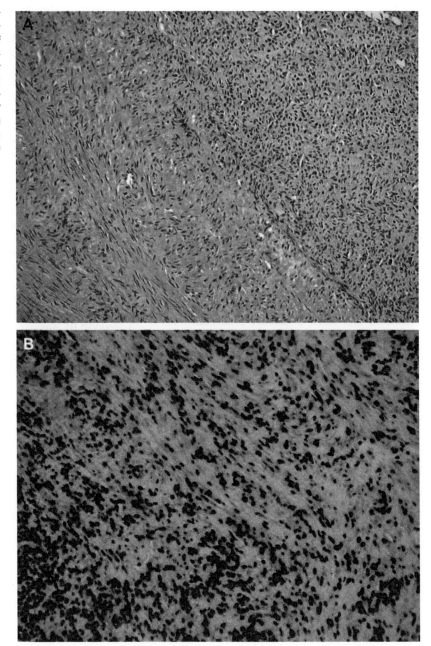

Fig. 11. (*A*) Epstein-Barr virus smooth muscle tumor composed of fascicles of spindled cells sharply separated from a more cellular nodule with round cell features. (*B*) In situ hybridization for Epstein-Barr early mRNAs, supporting the diagnosis of an Epstein-Barr virus smooth muscle tumor.

MICROSCOPIC FEATURES OF METASTATIC SARCOMA

As with carcinomas, the microscopic appearance correlates with the line of differentiation of the primary sarcoma. Immunohistochemical analysis is critical for confirming the line of differentiation and, depending on the tumor morphology, skeletal markers (desmin, myogenin, MyoD1, and smooth muscle actin), translocation-specific markers (TFE3 and carboxy-terminus of WT1), and neural markers (S-100 protein) should be considered.

DIFFERENTIAL DIAGNOSIS OF METASTATIC SARCOMA

Of the primary sarcomas of bone that must be excluded, osteosarcoma has the highest incidence. Other primary sarcomas of bone are rare and include fibrosarcoma/malignant fibrous histiocytoma of bone, angiosarcoma, leiomyosarcoma, and liposarcoma. Other sarcomas that typically present in soft tissue have been documented in isolated case reports.[55,56]

Leiomyosarcoma of bone is well described and typically involves the long tubular bones of the lower extremity. Craniofacial location has been associated with previous radiation therapy.[57–59] These are rare tumors, however, and careful exclusion of a metastatic source is critical, particularly in female patients.

Epstein-Barr virus–associated smooth muscle tumors are rare tumors that arise in the setting of immunosuppression. These tumors are often multifocal and have a distinct predilection for bone and may, therefore, raise the possibility of metastatic leiomyosarcoma (Fig. 11A).[60] Unlike metastatic leiomyosarcoma, however, Epstein-Barr virus–associated smooth muscle tumors are not clinically aggressive and rarely are a direct cause of death. Clinical history and in situ

Pitfalls
METASTATIC SARCOMA

! Multifocal skeletal smooth muscle tumors may represent Epstein-Barr virus–associated smooth muscle tumors and not metastatic leiomyosarcoma.

! Imaging evaluation of the pediatric population is complicated by a variety of factors that may result in higher rates of false-positive and false-negative results.

hybridization assays for Epstein-Barr early mRNAs (see Fig. 11B) are helpful in arriving at the correct diagnosis.

Even less common are tumors that are considered benign (eg, leiomyoma, giant cell tumor of bone, and pleomorhic adenoma) that metastasize to bone, even in cases without evidence of histologic progression to an aggressive lesion.[61–63] These instances are primarily of academic interest.

Differential Diagnosis
METASTATIC SARCOMA

• Metastatic osteosarcoma may mimic a primary osteosarcoma.

• If a diagnosis of leiomyosarcoma is under consideration, metastasis from the gynecologic tract should be excluded in women.

• In the setting of multifocal smooth muscle tumors, Epstein-Barr virus–associated smooth muscle tumor should be ruled out.

REFERENCES

1. Batson OV. The Function of the vertebral veins and their role in the spread of metastases. Ann Surg 1940;112:138–49.
2. Krishnan C, George TI, Arber DA. Bone marrow metastases: a survey of nonhematologic metastases with immunohistochemical study of metastatic carcinomas. Appl Immunohistochem Mol Morphol 2007; 15:1–7.
3. Rougraff BT, Kneisl JS, Simon MA. Skeletal metastases of unknown origin. A prospective study of a diagnostic strategy. J Bone Joint Surg Am 1993; 75:1276–81.
4. Asanuma H, Nakai H, Takeda M, et al. Renal cell carcinoma in children: experience at a single institution in Japan. J Urol 1999;162:1402–5.
5. Kutluk MT, Yalcin B, Buyukpamukcu N, et al. Fibrolamellar hepatocellular carcinoma with skeletal metastases. Pediatr Hematol Oncol 2001;18:273–8.
6. Lucarini S, Fortier M, Leaker M, et al. Hepatocellular carcinoma bone metastasis in an 11-year-old boy. Pediatr Radiol 2008;38:111–4.
7. McDermott M, Gamis AS, el-Mofty S, et al. Adenocarcinoma of minor salivary gland origin with skeletal metastasis in a child. Pediatr Pathol Lab Med 1996; 16:89–98.
8. Rosenthal DI. Radiologic diagnosis of bone metastases. Cancer 1997;80:1595–607.
9. Rouleau P, Wenger D. Radiologic evaluation of metastatic bone disease. Rosemont (IL): American Academy of Orthopaedic Surgeons; 2002. p. 313–22.

10. Healey JH, Turnbull AD, Miedema B, et al. Acrometastases. A study of twenty-nine patients with osseous involvement of the hands and feet. J Bone Joint Surg Am 1986;68:743–6.

11. Libson E, Bloom RA, Husband JE, et al. Metastatic tumours of bones of the hand and foot. A comparative review and report of 43 additional cases. Skeletal Radiol 1987;16:387–92.

12. Gosfield E 3rd, Alavi A, Kneeland B. Comparison of radionuclide bone scans and magnetic resonance imaging in detecting spinal metastases. J Nucl Med 1993;34:2191–8.

13. Ito S, Kato K, Ikeda M, et al. Comparison of 18F-FDG PET and bone scintigraphy in detection of bone metastases of thyroid cancer. J Nucl Med 2007;48: 889–95.

14. Munk PL, Poon PY, O'Connell JX, et al. Osteoblastic metastases from breast carcinoma with false-negative bone scan. Skeletal Radiol 1997;26: 434–7.

15. Traill ZC, Talbot D, Golding S, et al. Magnetic resonance imaging versus radionuclide scintigraphy in screening for bone metastases. Clin Radiol 1999; 54:448–51.

16. Rubin BP, Skarin AT, Pisick E, et al. Use of cytokeratins 7 and 20 in determining the origin of metastatic carcinoma of unknown primary, with special emphasis on lung cancer. Eur J Cancer Prev 2001; 10:77–82.

17. Athanasou NA, Quinn J, Heryet A, et al. Effect of decalcification agents on immunoreactivity of cellular antigens. J Clin Pathol 1987;40:874–8.

18. Bussolati G, Leonardo E. Technical pitfalls potentially affecting diagnoses in immunohistochemistry. J Clin Pathol 2008;61:1184–92.

19. Deshpande V, Rosenberg AE, O'Connell JX, et al. Epithelioid angiosarcoma of the bone: a series of 10 cases. Am J Surg Pathol 2003;27:709–16.

20. Hasegawa T, Fujii Y, Seki K, et al. Epithelioid angiosarcoma of bone. Hum Pathol 1997;28:985–9.

21. O'Connell JX, Kattapuram SV, Mankin HJ, et al. Epithelioid hemangioma of bone. A tumor often mistaken for low-grade angiosarcoma or malignant hemangioendothelioma. Am J Surg Pathol 1993;17: 610–7.

22. Santeusanio G, Bombonati A, Tarantino U, et al. Multifocal epithelioid angiosarcoma of bone: a potential pitfall in the differential diagnosis with metastatic carcinoma. Appl Immunohistochem Mol Morphol 2003;11:359–63.

23. Wenger DE, Wold LE. Malignant vascular lesions of bone: radiologic and pathologic features. Skeletal Radiol 2000;29:619–31.

24. Adams H, Schmid P, Dirnhofer S, et al. Cytokeratin expression in hematological neoplasms: a tissue microarray study on 866 lymphoma and leukemia cases. Pathol Res Pract 2008;204:569–73.

25. Stewart WR, Gelberman RH, Harrelson JM, et al. Skeletal metastases of melanoma. J Bone Joint Surg Am 1978;60:645–9.

26. Patten RM, Shuman WP, Teefey S. Metastases from malignant melanoma to the axial skeleton: a CT study of frequency and appearance. AJR Am J Roentgenol 1990;155:109–12.

27. Muller-Horvat C, Radny P, Eigentler TK, et al. Prospective comparison of the impact on treatment decisions of whole-body magnetic resonance imaging and computed tomography in patients with metastatic malignant melanoma. Eur J Cancer 2006;42:342–50.

28. McNeer G, Dasgupta T. Life history of melanoma. Am J Roentgenol Radium Ther Nucl Med 1965;93: 686–94.

29. Selby HM, Sherman RS, Pack GT. A roentgen study of bone metastases from melanoma. Radiology 1956;67:224–8.

30. Fon GT, Wong WS, Gold RH, et al. Skeletal metastases of melanoma: radiographic, scintigraphic, and clinical review. AJR Am J Roentgenol 1981; 137:103–8.

31. Premkumar A, Marincola F, Taubenberger J, et al. Metastatic melanoma: correlation of MRI characteristics and histopathology. J Magn Reson Imaging 1996;6:190–4.

32. Giuliano AE, Moseley HS, Morton DL. Clinical aspects of unknown primary melanoma. Ann Surg 1980;191:98–104.

33. Jain D, Singh T, Kumar N, et al. Metastatic malignant melanoma in bone marrow with occult primary site– a case report with review of literature. Diagn Pathol 2007;2:38.

34. Torii I, Kondo N, Takuwa T, et al. Perivascular epithelioid cell tumor of the rib. Virchows Arch 2008;452: 697–702.

35. Banerjee SS, Harris M. Morphological and immunophenotypic variations in malignant melanoma. Histopathology 2000;36:387–402.

36. Leader M, Patel J, Makin C, et al. An analysis of the sensitivity and specificity of the cytokeratin marker CAM 5.2 for epithelial tumours. Results of a study of 203 sarcomas, 50 carcinomas and 28 malignant melanomas. Histopathology 1986;10:1315–24.

37. Zarbo RJ, Gown AM, Nagle RB, et al. Anomalous cytokeratin expression in malignant melanoma: one- and two-dimensional western blot analysis and immunohistochemical survey of 100 melanomas. Mod Pathol 1990;3:494–501.

38. Lian DW, Chuah KL, Cheng MH, et al. Malignant perivascular epithelioid cell tumour of the fibula: a report and a short review of bone perivascular epithelioid cell tumour. J Clin Pathol 2008;61: 1127–9.

39. DeBoer DK, Schwartz HS, Thelman S, et al. Heterogeneous survival rates for isolated skeletal metastases

from melanoma. Clin Orthop Relat Res 1996;(323): 277–83.

40. Steiner GM, MacDonald JS. Metastases to bone from malignant melanoma. Clin Radiol 1972;23:52–7.

41. Gustafson P. Soft tissue sarcoma. Epidemiology and prognosis in 508 patients. Acta Orthop Scand Suppl 1994;259:1–31.

42. Vezeridis MP, Moore R, Karakousis CP. Metastatic patterns in soft-tissue sarcomas. Arch Surg 1983; 118:915–8.

43. Yoshikawa H, Ueda T, Mori S, et al. Skeletal metastases from soft-tissue sarcomas. Incidence, patterns, and radiological features. J Bone Joint Surg Br 1997;79:548–52.

44. Schwab JH, Boland P, Guo T, et al. Skeletal metastases in myxoid liposarcoma: an unusual pattern of distant spread. Ann Surg Oncol 2007;14:1507–14.

45. Schwab JH, Boland PJ, Antonescu C, et al. Spinal metastases from myxoid liposarcoma warrant screening with magnetic resonance imaging. Cancer 2007;110:1815–22.

46. Disler DG, Rosenberg AE, Springfield D, et al. Extensive skeletal metastases from chondrosarcoma without pulmonary involvement. Skeletal Radiol 1993;22:595–9.

47. Strina C, Zannoni M, Parolin V, et al. Bone metastases from primary cardiac sarcoma: case report. Tumori 2009;95:251–3.

48. Leeson MC, Makley JT, Carter JR. Metastatic skeletal disease in the pediatric population. J Pediatr Orthop 1985;5:261–7.

49. Argani P, Perlman EJ, Breslow NE, et al. Clear cell sarcoma of the kidney: a review of 351 cases from the National Wilms Tumor Study Group Pathology Center. Am J Surg Pathol 2000;24:4–18.

50. Daldrup-Link HE, Franzius C, Link TM, et al. Whole-body MR imaging for detection of bone metastases in children and young adults: comparison with skeletal scintigraphy and FDG PET. AJR Am J Roentgenol 2001;177:229–36.

51. Franzius C, Sciuk J, Daldrup-Link HE, et al. FDG-PET for detection of osseous metastases from malignant primary bone tumours: comparison with bone scintigraphy. Eur J Nucl Med 2000;27: 1305–11.

52. Gyorke T, Zajic T, Lange A, et al. Impact of FDG PET for staging of Ewing sarcomas and primitive neuro-ectodermal tumours. Nucl Med Commun 2006;27: 17–24.

53. Siegel MJ, Ishwaran H, Fletcher BD, et al. Staging of neuroblastoma at imaging: report of the radiology diagnostic oncology group. Radiology 2002;223: 168–75.

54. Noble JL, Moskovic E, Fisher C, et al. Imaging of skeletal metastases in myxoid liposarcoma. Sarcoma 2010;2010:262361.

55. Gelczer RK, Wenger DE, Wold LE. Primary clear cell sarcoma of bone: a unique site of origin. Skeletal Radiol 1999;28:240–3.

56. Park YK, Unni KK, Kim YW, et al. Primary alveolar soft part sarcoma of bone. Histopathology 1999;35:411–7.

57. Antonescu CR, Erlandson RA, Huvos AG. Primary leiomyosarcoma of bone: a clinicopathologic, immunohistochemical, and ultrastructural study of 33 patients and a literature review. Am J Surg Pathol 1997;21:1281–94.

58. Shen SH, Steinbach LS, Wang SF, et al. Primary leiomyosarcoma of bone. Skeletal Radiol 2001;30: 600–3.

59. Sundaram M, Akduman I, White LM, et al. Primary leiomyosarcoma of bone. AJR Am J Roentgenol 1999;172:771–6.

60. Deyrup AT, Lee VK, Hill CE, et al. Epstein-Barr virus-associated smooth muscle tumors are distinctive mesenchymal tumors reflecting multiple infection events: a clinicopathologic and molecular analysis of 29 tumors from 19 patients. Am J Surg Pathol 2006;30:75–82.

61. Alessi G, Lemmerling M, Vereecken L, et al. Benign metastasizing leiomyoma to skull base and spine: a report of two cases. Clin Neurol Neurosurg 2003; 105:170–4.

62. Qureshi AA, Gitelis S, Templeton AA, et al. "Benign" metastasizing pleomorphic adenoma. A case report and review of literature. Clin Orthop Relat Res 1994;(308):192–8.

63. Takahashi T, Katano S, Ishikawa H, et al. Aggressive clinical course of giant cell tumor arising from thoracic vertebra after a long latent period. Radiat Med 2006;24:534–7.

TREATMENT OF BONE TUMORS

Rajiv Rajani, MD, C. Parker Gibbs, MD*

KEYWORDS

• Bone tumor • Ewing sarcoma • Osteosarcoma • Chondrosarcoma

ABSTRACT

This article summarizes the state of the art and future potential in the management of osteosarcoma, Ewing sarcoma, and chondrosarcoma. It covers systemic therapy, surgical therapy, and radiotherapy along with targeted therapies to inhibit signal transduction pathways. It discusses staging and the role of imaging evaluation to provide an overview of bone tumor treatment. Images presenting pathologic-radiologic correlations are included.

Malignant bone tumors are rare neoplasms that cause significant morbidity and mortality. Despite advances in both surgical and medical oncology, few significant positive changes in function or survival have occurred for patients with these diseases during the past 30 years.

OSTEOSARCOMA

OVERVIEW

Osteosarcoma is a highly malignant mesenchymal tumor of bone in which the malignant cells produce osteoid. It is the most common primary, nonhematologic bone malignancy in children, occurring most frequently in patients between the ages of 10 and 25.[1] Before the advent of multiagent chemotherapy, amputation provided a long-term survival rate of approximately 20%. The use of multiagent chemotherapy combined with aggressive surgery has improved long-term survival in these patients to approximately 60%.[2] Survival of patients treated with chemotherapy alone is only 20%,[3] suggesting that populations of tumor cells in a large percentage of osteosarcomas are highly resistant to chemotherapy. Despite intensive efforts in both surgical and medical management, the survival rate has not improved during the past 30 years and 40% of osteosarcoma patients die of their disease.

Osteosarcoma can arise in any bone but occurs primarily in the juxtaepiphyseal regions of rapidly growing long bones. The histopathologic appearance of high-grade intramedullary osteosarcoma is one of malignant spindle cells producing osteoid and immature bone (Fig. 1D, E). The bone structure is disorganized and can appear as a fine lacey trabecular pattern or as irregular clumps of osteoid, distinctly unlike normal bone formation. Classic osteosarcoma may also appear predominantly fibrous or chondroid with only small areas of osteoid formation.[1] Grossly, osteosarcoma begins as a process destructive of medullary bone that progresses to destroying cortical bone, often with a large associated soft tissue component (see Fig. 1A). The natural history of osteosarcoma is one of relentless local progression with loss of the function of the affected extremity and distant metastasis, most often to the lung.[2,4] A small percentage of patients develop bone metastases, which are almost always fatal.[5]

ETIOLOGY

Cytogenetic evaluation has revealed many complex chromosomal abnormalities that vary both within and between individual tumors in osteosarcoma. Different from other sarcomas, such as Ewing sarcoma, synovial sarcoma, and alveolar rhabdomyosarcoma, osteosarcoma has not been

The authors have no conflicts of interest.

The authors acknowledge support of a grant from the National Cancer Institute (NCI) in the formation of this article: RO1 CA 137186. PI: CP Gibbs.

Department of Orthopaedics and Rehabilitative Medicine, Division of Oncology, University of Florida, 3450 Hull Road, PO Box 112727, Gainesville, FL 32611, USA

* Corresponding author.

E-mail address: gibbscp@ortho.ufl.edu

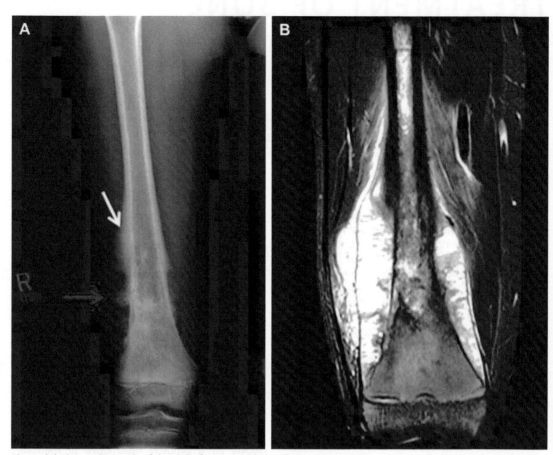

Fig. 1. (*A*) Plain radiograph of the right femur in a skeletally immature patient shows a destructive, bone-forming lesion that involves the entire metaphysis. Small white arrow designates a Codman triangle, periosteal new bone formed in response to tumor. This is contrasted to the less organized malignant bone denoted by the red arrow. (*B*) A coronal T2-weighted image shows a large soft tissue mass with new bone formation and periosteal elevation. Note the intramedullary and extramedullary tumor extension.

associated with a specific recurrent chromosomal rearrangement.[6] Molecular analyses have revealed a variety of genetic alterations in osteosarcoma, including inactivation of p53 and retinoblastoma tumor suppressor genes and overexpression of oncogenes, such as MDM2.[7] For example, alterations of the RB1 gene have been shown in up to 70% of reported cases, and loss of heterozygosity for RB1 has been shown a marker of poor prognosis. Patients with retinoblastoma develop osteosarcoma at a rate 500 times the general population.[8]

Osteosarcoma is the second most common malignancy associated with Li-Fraumeni syndrome, characterized by p53 mutations at chromosome 17p13 and the development of many and varied cancers.[9] Although this information has provided insight into aspects of the molecular dysregulation of osteosarcoma and its

heterogeneous nature, to date these types of studies have been of limited value in establishing the molecular determinants of tumorigenesis or in the development of effective therapies.[10] In recognition of this, recently some investigators have postulated a role for tumor initiating cells in the pathogenesis of osteosarcoma. The existence of these so-called cancer stem cells was first suggested by the observation that osteosarcoma cells grown in media developed to isolate neural stem cells expressed primitive transcription factors normally restricted to embryonic stem cells.[11] Wu and colleagues[12] noted that sarcoma cells isolated based on the ability to exclude Hoechst dye (side population) seemed to exhibit increased tumorigenic potential relative to those cells that could not. Most recently, Levings and colleagues[13] demonstrated the ability to prospectively identify a highly tumorigenic subpopulation of cells within

Fig. 1. (*C*) Axial T1-weighted images, used for surgical planning, show the nearby superficial femoral artery, vein, and sciatic nerve. Periosteal new bone is appreciated in a circumferential pattern around the femoral shaft as designated by the arrow. (*D*) A low-power photomicrograph shows a highly cellular lesion with osteoid formation. (*E*) Higher power reveals densely staining chromatin and significant nuclear pleomorphism.

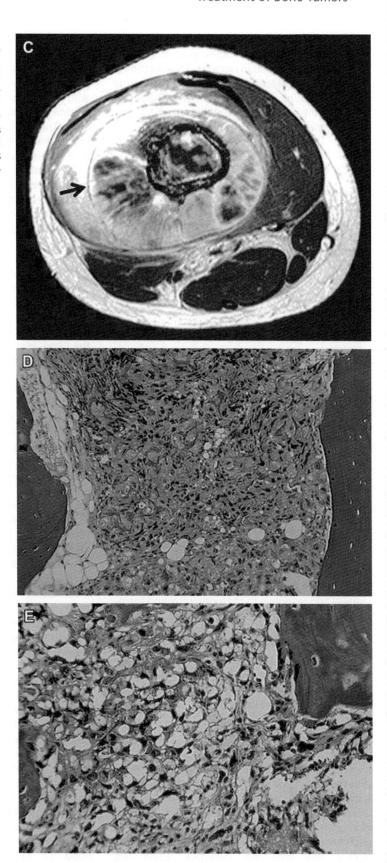

an individual osteosarcoma by its ability to transcriptionally activate an Oct-4 promoter–driven green fluorescent protein reporter. Their data suggested that the osteosarcoma-initiating cell might be regulated at an epigenetic level. Together, these recent reports offer further insight into the origin of this aggressive malignancy.

IMAGING

Appropriate local and distant imaging continues to be critical for the accurate staging of osteosarcoma patients. The diagnosis is most often strongly suggested by plain radiography. Radiographs of the entire bone are obtained and classically demonstrate a metaphyseal lesion destructive of both cortical and medullary bone with an ossified extraosseous soft tissue mass (see Fig. 1A). More than 50% of osteosarcomas occur about the knee. Although plain radiographs are almost diagnostic, MRI is the gold standard for determining the anatomic extent of the tumor and preoperative planning. An MRI of the entire involved bone is used to determine the intraosseous and the extraosseous extent of the tumor. MRI reveals the proximity of vital neurovascular structures as well as the presence of skip metastases and intraarticular involvement (see Fig. 1B, C). Technetium bone scans are used to detect both skip and distant bone metastases.[14] CT scans are used for determining the presence of pulmonary metastases and less so for the assessment of the primary tumor. The vast majority of metastases from osteosarcoma occur to the lungs.

Positron emission tomography (PET) is currently being evaluated as an imaging modality in osteosarcoma. The potential advantage of PET scanning is that it may be able to demonstrate tumor viability and response to chemotherapy and therefore help guide therapy. One study has reported that high standardized uptake values either before or after chemotherapy portend a worse prognosis.[15] Although the role of PET scans in the staging of osteosarcomas in unknown at present, as more data are collected, the benefit of PET scans may become elucidated.

SURGICAL MANAGEMENT

In most cases of osteosarcoma, the treatment protocol includes surgical resection of the primary tumor and any bony metastasis. The surgical margin, reconstruction, and adjuvant therapy plan are further delineated by the subtype of osteosarcoma. These include juxtacortical, intramedullary, and periosteal subtypes. Each has

a different local recurrence, metastatic, and survival rate.

High-grade intramedullary osteosarcoma is the prototypical bone sarcoma. It usually presents with not only cancellous and cortical bone destruction but also significant soft tissue extension. Therapy normally consists of neoadjuvant chemotherapy followed by wide surgical resection and subsequent adjuvant chemotherapy. The resulting skeletal defect is most commonly managed by reconstruction with modular metallic prostheses, allogeneic bone grafts, or a combination of both. Parosteal osteosarcoma is typically a low-grade lesion that occurs on the posterior aspect of the distal femur, although it can occur on the cortical surface of any bone. The mainstay of treatment is wide surgical excision. Chemotherapy can be used in patients with dedifferentiated high-grade lesions. Radiographically, it appears as a lobular ossified mass with well-marginated borders pasted onto the surface of the bone. Histologically, it has the appearance of a well-differentiated spindle cell sarcoma with minimal atypia. This tumor typically arises from the periosteum and survival rates are greater than 80% at 5 years.[16]

Low-grade intramedullary osteosarcoma accounts for approximately 1% to 2% of osteosarcomas and also is generally a low-grade lesion. It occurs in the metaphysis and diaphysis of long bones. Radiographically, it appears as an intramedullary lesion with variable density and poorly defined margins. It may be radiodense, lucent, or mixed. Often it is mistaken for a benign lesion. Histologically, it is similar to parosteal osteosarcoma in that it is low grade and predominantly fibrous. Overall, the cellularity is low and can be confused with fibrous dysplasia. Management of most lesions is surgical with wide excision and reconstruction, depending on the location and extent of the lesion. Chemotherapy is not commonly used. Schwab and colleagues[17] reviewed 59 patients with these two diseases and showed that the rates of local recurrence, dedifferentiation, distant metastases, and survival were the same. Although the physical location of these lesions is different (endosteal vs parosteal), the investigators thought they represented similar entities and should be treated similarly.

Periosteal osteosarcoma often presents as another surface variant of osteosarcoma with erosion of the cortex usually apparent on plain radiographs. Histologically, these tumors are largely chondroblastic with some areas of osteoid formation. There is a high level of variability with most lesions low grade but with a greater likelihood of high-grade lesions than parosteal osteosarcomas. Treatment still consists of wide surgical resection with chemotherapy reserved for high-grade and metastatic lesions.

SYSTEMIC THERAPY

The most dramatic improvement in survival for osteosarcoma occurred in the late 1970s and early 1980s with the development of multiagent chemotherapy. Before the use of chemotherapy, amputation alone provided only a 20% chance of survival. Some early benefit was seen with single-agent doxorubicin. This early success was improved with the addition of methotrexate and reported survivals of up to 60%.[18,19] As limb salvage surgery became more common with effective chemotherapeutic agents, the drugs were given most often in a neoadjuvant manner. This provided the theoretic benefits of killing microscopic metastatic disease and facilitating surgical resection by decreasing the tumor in the reactive zone about the primary tumor. In reality, however, the practice was started to provide surgeons the 6 to 8 weeks required to fabricate custom prostheses for these patients. Today, in the age of modular readily available prostheses, most surgeons and oncologists still prefer neoadjuvant therapy although no survival data exist supporting its use over that in the adjuvant setting.

Current chemotherapy regimens include doxorubicin, high-dose methotrexate, cisplatin, and sometimes ifosfamide. This multidrug approach yields survival rates of approximately 70% in those patients with no evidence of metastasis at diagnosis.[20] Those patients presenting with metastases, however, enjoy only a 20% survival rate. It has been shown that those patients who exhibit greater than 90% necrosis of their primary tumor on resection after neoadjuvant therapy have a significant survival advantage.[21] Although this suggests changing agents in those patients who responded poorly to induction therapy, no studies to date have demonstrated this to be of benefit. To study this further, the European and American Osteosarcoma Study Group 1 in a collaborative effort with the Children's Oncology Group has an ongoing multinational study to determine the effectiveness of adding ifosfamide and etoposide after resection in poor responders.

NEW DIRECTIONS

Agents that inhibit signal transduction pathways are among the few promising therapeutics being developed in sarcoma. The most studied in osteosarcoma are those that inhibit mammalian target of rapamycin (mTOR). mTOR, a member of the phosphatidylinositol 3 (PI3) kinase family, is a serine/threonine kinase that phosphorylates various downstream targets that have an impact on cellular proliferation and mRNA translation among other functions. It is a critical component of the cell cycle progression from G1 to S phase. Altered mTOR signaling has been demonstrated in various malignancies and has been linked to a worse prognosis in osteosarcoma.[22] Direct inhibition of mTOR with rapamycin or its analogs has shown promise in vitro and in vivo. In one phase II trial, partial response or stability was demonstrated in 30% of patients treated with AP23573, an analog of rapamycin.[23]

Current data suggest that the benefit of the mTOR inhibitors will largely be disease stabilization and that inroads toward increased survival will require combination therapy.[24] Along these lines, their efficacy seems potentiated in vitro by the addition of zolendronate sodium, a commonly used bisphosphonate.[25]

Transmembrane tyrosine kinase inhibitors, such as imatinib, have been a popular and sometimes effective target for novel therapies in several malignancies.[26] Their surface location and effect on downstream signal transduction cascades make them particularly attractive when designing targeted therapies. The insulinlike growth factor (IGF) receptors have been extensively studied in osteosarcoma. IGF-1, IGF-2, and IGF-3 have all been found overexpressed in sarcomas.[27] One of the normal functions of IGF-1 is the regulation of longitudinal skeletal growth.[28] Thus, dysregulation of IGF-1 and its receptor might be involved in osteosarcomagenesis.[29] The IGF-1 receptor (IGF-1R) dimerically functions by binding IGF-1 and IGF-2 affecting intracellular signaling of PI3 kinase and mitogen-activated protein kinase (MAPK). The developments of monoclonal antibodies to IGF-1R have met with some preclinical success. In animal models with osteosarcoma xenografts, an antibody alone induced complete responses in two tumors.[30] Rapamycin in combination with a different anti–IGF-R antibody induced reduction of xenografts in 3 of 4 animals.[31] Clinical trials of monoclonal antibodies are ongoing. The development of small molecule inhibitors to IGF-R 1 has been limited by the toxicity of these agents.

Muramyl tripeptide phosphatidylethanolamine (MTP-PE) is a nonspecific immune modulator that is a synthetic analog of bacterial cell wall components. It is delivered encapsulated in liposomes, facilitating delivery to lung tissue where micrometastases exist. MTP-PE is believed to activate macrophages and monocytes against nearby tumor cells. MTP-PE has been shown to have a positive impact on survival when given in combination with standard chemotherapy in non-metastatic patients.[32] Although not as clear, its potential role in the treatment of patients who present with metastases is encouraging.[33]

CHONDROSARCOMA

OVERVIEW

Chondrosarcoma is a malignant mesenchymal tumor characterized by variously differentiated cells producing chondroid matrix. Unlike osteosarcoma and Ewing sarcoma, it is usually a malignancy of adulthood with most cases occurring in patients over age 40.[1] Primary chondrosarcomas are neoplasms that arise de novo from pre-existing normal bone. Secondary chondrosarcomas most often arise in the setting of an underlying pre-existing benign cartilaginous tumor, such as enchondromas, multiple enchondromatosis, and multiple hereditary exostoses. They can, however, also occur in conditions, such as Paget disease, fibrous dysplasia, irradiated bone, chondroblastoma, and, although extremely rare, unicameral bone cysts and synovial chondromatosis.

Anatomically, the majority of cases occur in the pelvis, hip girdle, and shoulder girdle. The anatomic depth of these lesions often leads to a late diagnosis, potentially leading to poorer prognoses.[34] Most frequently, the presenting symptom is pain referable directly to the site of the lesion. Often, a palpable mass can be appreciated as growing while causing an external pressure effect leading to pain. Neurovascular compromise is uncommon.

The histopathologic appearance of cartilaginous tumors exhibit a continuum from well-differentiated hyaline like hypocellular chondroid lesions with little or no mitotic activity to high-grade pleomorphic chondrosarcomas that may have little chondroid at all. The prevailing appearance, however, is one of malignant spindle cells producing chondroid matrix. Grade I chondrosarcomas have little to no cellular atypia with an abundance of hyaline cartilage (Fig. 2D, E). Encasement of trabecular bone by the cartilage matrix can help to differentiate benign from low-grade cartilage malignancy. Grade II chondrosarcomas have few mitoses and increased cellularity and may have mild cellular atypia. Grade III chondrosarcomas contain several mitotic figures and a myxoid cartilaginous matrix along with many atypical malignant spindle cells. The most highly malignant is dedifferentiated chondrosarcoma, characterized by the classic finding of low-grade or intermediate-grade cartilage tissue juxtaposed to a high-grade spindle cell neoplasm. Grossly, high-grade central chondrosarcomas usually demonstrate significant cortical destruction and a soft tissue mass. In secondary tumors, the pre-existing lesion, such as an osteochondroma or enchondroma, can often be appreciated.[35]

The natural progression of chondrosarcomas is generally slow, local growth with subsequent distant metastasis, most commonly to the lung. Five-year survival rates vary significantly based on size and histologic grade. Low-grade lesions have greater than 90% survival at 5 years whereas high-grade dedifferentiated chondrosarcomas have less than 20% survival in the same time frame.[1] Distant metastasis at diagnosis, as with all sarcomas, portends a worse prognosis.[36]

ETIOLOGY

Hedgehog signaling has been implicated in the development of benign and malignant cartilage lesions. Experiments blocking hedgehog signaling, in vitro and in vivo, have shown decreased growth of chondrosarcoma.[37] p53 and RB alterations seem more correlated with high-grade chondrosarcomas, with approximately 96% having involvement of one or the other.[38] In support of this, amplifications of 12q13 and loss of 9p21, both associated with p53 pathways, are seen consistently in chondrosarcoma.[39] Loss of INK4, which inhibits the cell cycle by causing arrest at G1, has also been associated with increasing histologic grade.[40] CDK4 has also been implicated as a driver of chondrosarcomagenesis, and its knockdown by short hairpin RNAs has resulted in decreased colony formation in culture.[38] Some investigators have suggested an epigenetic component to the pathogenesis of chondrosarcoma. This has been supported by the demonstration of differentiation induction by histone deacetylase inhibitors in vitro.[41,42] Further work looking at differences between benign cartilage and the progression of malignant cartilage from low grade to high grade may yield even more clues as to the origin of this group of tumors.

IMAGING

Plain radiographs in orthogonal planes are the initial radiologic study of choice. Primary chondrosarcomas appear as destructive lesions of bone often containing punctate calcification (see Fig. 2A). The zone between the tumor and normal bone is often ill defined. The radiographic hallmarks of a malignant cartilage tumor include endosteal scalloping, frank cortical destruction, periosteal new bone, cortical thickening, and often soft tissue extension. In the setting of a pre-existing

Fig. 2. (*A*) An anteroposterior radiograph of a skeletally mature patient shows a large soft tissue mass in the right hemipelvis with punctate calcifications characteristic of cartilage (*arrow*). (*B*) Axial CT scan image shows the anterior and posterior extent of the tumor extension into surrounding soft tissue. Punctate or stippled calcifications are readily apparent as indicated by white arrow.

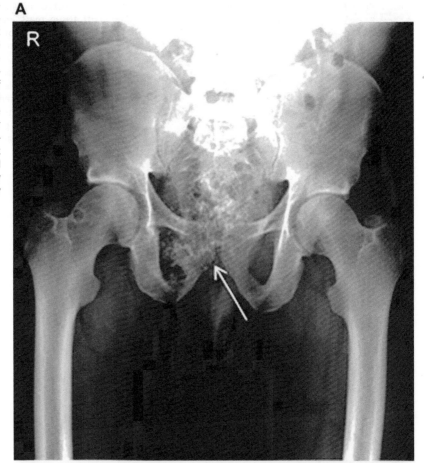

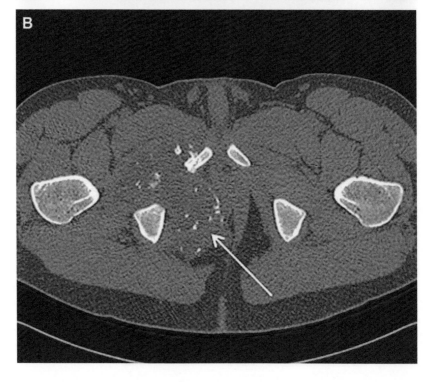

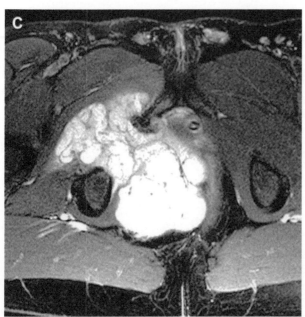

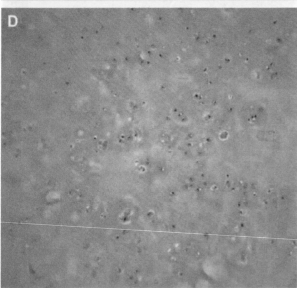

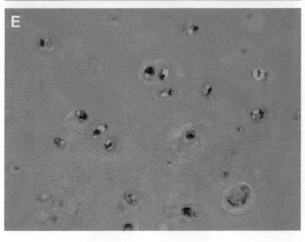

Fig. 2. (*C*) Axial T2-weighted MRI shows a large soft tissue mass arising from the bone that extends into the soft tissues. Proximity to neurovascular structures is demonstrated. Bright signal is indicative of high water content. (*D*) Low-powered photomicrograph shows low cellularity and nuclear atypia. Abundant chondroid matrix is seen on hematoxylin-eosin staining. (*E*) Higher power shows minimal cellular atypia and pleomorphism, most consistent with a low-grade chondrosarcoma.

enchondroma, new areas of radiolucency may become apparent.[43]

MRI and CT have been shown to have greater sensitivity when differentiating chondrosarcomas from enchondromas.[44] Soft tissue and intramedullary extent can be measured for planned surgical resection (see **Fig.** 2C). In lesions arising from osteochondromas, the thickness of the cartilaginous cap can be measured as a determinant of malignancy.

CT also can be used to distinguish between benign and malignant lesions. Specifically, CT is recommended in the pelvis and other flat bones to distinguish the pattern of bone destruction, extent of mineralization, and cartilage thickness (see **Fig.** 2B). CT is also used during staging to evaluate for the presence of pulmonary metastases.

The role of PET scanning in chondrosarcoma is evolving. Small case series have demonstrated some usefulness of PET in differentiating benign from malignant cartilaginous lesions when correlated with pathology.[45] Other investigators have suggested that PET can be used to predict histologic grade and outcomes in patients with chondrosarcoma.[46] The accuracy of histopathology in determining the malignancy of low-grade cartilage lesions, however, is not high; therefore, using it as a standard may not be appropriate.

RADIATION THERAPY

Radiotherapy traditionally has not been useful for local or distant control of chondrosarcoma. It is resistant to radiation and chemotherapy because of its low oxygen tension, low vascularity, and low rate of cell division.[47] Dosages of greater than 70 Gy are required and even at this dose, recurrence is common. Surrounding joints and neurovascular and viscus structures are at risk for adhesion, fibrosis, and necrosis. Proton beam therapy has been found beneficial in the setting of incompletely resected tumors around the skull base and spine and has been used with reasonable outcomes in unresectable tumors.[48]

SYSTEMIC THERAPY

Similar to radiotherapy, chemotherapy is generally not effective in chondrosarcomas. In addition to prolonged doubling time and limited vascularity, it has been suggested that the multidrug resistance 1 gene (MDR-1) P-glycoprotein may play a role in chemotherapy resistance.[49,50] For conventional chondrosarcoma, current recommendations do not include use of adjuvant or neoadjuvant chemotherapy.

In the specific setting of dedifferentiated chondrosarcomas containing a high-grade spindle cell component, some investigators have suggested efficacy for chemotherapeutic agents. Mitchell and colleagues[51] showed a small improvement in 22 patients but with median survival of only 9 months and only 18% alive at 5 years. Dickey and colleagues,[52] looking at 45 patients, showed poor results with median survival of 7.5 months and a 5-year survival of only 7.1%. Similarly, in a large multi-institutional European study of 337 patients, no benefit of chemotherapy could be demonstrated.[53] Better therapies need to be elucidated.

FUTURE STRATEGIES

Unlike osteosarcoma and Ewing sarcoma, currently there are no proved effective adjuvant therapies for chondrosarcoma, although early experimental results suggest possibilities. One such group of agents is those that inhibit heat shock protein 90 (HSP90). HSP90 is a chaperone that ensures proper folding of attendant proteins, such as the oncogenic proteins, BRAF, ERBB2, and CDK4.[54,55] Agents that inhibit HSP90 function then allow the depletion of the attendant oncoproteins and are thus attractive as anticancer drugs.[56]

Recent phase I work has shown stable disease in a few sarcomas, including a single chondrosarcoma, when patients were treated with the HSP90 inhibitor, 17-(dimethylaminoethylamino)-17-demethoxygeldanamycin (17-DMAG).[57] Oncostatin, a proapoptotic, cytostatic cytokine shown to have some efficacy against osteosarcoma cells has recently been evaluated in chondrosarcoma.[58] The investigators noted that oncostatin blocked cell cycle progression in 4 of 5 human cell lines examined and demonstrated induced differentiation as measured by an increased Cbfa1/SOX9 ratio and induced expression of collagen 10, matrix metalloproteinase 13, and RANKL (receptor activator of nuclear factor kB ligand). They proposed that the effect is mediated by the JAK/STAT signaling pathway. Because of severe inflammatory side effects when given systemically, the investigators noted that the delivery of oncostatin would likely have to be injected directly into a patient's tumor, perhaps limiting its usefulness in the typically large tumors seen in human chondrosarcoma.

Perhaps one of the more promising agents is recombinant human apoptosis ligand 2/tumor necrosis factor–related apoptosis-inducing ligand (Apo2L/TRAIL). It is a proapoptotic member of the tumor necrosis factor cytokine family and activates the extrinsic apoptotic pathway by the death receptors DR4 and DR5. In a phase I dose escalation trial of Apo2L/TRAIL in 71 advanced cancer patients, 5 had chondrosarcoma and 2 of these demonstrated prolonged (>3 years) partial response to the continued administration of the agent.[59] Additionally, marked necrosis was observed at time of surgical resection in an additional 2. Although encouraging, it must be remembered that these strategies are in early stages of evaluation.

Although there are many agents reported that are effective against chondrosarcoma in culture, delivery of these to real tumors will always be a technical hurdle because of the low vascular penetration and abundant matrix encasing the malignant cells.

SURGICAL MANAGEMENT

Standard management of chondrosarcoma consists of wide surgical resection without the benefit of adjuvant radiation or chemotherapy. As with all bone sarcomas, skeletal reconstruction is usually necessary and is most often in the form of metallic endoprostheses, allografts, or alloprosthetic composites.[1] Recently, however, in cases of low-grade lesions, some support has arisen for curettage with the use of an adjuvant, such as phenol, cryosurgery, or argon laser. Mohler and colleagues[60] reviewed 46 patients who had intralesional curettage and cryotherapy for atypical enchondromas and low-grade chondrosarcomas and demonstrated a 4.3% local recurrence rate. The two recurrences underwent wide re-excision and were disease-free at 30 and 36 months, respectively.

The Istituto Rizzoli reviewed patients who had undergone intralesional curettage of low-grade chondrosarcomas and compared them with those who had wide resection. They found no recurrences in the resection group and 2 recurrences in 15 patients in the curretage group. The 2 recurrences were managed with re-excision and no patient developed distant disease. The functional score was higher in those patients undergoing curettage.[61] Although these studies are encouraging for using lesser surgery in low-grade chondrosarcoma, further study with larger patient cohorts are needed to determine the safety and efficacy of intralesional curettage. In the setting of secondary chondrosarcomas arising from osteochondromas, wide excision of the entire lesion is recommended, including the associated cartilaginous cap.

The local recurrence and metastasis rate for low-grade and intermediate-grade chondrosarcomas are extremely low if complete excision is achieved. Overall survival rates are still disappointingly low in high-grade tumors, with 50% long-term survival. Dedifferentiated chondrosarcomas

are worse, having 20% survival rates at 5 years.[62] As with most other sarcomas, it is apparent that novel breakthrough therapies are needed.

EWING SARCOMA

OVERVIEW

Ewing sarcoma is a small, round, blue cell malignancy that is the second most common primary bone malignancy in children and adolescents. It typically affects individuals in the first 3 decades of life. The long tubular bones are the most common location, with the femur (25%) the single most common followed by the tibia, fibula, pelvic girdle, and ribs.[1] Although commonly described as a diaphyseal lesion, metadiaphyseal and metaphyseal involvement is twice as common. Histologically, uniform, small round blue, undifferentiated cells with scant cytoplasm are visualized (Fig. 3D, E).

Immunohistochemical, anlalysis of Ewing sarcoma demonstrates nonspecific but strong staining for vimentin and S-100. The vast majority of tumors are positive for the surface antigen, CD99/MIC2.[63] CD99 is not specific to Ewing sarcoma, however, and is seen in various other malignancies, such as lymphomas, leukemias, and rhabdomyosarcoma. Thus, the diagnosis often rests on the demonstration of the characteristic t(11;22) translocation by either cytogenetics or fluorescence in situ hybridization.[64] Poor prognostic factors in Ewing sarcoma include axial skeletal location (in particular the pelvis) size greater than 8 cm and metastatic disease at diagnosis. Unlike other sarcomas, staging includes bone marrow biopsy as occult bone metastases are not uncommon.

ETIOLOGY

Most cases of Ewing sarcoma contain the (11;22)(q24;q12) chromosomal translocation that encodes the EWS/FLI oncoprotein. The oncogenic potential of this fusion product has been demonstrated by transforming immortalized murine NIH3T3 cells.[65] Although persistent EWS/FLI1 expression is needed to maintain the malignant phenotype of Ewing sarcoma cells, no normal human cells have been transformed in this fashion to date.[66,67] The tissue or cell of origin is not known. Prevailing thought implicates either neural ectoderm or mesenchymal stem cells.[68] A neuroectodermal origin is supported by the expression of neuroectodermal surface antigens on Ewing cells; the entity, primitive neuroectodermal tumor, and Ewing sarcoma sharing the same t(11;22) translocation; and neuronal developmental genes

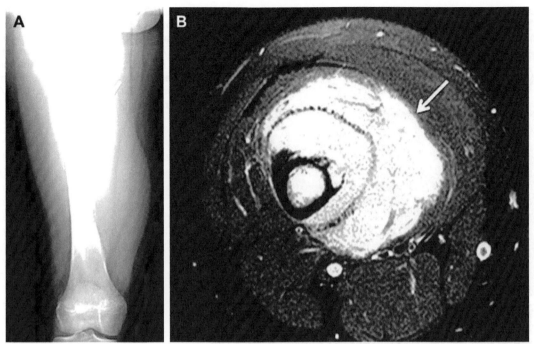

Fig. 3. (*A*) An anteroposterior radiograph of a femoral Ewing sarcoma showing a diaphyseal-based lesion with an associated Codman triangle (*arrow*). (*B*) Axial T2-weighted image before neoadjuvant therapy shows a large soft tissue mass (*white arrow*) with little bone destruction typical of Ewing sarcoma.

expression, in Ewing cells.[69,70] More recently, using a tetracycline-inducible EWS/FLI1 expression system in a rhabdomyosarcoma cell line, it has been shown that the presence of EWS/FLI induces the expression of genes normally associated with neural crest development. The investigators suggested that the neuroectodermal phenotype of Ewing sarcoma might more accurately reflect aberrant transcription rather than suggesting a neural cell of origin.[71–73]

Other studies have suggested that Ewing sarcoma is derived from a mesenchymal stem or progenitor cell. Introducing EWS/FLI into primary murine bone marrow cells or mesenchymal progenitor cells resulted in tumors with small round cell morphology and expression of CD99.[74] Gene expression profiles of these tumors displayed marked similarities to human Ewing sarcoma.[66,75] Moreover, in a complementary assay, RNA interference (RNAi) silencing of EWS/FLI expression in Ewing sarcoma cell lines resulted in mesenchymal stem cell gene expression profile and inducibility of osteogenic and adipogenic lineages consistent with a base mesenchymal stem cell–like state.[76] Despite these intriguing data, the cell of origin remains unknown.

IMAGING

The imaging evaluation for Ewing sarcoma is similar to that for osteosarcoma. Plain radiographs in 2 orthogonal planes usually reveal a permeative destructive bone lesion along with the shadow from an associated soft tissue mass (see **Fig. 3**A). Radiographs of the entire bone commonly identify a metaphyseal or diaphyseal lesion with classic features, including onion skinning of the periosteum. Expansion of the tumor and rapid remodeling of the overlying periosteum with associated mineralization lead to this characteristic finding. Ewing sarcoma, however, is not the only cause that has rapid periosteal remodeling—this can be seen in osteomyelitis, osteosarcoma, and other aggressive lesions.

The gold standard for detailed imaging is MRI. MRI allows determination of both intramedullary and extramedullary extent of disease. Classically, Ewing sarcoma exhibits a large soft tissue mass out of proportion to the amount of bone destruction (see **Fig. 3**B). MRI allows accurate surgical and/or radiotherapy planning. Skip metastases can be visualized and for this reason the entire involved bone should be included on the scan. Additionally, recent data suggest that a change

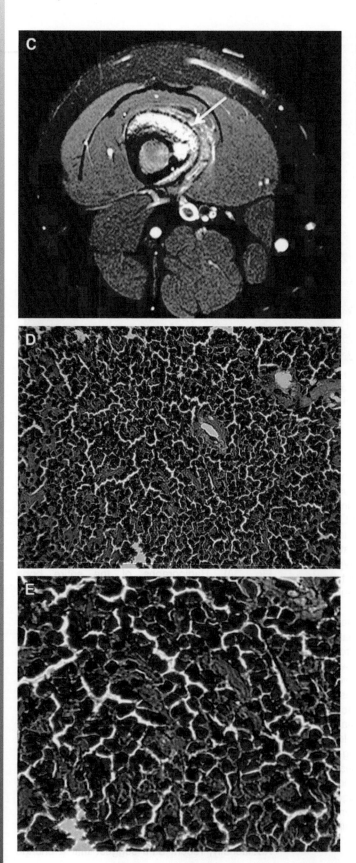

Fig. 3. (*C*) Postchemotherapy axial T2-weighted image shows a significant decrease in the size of the soft tissue mass. Arrow designate the extent of soft tissue mass. (*D*) A low-powered photomicrograph shows a highly cellular neoplasm predominantly small round blue cells. (*E*) A higher-power photomicrograph.

in the size and signal of the tumor postchemotherapy may predict local recurrence and survival (see Fig. 3C).[77]

Technitium bone scans are recommended to assess for local activity or distant bony metastasis. A CT scan of the chest is performed to assess for metastatic disease in the lung parenchyma, which is the most common distant site.

Currently, the benefit of a PET scan is unknown and not part of the standardized initial staging protocol. PET scans have been combined with CT scans with good results for restaging and surveillance of metastasis. The use of fluorodeoxyglucose F 18 has been useful for the detection of local recurrence and distant metastasis.[78] It does, however, carry a significant false-positive rate and larger studies are under way to address its specificity and sensitivity.

SYSTEMIC THERAPY

The standard neoadjuvant chemotherapy regimen consists of cyclophosphamide, vincristine, and doxorubicin alternating with etoposide and ifosfamide. This can be combined with radiation, surgery, or both. Current event-free survival and overall survival have been reported as high as 65% and 82% with localized disease and 25% and 39% in those with detectable metastatic disease.[79–81]

Current studies focus on intensifying the alkylating agents and administering more intense chemotherapy over a shorter time-period. Picci and colleagues,[82] in a review of the experience at the Istituto Rizzoli, found significantly improved survival when there was a good histologic response to neoadjuvant chemotherapy.[83]

SURGICAL MANAGEMENT

Surgical management of Ewing sarcoma includes wide resection of lesions in the appendicular skeleton and selected resection for lesions in the axial skeleton. Appropriate surgical treatment results in less than a 10% local recurrence rate.[84,85]

The benefits of surgical resection and reconstruction after neoadjuvant chemotherapy include complete removal of all tumor cells, including potentially drug resistant cells, thus minimizing local recurrence while also providing a stable construct for ambulation or upper-extremity function. As with osteosarcoma, histologic determination of the percent necrosis within the tumor allows for prognoses stratification. Adjuvant chemotherapy may be altered if a poor response is seen. A recent French Society of Pediatric Oncology study showed that event-free survival

at 5 years for patients with less than 5% viable tumor, 5% to 30% viable tumor, and greater than 30% viable tumor were 75%, 48%, and 20%, respectively.[86]

Positive surgical margins are correlated with local recurrence. Patients with appropriate margins have improved 5-year event-free survival compared with those with intralesional or marginal resections.[87] In cases with positive margins, repeat resection should be undertaken along with possible adjuvant radiation therapy. In cases of planned intralesional debulking followed by radiation therapy, however, the local control rates are not improved by radiotherapy.[84,88] Therefore, in instances where complete surgical extirpation cannot be achieved, consideration should be given to local management with radiation alone. Surgical resection must be weighed against its morbidity and the ability to preserve or reconstruct skeletal function. Significant controversy exists over the definitive local control modality for Ewing's sarcoma of the pelvis and spine, and collaborative studies are ongoing to help determine the relative benefits of surgical resection and radiation in this setting.

The vast majority of patients can be managed with limb salvage surgery, avoiding amputation. Prerequisites for limb salvage include complete tumor resection, the ability to retain the critical neurovascular structures of the extremity, and the creation of a stable construct for ambulation. Although previously considered a contraindication to limb salvage, pathologic fracture has not been found to have higher incidence of recurrence after limb salvage. Resections that involve neurologic structures, including the sciatic, tibial, or peroneal nerves, are no longer considered absolute indications for amputation because these patients can do well with gait training and bracing. Typically, lesions in the foot or distal leg are more often considered for amputation because of the high morbidity associated with flap coverage and the excellent function of modern orthoses.

Reconstructive options are similar to those for osteosarcoma, including osteoarticular allografts, allograft prosthetic composites, megaprosthetic implants, amputation, rotationplasty, and free tissue transfer.

RADIOTHERAPY

Ewing sarcoma is the most radiosensitive of the bone sarcomas. Radiotherapy may be used as the primary local control modality or combined with surgery.[89,90] Indications for radiotherapy include unplanned positive margins in resected tumors, unresectable tumors, tumors for which resection would cause unacceptable morbidity (eg, acetabulum and spine), and tumors that have poor chemotherapeutic response.[91] Additionally, radiation is often used in addition to surgery and chemotherapy in a neoadjuvant fashion.

Treatment protocols include the use of external beam radiotherapy that incorporates the gross tumor volume with an adequate margin, usually 5 cm to 10 cm. Typical treatments include 55.8 Gy to 60.0 Gy for primary local control, without surgery. In cases with surgical intervention, 45 Gy is administered preoperatively. Postoperative doses are higher secondary to local tissue hypoxia. Most treatment is given by either 3-D conformal or intensity-modulated radiation therapy. The role of proton beam radiation in the spine and skull is well accepted; its role in more accessible sites remains to be determined.

The long-term complications from radiotherapy have become more apparent as neoadjuvant chemotherapy has resulted in higher survival rates. In addition, because most patients are skeletally immature, these complications include arthrofibrosis, leg-length discrepancy, pathologic fracture, and secondary malignancies.[92]

FUTURE STUDIES

Future treatment protocols are likely to be derived from elucidation of the molecular abnormalities driving Ewing sarcoma. The most obvious target is EWS/FLI-1 function itself, which is necessary but not sufficient for the malignant phenotype of Ewing sarcoma. Preclinical work blocking the oncogenic protein interaction of EWS-FLI-1 with RNA helicase A using a small molecule inhibitor inhibited tumor growth in an orthotopic xenograft model.[93] Furthermore, it has been shown that administration of EWS/FLI-1 antisense oligonucleotides and rapamycin induced apotosis of Ewing cells in culture.[94] This in vitro work was subsequently supported by demonstration of a decreased tumor growth in a small interfering RNA (siRNA) knockdown murine model.[95] Unfortunately, direct interference with EWS/FLI-1 has proved difficult to evaluate beyond in vitro and rodent models.

In 1990, Yee and colleagues[96] first demonstrated that Ewing cell lines expressed IGF-1 and its receptor, IGF-1R. They further showed that antibodies blocking IGF-1R slowed cell growth in culture. Subsequent work by other investigators has shown that the IGF pathway may be regulated by EWS/FLI-1, making it an intriguing therapeutic target. Several preclinical experiments and early-phase clinical trials have shown promise using small molecule and antibody inhibitors of the IGF pathway.[97–99] IGF signaling inhibition alone, however, has benefited only a few patients in these studies. It has recently been demonstrated that failure of monotherapy with IGF-1R inhibitors may be due the cells' ability to switch pathways from IGF-1 to IGF-2 and its associated enhanced receptor, IR-A.[100] Another potential mode of failure in single agent IGF-1 blockade is that mTOR expression may be induced when IGF-1R is blocked. Thus combination therapy with an mTOR inhibitor may be beneficial.[101] Because the PI3 kinase and MAPK pathways are constitutively activated in Ewing sarcoma secondary to IGF-1R autocrine feedback loops, PI3 kinase inhibitors being developed in other malignancies may also offer benefit.[102]

Although CD99 is not specific to Ewing sarcoma, its blockade has been suggested as a target for therapy. Antibody inhibition induces apoptosis in culture, slows tumor formation in vivo, and acts synergistically with doxorubicin and vincristine in vitro.[103,104] Recent work has suggested that CD99 may have some role in pathogenesis. Rocchi and colleagues,[105] in knockdown experiments using Ewing sarcoma cell lines, demonstrated that knockdown of CD99 resulted in decreased cell growth as well as smaller tumors with fewer metastases in a mouse model.

Immunotherapy has had a checkered past in the treatment of sarcomas. Recently, however, investigators have shown data in support of the use of expanded ex vivo natural killer (NK) cells in Ewing sarcoma.[106] NK cytotoxicity is induced via activating receptors, the most studied of which is NKG2D. The investigators were able to expand NK cells in culture and demonstrated significant cytotoxicity against Ewing cells mediated by the NKG2D ligand and receptor. Furthermore, they were able to increase the cytotoxic effect when the cells were treated with radiation that purportedly increased the expression of the NKG2D ligand in response to stress. These and experiments like them offer some optimism for the development of complementary therapies to augment the current cyotoxic agents.

In summary, there have been large strides in understanding the molecular and cellular underpinnings of these 3 bony malignancies. These have not yet led to the hoped-for changes in survival for patients. Further study, perhaps focusing on intratumoral and intertumoral heterogeneity, may yield more useful data on which to build more effective therapies.

REFERENCES

1. Gibbs CP Jr, Weber K, Scarborough MT. Malignant bone tumors. Instr Course Lect 2002;51:413–28.

2. Meyers PA, Schwartz CL, Krailo M, et al. Osteosarcoma: a randomized, prospective trial of the addition of ifosfamide and/or muramyl tripeptide to cisplatin, doxorubicin, and high-dose methotrexate. J Clin Oncol 2005;23(9):2004–11.

3. Jaffe N, Carrasco H, Raymond K, et al. Can cure in patients with osteosarcoma be achieved exclusively with chemotherapy and abrogation of surgery? Cancer 2002;95(10):2202–10.

4. Chi SN, Conklin LS, Qin J, et al. The patterns of relapse in osteosarcoma: the Memorial Sloan-Kettering experience. Pediatr Blood Cancer 2004; 42(1):46–51.

5. Wuisman P, Enneking WF. Prognosis for patients who have osteosarcoma with skip metastasis. J Bone Joint Surg Am 1990;72(1):60–8.

6. Sandberg AA, Bridge JA. Updates on the cytogenetics and molecular genetics of bone and soft tissue tumors: osteosarcoma and related tumors. Cancer Genet Cytogenet 2003;145(1):1–30.

7. Miller CW, Aslo A, Won A, et al. Alterations of the p53, Rb and MDM2 genes in osteosarcoma. J Cancer Res Clin Oncol 1996;122(9):559–65.

8. Feugeas O, Guriec N, Babin-Boilletot A, et al. Loss of heterozygosity of the RB gene is a poor prognostic factor in patients with osteosarcoma. J Clin Oncol 1996;14(2):467–72.

9. Siddiqui NH, Jani J. Osteosarcoma metastatic to adrenal gland diagnosed by fine-needle aspiration. Diagn Cytopathol 2005;33(3):201–4.

10. Ragland BD, Bell WC, Lopez RR, et al. Cytogenetics and molecular biology of osteosarcoma. Lab Invest 2002;82(4):365–73.

11. Gibbs CP, Kukekov VG, Reith JD, et al. Stem-like cells in bone sarcomas: implications for tumorigenesis. Neoplasia 2005;7(11):967–76.

12. Wu C, Wei Q, Utomo V, et al. Side population cells isolated from mesenchymal neoplasms have tumor initiating potential. Cancer Res 2007;67(17):8216–22.

13. Levings PP, McGarry SV, Currie TP, et al. Expression of an exogenous human Oct-4 promoter identifies tumor-initiating cells in osteosarcoma. Cancer Res 2009;69(14):5648–55.

14. Stokkel MP, Linthorst MF, Borm JJ, et al. A reassessment of bone scintigraphy and commonly tested pretreatment biochemical parameters in newly diagnosed osteosarcoma. J Cancer Res Clin Oncol 2002;128(7):393–9.

15. Costelloe CM, Macapinlac HA, Madewell JE, et al. 18F-FDG PET/CT as an indicator of progression-free and overall survival in osteosarcoma. J Nucl Med 2009;50(3):340–7.

16. Okada K, Frassica FJ, Sim FH, et al. Parosteal osteosarcoma. A clinicopathological study. J Bone Joint Surg Am 1994;76(3):366–78.

17. Schwab JH, Antonescu CR, Athanasian EA, et al. A comparison of intramedullary and juxtacortical low-grade osteogenic sarcoma. Clin Orthop Relat Res 2008;466(6):1318–22.

18. Eilber FR, Rosen G. Adjuvant chemotherapy for osteosarcoma. Semin Oncol 1989;16(4):312–22.

19. Link MP, Goorin AM, Miser AW, et al. The effect of adjuvant chemotherapy on relapse-free survival in patients with osteosarcoma of the extremity. N Engl J Med 1986;314(25):1600–6.

20. Ferrari S, Smeland S, Mercuri M, et al. Neoadjuvant chemotherapy with high-dose Ifosfamide, high-dose methotrexate, cisplatin, and doxorubicin for patients with localized osteosarcoma of the extremity: a joint study by the Italian and Scandinavian Sarcoma Groups. J Clin Oncol 2005;23(34): 8845–52.

21. Glasser DB, Lane JM, Huvos AG, et al. Survival, prognosis, and therapeutic response in osteogenic sarcoma. The Memorial Hospital experience. Cancer 1992;69(3):698–708.

22. Zhou Q, Deng Z, Zhu Y, et al. mTOR/p70S6K signal transduction pathway contributes to osteosarcoma progression and patients' prognosis. Med Oncol 2010;27(4):1239–45.

23. Vemulapalli S, Mita A, Alvarado Y, et al. The emerging role of mammalian target of rapamycin inhibitors in the treatment of sarcomas. Target Oncol 2011;6(1):29–39.

24. Mita MM, Mita AC, Chu QS, et al. Phase I trial of the novel mammalian target of rapamycin inhibitor deforolimus (AP23573; MK-8669) administered intravenously daily for 5 days every 2 weeks to patients with advanced malignancies. J Clin Oncol 2008;26(3):361–7.

25. Moriceau G, Ory B, Mitrofan L, et al. Zoledronic acid potentiates mTOR inhibition and abolishes the resistance of osteosarcoma cells to RAD001 (Everolimus): pivotal role of the prenylation process. Cancer Res 2010;70(24):10329–39.

26. Cirocchi R, Farinella E, La Mura F, et al. Efficacy of surgery and imatinib mesylate in the treatment of advanced gastrointestinal stromal tumor: a systematic review. Tumori 2010;96(3):392–9.

27. Scotlandi K, Picci P, Kovar H. Targeted therapies in bone sarcomas. Curr Cancer Drug Targets 2009; 9(7):843–53.

28. Ahmed SF, Farquharson C. The effect of GH and IGF1 on linear growth and skeletal development and their modulation by SOCS proteins. J Endocrinol 2010;206(3):249–59.

29. Scotlandi K, Picci P. Targeting insulin-like growth factor 1 receptor in sarcomas. Curr Opin Oncol 2008;20(4):419–27.

30. Kolb EA, Gorlick R, Houghton PJ, et al. Initial testing (stage 1) of a monoclonal antibody (SCH 717454) against the IGF-1 receptor by the pediatric preclinical testing program. Pediatr Blood Cancer 2008;50(6):1190–7.

31. Kurmasheva RT, Dudkin L, Billups C, et al. The insulin-like growth factor-1 receptor-targeting antibody, CP-751,871, suppresses tumor-derived VEGF and synergizes with rapamycin in models of childhood sarcoma. Cancer Res 2009;69(19): 7662–71.

32. Meyers PA, Schwartz CL, Krailo MD, et al. Osteosarcoma: the addition of muramyl tripeptide to chemotherapy improves overall survival–a report from the Children's Oncology Group. J Clin Oncol 2008;26(4):633–8.

33. Chou AJ, Kleinerman ES, Krailo MD, et al. Addition of muramyl tripeptide to chemotherapy for patients with newly diagnosed metastatic osteosarcoma: a report from the Children's Oncology Group. Cancer 2009;115(22):5339–48.

34. Shin KH, Rougraff BT, Simon MA. Oncologic outcomes of primary bone sarcomas of the pelvis. Clin Orthop Relat Res 1994;(304):207–17.

35. Brien EW, Mirra JM, Kerr R. Benign and malignant cartilage tumors of bone and joint: their anatomic and theoretical basis with an emphasis on radiology, pathology and clinical biology. I. The intramedullary cartilage tumors. Skeletal Radiol 1997; 26(6):325–53.

36. Bruns J, Elbracht M, Niggemeyer O. Chondrosarcoma of bone: an oncological and functional follow-up study. Ann Oncol 2001;12(6):859–64.

37. Tiet TD, Hopyan S, Nadesan P, et al. Constitutive hedgehog signaling in chondrosarcoma upregulates tumor cell proliferation. Am J Pathol 2006;168(1):321–30.

38. Schrage YM, Lam S, Jochemsen AG, et al. Central chondrosarcoma progression is associated with pRb pathway alterations: CDK4 down-regulation and p16 overexpression inhibit cell growth in vitro. J Cell Mol Med 2009;13(9A):2843–52.

39. Larramendy ML, Tarkkanen M, Valle J, et al. Gains, losses, and amplifications of DNA sequences evaluated by comparative genomic hybridization in chondrosarcomas. Am J Pathol 1997;150(2):685–91.

40. van Beerendonk HM, Rozeman LB, Taminiau AH, et al. Molecular analysis of the INK4A/INK4A-ARF gene locus in conventional (central) chondrosarcomas and enchondromas: indication of an important gene for tumour progression. J Pathol 2004;202(3): 359–66.

41. Okada T, Tanaka K, Nakatani F, et al. Involvement of P-glycoprotein and MRP1 in resistance to cyclic tetrapeptide subfamily of histone deacetylase inhibitors in the drug-resistant osteosarcoma and Ewing's sarcoma cells. Int J Cancer 2006;118(1): 90–7.

42. Sakimura R, Tanaka K, Yamamoto S, et al. The effects of histone deacetylase inhibitors on the induction of differentiation in chondrosarcoma cells. Clin Cancer Res 2007;13(1):275–82.

43. Marco RA, Gitelis S, Brebach GT, et al. Cartilage tumors: evaluation and treatment. J Am Acad Orthop Surg 2000;8(5):292–304.

44. Murphey MD, Flemming DJ, Boyea SR, et al. Enchondroma versus chondrosarcoma in the appendicular skeleton: differentiating features. Radiographics 1998;18(5):1213–37 [quiz: 1244–5].

45. Feldman F, Van Heertum R, Saxena C, et al. 18FDG-PET applications for cartilage neoplasms. Skeletal Radiol 2005;34(7):367–74.

46. Brenner W, Conrad EU, Eary JF. FDG PET imaging for grading and prediction of outcome in chondrosarcoma patients. Eur J Nucl Med Mol Imaging 2004;31(2):189–95.

47. Jamil N, Howie S, Salter DM. Therapeutic molecular targets in human chondrosarcoma. Int J Exp Pathol 2010;91(5):387–93.

48. Nguyen QN, Chang EL. Emerging role of proton beam radiation therapy for chordoma and chondrosarcoma of the skull base. Curr Oncol Rep 2008; 10(4):338–43.

49. Wyman JJ, Hornstein AM, Meitner PA, et al. Multidrug resistance-1 and p-glycoprotein in human chondrosarcoma cell lines: expression correlates with decreased intracellular doxorubicin and in vitro chemoresistance. J Orthop Res 1999; 17(6):935–40.

50. Terek RM, Healey JH, Garin-Chesa P, et al. p53 mutations in chondrosarcoma. Diagn Mol Pathol 1998;7(1):51–6.

51. Mitchell AD, Ayoub K, Mangham DC, et al. Experience in the treatment of dedifferentiated chondrosarcoma. J Bone Joint Surg Br 2000;82(1): 55–61.

52. Dickey ID, Rose PS, Fuchs B, et al. Dedifferentiated chondrosarcoma: the role of chemotherapy with updated outcomes. J Bone Joint Surg Am 2004; 86(11):2412–8.

53. Grimer RJ, Gosheger G, Taminiau A, et al. Dedifferentiated chondrosarcoma: prognostic factors and outcome from a European group. Eur J Cancer 2007;43(14):2060–5.

54. Workman P, Burrows F, Neckers L, et al. Drugging the cancer chaperone HSP90: combinatorial therapeutic exploitation of oncogene addiction and tumor stress. Ann N Y Acad Sci 2007;1113:202–16.

55. Hollingshead M, Alley M, Burger AM, et al. In vivo antitumor efficacy of 17-DMAG (17-dimethylaminoethylamino-17-demethoxygeldanamycin hydrochloride), a water-soluble geldanamycin derivative. Cancer Chemother Pharmacol 2005;56(2):115–25.

56. Trepel J, Mollapour M, Giaccone G, et al. Targeting the dynamic HSP90 complex in cancer. Nat Rev Cancer 2010;10(8):537–49.

57. Pacey S, Wilson RH, Walton M, et al. A phase I study of the heat shock protein 90 inhibitor alvespimycin (17-DMAG) given intravenously to patients

with advanced solid tumors. Clin Cancer Res 2011; 17(6):1561–70.

58. David E, Guihard P, Brounais B, et al. Direct anti-cancer effect of oncostatin M on chondrosarcoma. Int J Cancer 2011;128(8):1822–35.

59. Herbst RS, Eckhardt SG, Kurzrock R, et al. Phase I dose-escalation study of recombinant human Apo2L/TRAIL, a dual proapoptotic receptor agonist, in patients with advanced cancer. J Clin Oncol 2010;28(17):2839–46.

60. Mohler DG, Chiu R, McCall DA, et al. Curettage and cryosurgery for low-grade cartilage tumors is associated with low recurrence and high function. Clin Orthop Relat Res 2010;468(10):2765–73.

61. Donati D, Colangeli S, Colangeli M, et al. Surgical treatment of grade I central chondrosarcoma. Clin Orthop Relat Res 2010;468(2):581–9.

62. Bruns J, Fiedler W, Werner M, et al. Dedifferenti-ated chondrosarcoma—a fatal disease. J Cancer Res Clin Oncol 2005;131(6):333–9.

63. Franchi A, Pasquinelli G, Cenacchi G, et al. Immu-nohistochemical and ultrastructural investigation of neural differentiation in Ewing sarcoma/PNET of bone and soft tissues. Ultrastruct Pathol 2001; 25(3):219–25.

64. Taylor C, Patel K, Jones T, et al. Diagnosis of Ew-ing's sarcoma and peripheral neuroectodermal tumour based on the detection of t(11;22) using fluorescence in situ hybridisation. Br J Cancer 1993;67(1):128–33.

65. Zwerner JP, Guimbellot J, May WA. EWS/FLI func-tion varies in different cellular backgrounds. Exp Cell Res 2003;290(2):414–9.

66. Riggi N, Suva ML, Suva D, et al. EWS-FLI-1 expres-sion triggers a Ewing's sarcoma initiation program in primary human mesenchymal stem cells. Cancer Res 2008;68(7):2176–85.

67. Kinsey M, Smith R, Lessnick SL. NR0B1 is required for the oncogenic phenotype mediated by EWS/FLI in Ewing's sarcoma. Mol Cancer Res 2006;4(11): 851–9.

68. Toomey EC, Schiffman JD, Lessnick SL. Recent advances in the molecular pathogenesis of Ewing's sarcoma. Oncogene 2010;29(32):4504–16.

69. Kovar H. Ewing's sarcoma and peripheral primitive neuroectodermal tumors after their genetic union. Curr Opin Oncol 1998;10(4):334–42.

70. Staege MS, Hutter C, Neumann I, et al. DNA micro-arrays reveal relationship of Ewing family tumors to both endothelial and fetal neural crest-derived cells and define novel targets. Cancer Res 2004;64(22): 8213–21.

71. Hu-Lieskovan S, Zhang J, Wu L, et al. EWS-FLI1 fusion protein up-regulates critical genes in neural crest development and is responsible for the observed phenotype of Ewing's family of tumors. Cancer Res 2005;65(11):4633–44.

72. Lessnick SL, Dacwag CS, Golub TR. The Ewing's sarcoma oncoprotein EWS/FLI induces a p53-dependent growth arrest in primary human fibro-blasts. Cancer Cell 2002;1(4):393–401.

73. Rorie CJ, Thomas VD, Chen P, et al. The Ews/Fli-1 fusion gene switches the differentiation program of neuroblastomas to Ewing sarcoma/peripheral primitive neuroectodermal tumors. Cancer Res 2004;64(4):1266–77.

74. Castillero-Trejo Y, Eliazer S, Xiang L, et al. Expres-sion of the EWS/FLI-1 oncogene in murine primary bone-derived cells Results in EWS/FLI-1-dependent, ewing sarcoma-like tumors. Cancer Res 2005;65(19):8698–705.

75. Miyagawa Y, Okita H, Nakaijima H, et al. Inducible expression of chimeric EWS/ETS proteins confers Ewing's family tumor-like phenotypes to human mesenchymal progenitor cells. Mol Cell Biol 2008; 28(7):2125–37.

76. Tirode F, Laud-Duval K, Prieur A, et al. Mesen-chymal stem cell features of Ewing tumors. Cancer Cell 2007;11(5):421–9.

77. Lemmi MA, Fletcher BD, Marina NM, et al. Use of MR imaging to assess results of chemotherapy for Ewing sarcoma. AJR Am J Roentgenol 1990; 155(2):343–6.

78. Hawkins DS, Schuetze SM, Butrynski JE, et al. [18F]Fluorodeoxyglucose positron emission tomography predicts outcome for Ewing sarcoma family of tumors. J Clin Oncol 2005;23(34): 8828–34.

79. Rodriguez-Galindo C, Navid F, Liu T, et al. Prog-nostic factors for local and distant control in Ewing sarcoma family of tumors. Ann Oncol 2008;19(4): 814–20.

80. Esiashvili N, Goodman M, Marcus RB Jr. Changes in incidence and survival of Ewing sarcoma patients over the past 3 decades: surveillance epidemiology and end results data. J Pediatr Hem-atol Oncol 2008;30(6):425–30.

81. Grier HE, Krailo MD, Tarbell NJ, et al. Addition of ifosfamide and etoposide to standard chemo-therapy for Ewing's sarcoma and primitive neuroec-todermal tumor of bone. N Engl J Med 2003;348(8): 694–701.

82. Picci P, Rougraff BT, Bacci G, et al. Prognostic significance of histopathologic response to chemo-therapy in nonmetastatic Ewing's sarcoma of the extremities. J Clin Oncol 1993;11(9):1763–9.

83. Wunder JS, Paulian G, Huvos AG, et al. The histo-logical response to chemotherapy as a predictor of the oncological outcome of operative treatment of Ewing sarcoma. J Bone Joint Surg Am 1998; 80(7):1020–33.

84. Bacci G, Forni C, Longhi A, et al. Long-term outcome for patients with non-metastatic Ewing's sarcoma treated with adjuvant and neoadjuvant

chemotherapies. 402 patients treated at Rizzoli between 1972 and 1992. Eur J Cancer 2004; 40(1):73–83.

85. Bacci G, Longhi A, Briccoli A, et al. The role of surgical margins in treatment of Ewing's sarcoma family tumors: experience of a single institution with 512 patients treated with adjuvant and neoadjuvant chemotherapy. Int J Radiat Oncol Biol Phys 2006;65(3):766–72.

86. Oberlin O, Deley MC, Bui BN, et al. Prognostic factors in localized Ewing's tumours and peripheral neuroectodermal tumours: the third study of the French Society of Paediatric Oncology (EW88 study). Br J Cancer 2001;85(11):1646–54.

87. Sluga M, Windhager R, Lang S, et al. The role of surgery and resection margins in the treatment of Ewing's sarcoma. Clin Orthop Relat Res 2001;(392):394–9.

88. Laskar S, Mallick I, Gupta T, et al. Post-operative radiotherapy for Ewing sarcoma: when, how and how much? Pediatr Blood Cancer 2008;51(5):575–80.

89. Indelicato DJ, Keole SR, Shahlaee AH, et al. Definitive radiotherapy for ewing tumors of extremities and pelvis: long-term disease control, limb function, and treatment toxicity. Int J Radiat Oncol Biol Phys 2008;72(3):871–7.

90. Shi W, Indelicato DJ, Keole SR, et al. Radiation treatment for Ewing family of tumors in adults: the University of Florida experience. Int J Radiat Oncol Biol Phys 2008;72(4):1140–5.

91. Indelicato DJ, Keole SR, Shahlaee AH, et al. Impact of local management on long-term outcomes in Ewing tumors of the pelvis and sacral bones: the University of Florida experience. Int J Radiat Oncol Biol Phys 2008;72(1):41–8.

92. Davis AM, O'Sullivan B, Turcotte R, et al. Late radiation morbidity following randomization to preoperative versus postoperative radiotherapy in extremity soft tissue sarcoma. Radiother Oncol 2005;75(1):48–53.

93. Erkizan HV, Kong Y, Merchant M, et al. A small molecule blocking oncogenic protein EWS-FLI1 interaction with RNA helicase A inhibits growth of Ewing's sarcoma. Nat Med 2009;15(7):750–6.

94. Mateo-Lozano S, Tirado OM, Notario V. Rapamycin induces the fusion-type independent downregulation of the EWS/FLI-1 proteins and inhibits Ewing's sarcoma cell proliferation. Oncogene 2003;22(58):9282–7.

95. Hu-Lieskovan S, Heidel JD, Bartlett DW, et al. Sequence-specific knockdown of EWS-FLI1 by targeted, nonviral delivery of small interfering RNA inhibits tumor growth in a murine model of metastatic Ewing's sarcoma. Cancer Res 2005;65(19):8984–92.

96. Yee D, Favoni RE, Lebovic GS, et al. Insulin-like growth factor I expression by tumors of neuroectodermal origin with the t(11;22) chromosomal translocation. A potential autocrine growth factor. J Clin Invest 1990;86(6):1806–14.

97. Benini S, Manara MC, Baldini N, et al. Inhibition of insulin-like growth factor I receptor increases the antitumor activity of doxorubicin and vincristine against Ewing's sarcoma cells. Clin Cancer Res 2001;7(6):1790–7.

98. Toretsky JA, Gorlick R. IGF-1R targeted treatment of sarcoma. Lancet Oncol 2010;11(2):105–6.

99. Buck E, Gokhale PC, Koujak S, et al. Compensatory insulin receptor (IR) activation on inhibition of insulin-like growth factor-1 receptor (IGF-1R): rationale for cotargeting IGF-1R and IR in cancer. Mol Cancer Ther 2010;9(10):2652–64.

100. Garofalo C, Manara MC, Nicoletti G, et al. Efficacy of and resistance to anti-IGF-1R therapies in Ewing's sarcoma is dependent on insulin receptor signaling. Oncogene 2011;30(24):2730–40.

101. Salazar R, Reidy-Lagunes D, Yao J. Potential synergies for combined targeted therapy in the treatment of neuroendocrine cancer. Drugs 2011;71(7):841–52.

102. Ordonez JL, Osuna D, Herrero D, et al. Advances in Ewing's sarcoma research: where are we now and what lies ahead? Cancer Res 2009;69(18):7140–50.

103. Sohn HW, Choi EY, Kim SH, et al. Engagement of CD99 induces apoptosis through a calcineurin-independent pathway in Ewing's sarcoma cells. Am J Pathol 1998;153(6):1937–45.

104. Scotlandi K, Baldini N, Cerisano V, et al. CD99 engagement: an effective therapeutic strategy for Ewing tumors. Cancer Res 2000;60(18):5134–42.

105. Rocchi A, Manara MC, Sciandra M, et al. CD99 inhibits neural differentiation of human Ewing sarcoma cells and thereby contributes to oncogenesis. J Clin Invest 2010;120(3):668–80.

106. Cho HM, Rosenblatt JD, Tolba K, et al. Delivery of NKG2D ligand using an anti-HER2 antibody-NKG2D ligand fusion protein results in an enhanced innate and adaptive antitumor response. Cancer Res 2010;70(24):10121–30.

Index

Note: Page numbers of article titles are in **boldface** type.

surgpath.theclinics.com

Surgical Pathology 5 (2012) 319–326
doi:10.1016/S1875-9181(12)00010-4
1875-9181/12/$ – see front matter © 2012 Elsevier Inc. All rights reserved.

Printed and bound by CPI Group (UK) Ltd, Croydon, CR0 4YY

03/10/2024

01040350-0005